Effective Approaches to Patients' Behavior

GLADYS B. LIPKIN, A.R.N.P., M.S., C.S., F.A.A.N., was one of the first nurses certified by the American Nurses' Association (ANA) as a generalist and then as a specialist in adult psychiatric and mental health nursing, and by the ANA and the Nurses' Association of the American College of Obstetrics and Gynecology in maternal and neonatal nursing. In 1995, she received the Distinguished Alumnus Award from the Cornell University–New York Hospital School of Nursing. She has retired from her private psychotherapy practice and lives in Hollywood, Florida.

ROBERTA G. COHEN, R.N., M.S., C.S., is a clinical specialist at Mercy Medical Center, Rockville Centre, New York, and an independent nurse psychotherapist in private practice in North Bellmore, New York. She has been certified by the ANA as a specialist in adult psychiatric and mental health nursing, and is a past recipient of the ANA Council of Nurse Specialists Direct Practice in Psychiatric/Mental Health Nursing Award, the New York State Nurses Association Award for Clinical Practice, and the Nurses Association of Long Island District 14 Award for Clinical Practice.

Both authors are members of Sigma Theta Tau and were the corecipients of the Nassau County Medical Center Literary Award.

Effective Approaches to Patients' Behavior

Fifth Edition

A Guide Book For Health Care Professionals,
Patients, and Their Caregivers

Gladys B. Lipkin
Roberta G. Cohen

Springer Publishing Company

Springer Publishing Company, Inc.
536 Broadway
New York, NY 10012-3955

First edition, 1973
Second edition, 1980
Third edition, 1986
Fourth edition, 1992
Fifth edition, 1998

Cover design by Janet Joachim
Acquisitions Editor: Ruth Chasek
Production Editor: Kathleen Kelly

98 99 00 01 02 / 5 4 3 2 1

Library of Congress Cataloging-in-Publication Data

Lipkin, Gladys B.
    Effective approaches to patients' behavior : a guide book for
health care professionals, patients, and their caregivers / Gladys
B. Lipkin, Roberta G. Cohen. — 5th ed.
        p.   cm.
    Includes bibliographical references and index.
    ISBN 0-8261-1497-0 (hardcover); 0-8262-1498-9 (softcover)
    1. Psychiatric nursing.   2. Nurse and patient.   3. Patients—
Psychology.   4. Clinical health psychology.   I. Cohen, Roberta G.
II. Title.
    RC440.L568   1998
    610.73'06'99—dc21   97-52092
                                                              CIP

Printed in the United States of America

Once again, as we collaborated on this fifth edition, we realized how much we owe to friends, peers, patients, teachers, mentors, our associates at Springer Publishing, and our families. We have thanked them all privately, but as we have in the past, we want to especially thank our families for their support and patience. To Dr. Nathan J. Lipkin, Rebecca, Harriet (husband Chris and their children, Josh and Stephanie Sautter) and Dr. Alan Lipkin (wife Barbara and their children, Richard, Sam and Molly), plus Anne (husband Ohr and their children, Murray, Matanel and Tal) Cohen-Weinberg, and David (wife Karen and their son, Kevin) Cohen, we extend our thanks for being there when we needed support and love.

We dedicate this edition to all of you.

Contents

Part Three: Approaches to the Psychological Effects of Special Circumstances

Part Four: Approaches to the Psychological Effects of Physical Illness

Part Five: Working With Different Age Groups

Preface

Following the history of this book is a little like following the history of psychiatric care in the United States over the past 25 years.

When the first edition came out in 1974, 50% of all hospital beds in the United States were occupied by psychiatric patients. By 1980 this number had fallen to 40% and by the time the third edition was published in 1986 deinstitutionalization was in full swing and its sad after-effects were becoming evident. When the fourth edition was published in 1991 deinstitutionalization had resulted in the abandonment of the very population it was intended to help. The promised community services for the most part failed to materialize and many former patients found themselves among the homeless, unable to meet their own basic needs.

This fifth edition finds psychiatric care, and health care in general, in a state of profound flux. Managed care, with its emphasis on cost constraints, has come to dominate health care, and has also brought another "downsizing" of psychiatric care. Patients may find themselves limited to a finite number of therapist visits, if any, with psychiatric drugs viewed as a cheaper and easier alternative to "talk" therapy.

Yet throughout these 25 years of change there are many constants, and we feel that they make the book as needed now as it ever was. The chief constant is that individuals with emotional disturbances do not disappear—they still receive care, but often in nontraditional and often inadequate settings. This book is designed to meet the need for a short manual that describes problem behavior, offers a discussion of the dynamics involved, and suggests approaches to be used with the patient. It is a practical, concise, and informative guide for all health workers involved in the care of individuals who demonstrate some aspect of emotional disturbance, whether they be in the community, in the general hospital, or in a psychiatric setting.

Health workers in any setting are often confronted by patients with symptoms of emotional disturbances that may or may not be receiving treatment by a psychiatrist, yet are serious enough to require meaningful and assertive intervention on the worker's part. Health workers may shy away from such patients because they are not certain of what to say, how to say it, or when to initiate the approach to the patient. Often they fear that their actions may cause further deterioration in the patient's emotional or somatic state.

The purpose of this book is to present the problem areas in which health workers frequently become involved, and which necessitate on-the-spot action. The worker who is familiar with behavior patterns and the do's and don'ts of intervention will be able to function in this role with ease, understanding, and effectiveness. At the same time, the worker's action gives the patient an opportunity to learn how to cope with immediate stresses. Emotional growth is also fostered through these interactions.

As nurse psychotherapists, both authors have worked extensively with individuals who present difficulties manifested by changes in their emotional and/or physical states. Our experiences have reinforced our belief that the worker who is acquainted with basic psychiatric techniques and concepts is able to approach these individuals confidently and, we hope, successfully.

Patients once relied on receiving care in the hospital until they recovered fully from their illness. Now they are often told that they do not require admission to an inpatient area for many procedures, or are discharged from the hospital while still needing extensive care. As a result, reliance upon family members, the patient's significant others, and even patients themselves has become important for early intervention and the prevention of complications. For this reason the format of this edition has been changed, making it easier for the trained or untrained health care provider to intervene appropriately and effectively when mental health problems are present.

Although the need for continuity of care is evident, it is often unavailable. Medications needed to control psychiatric symptoms may not be taken properly, or their effectiveness not evaluated if supervision is inadequate. This leaves patients more vulnerable to regression or exacerbation of illnesses. It is therefore important that patients, their care providers and significant others be taught to recognize initial signs and symptoms of mental illness. They also need education to initiate the proper interventions that will prevent a downward cycle.

In some instances, the additional stress of emotional problems can prolong physical illness, just as physical illness can adversely affect an individual's psychiatric status. Either situation will add to the cost of care. It is more important than ever for every health care professional to be aware of the mental health status of all patients and to present information about appropriate psychiatric services, regardless of the care setting. It may be the lay assistant in the home or community who first recognizes the need for such help. If so, that person will need direction as to where to refer the patient.

To meet these needs, the book has been redesigned for ease of use, with each chapter offering an overview of a particular disorder or condition; case examples; information on self-management and short, intermediate, and long-term management; and common drugs prescribed. Introductory chapters give an overview of interpersonal dynamics and communication skills. Information on the changing health care system, managed care, and cultural concerns has been added to this section. This is followed by 29 specific psychiatric disorders and psychological conditions related to physical illness or psychosocial circumstances. The final section highlights important developmental milestones in the life span and their potential psychological ramifications.

We have deliberately used the term "health worker" throughout most of the book, in order to address the broadest possible audience. The health worker may be a nurse, a social worker, a physical therapist, a nursing assistant or home health aide—any person in the health care field who may encounter a patient undergoing psychological distress. We also believe that patients, their families, and interested lay readers can understand and benefit from the information in this book.

We have incorporated material from our own experiences in the attempt to increase the reader's understanding of various personality and behavior disturbances. Although we recognize that professional competence can be developed only through actual clinical practice, we hope the use of this book will expedite its acquisition.

Our goals will have been met if we give our readers a sense of *what* to do and *how* to do it, along with some comprehension of *why* we have found particular approaches to be helpful. We hope this edition will effectively meet the needs of all who approach the mentally ill, as well as those personally involved as recipients or providers of care.

Gladys B. Lipkin
Roberta G. Cohen

PART ONE

Overview

1

Looking at the Patient

Patients can be found in a variety of settings. In the past, the most likely place for the health worker to encounter those in need of psychiatric intervention was the hospital. However, fewer patients are hospitalized today, and earlier discharges may be mandated by insurance companies that set monetary limits on hospital care. As a result, nurses are often finding patients with psychiatric needs in community agencies, ambulatory settings, or in patients' homes. In some situations, the hospital stay is so short, and professional staffing so inadequate, that the need for any psychiatric input is not even recognized, particularly when the focus is on a physical illness.

THE PATIENT IN THE COMMUNITY

When patients are being cared for at home, regardless of the diagnosis, it may be that family therapy is required, for the caregivers may be family members feeling the stress as much (if not more) than the patient. Once again, it is imperative that care providers be tuned in to the patient's perception of what is happening. The individual who sees his own behavior as normal is unlikely to accept any intervention. If, however, his level of discomfort is high, he or she may welcome the help that is offered. If a family member is in charge of the care, that person may be too emotionally involved to recognize that the patient is having difficulty. It then behooves the professional to institute the necessary care. The initial meeting between patient and professional is crucial.

The professionals involved in these situations need to accept and recognize any cultural differences that may exist between themselves, the patient, and the family. It is important that the professionals understand certain behaviors that are distinctive to the patient's background.

If the care of the patient has been relegated to a family member, it may be up to the professional to provide support and guidance to that individual. Is that person angry at being thrust into a position with so much responsibility? Is there an underlying problem in the relationships within the home that requires exploration? Does the designated caregiver feel overwhelmed by the tasks at hand? Does that person feel abandoned by other family members who may keep their distance, choosing not to be involved with the patient's care? Or has the caregiver, knowingly or not, caused others to stay away in response to the way in which the care is being carried out? The professional has to evaluate the possibilities, and determine the most therapeutic approach without being judgmental or appearing to take sides.

Health care workers who set up appointments for psychotherapy within a hospital or other agency determine the hour, place, and length of the session. If, however, the patient or family is to be seen at home, the appointment must be scheduled to meet the needs within the home. The patient and all others in the household must cooperate in deciding when and where the meeting should occur. The length of the session must be determined in advance, so that all are aware that this therapeutic intervention is to be for professional, not social reasons. The professional must be the one to accept responsibility for determining how the session is to be run, who should be included, and how many sessions are to be held. All of this information must be shared with the patient and those providing his or her care, so that the intervention will be regarded seriously.

Some professionals are fearful of becoming involved on a psychiatric level, questioning whether their intervention will increase the patient's difficulty, perhaps affecting the course of the basic illness adversely. This fear can be put to rest if professionals realize that the patient's emotional disturbance did not start with the workers' involvement but rather may be substantially decreased by it. Patients can almost always accept the intervention of professionals who appear concerned, interested, and are truthful.

Professional care for psychiatric problems may be severely limited by the financial resources of the patient. More than ever, it becomes imperative for patients to be taught how to recognize symptoms of a flare-up and how to self-manage their own early symptoms. In some instances, medications have been discontinued against medical advice as patients feel better. They may not accept the importance of the medications and believe that they are "cured." In other cases, there may have been an increase in environmental stressors, perhaps in the family or at work, requiring an increase or change in the medications that have kept the symptoms under control. Most important, nurses can teach patients and significant others to become aware of changes as they begin, and provide them with techniques for self-management.

Early recognition of symptoms include an understanding of clues that may be recognized initially by only the patient, a sense that something is not quite right. This may be demonstrated by mild changes in behavior, perhaps based on a misinterpretation of ordinary cues that occur in daily living. If patients are taught to recognize the early symptoms of dysfunction, they may not progress to more serious aspects of their disorder. If the illness is seen as being on a continuum, starting with mild symptoms, that, if untreated, become worse, the need for early intervention becomes very apparent. Techniques for self-management may vary with the psychiatric diagnosis, but almost all include a lessening of stress, the ability to identify the troublesome initial symptom, and the use of skills to manage that symptom. The specific techniques will be presented in later chapters.

THE HOSPITALIZED PATIENT

Even without the problems of cultural diversity, those who require hospitalization may find themselves in an alien situation, requiring an understanding health provider. Determining whether the behavior of a patient is "normal" must include an evaluation of the circumstances in which that behavior occurs. For example, the person who wears a bathing suit to a barbecue held at a swimming area would be viewed as acting properly. However, if the same person wore a bathing suit to a formal dinner, he would certainly be looked at askance.

The patient's background is largely responsible for his daily actions and reactions while he is in the hospital. If hot water has been hard to come by throughout his life, and baths have been once-a-week affairs, the nurse is unlikely to be able to convince him that he really needs a full bed bath every day, unless she does some effective health teaching. If breakfast has always been bypassed, and between-meal snacks are a family habit, he will probably follow the same pattern in the hospital unless he can be made to realize that regular, well-balanced meals are a more healthful way of satisfying his hunger.

Reviewing the patient's background will help the nurse to understand that his behavior is not based on a desire to be dirty, and that he does not really want to be difficult at mealtime. However, there is a good chance that he may change his ingrained pattern of behavior if he can be convinced that other patterns are better for him. In any event, once the staff becomes conscious of his life style, it is improbable that they will continue to think of him as "that dirty old man who gives us so much trouble at mealtime."

The cultural factors that have shaped the sick person's behavior in the past will continue to affect his actions wherever he may be now. In some cultures, the sick or elderly have been traditionally cared for at home, and hospitals have been considered places only for the dying. The patient who is part of such a culture may feel abandoned when he is removed from his family and taken to the hospital for some minor procedure. In other cultures, the display of emotions is approved, so the patient may feel free to cry. In still other groups stoicism is encouraged, and the individual learns to maintain complete control—at least superficially. Discovering these background factors helps to improve understanding and leads to more meaningful relations between patients and the hospital staff.

Religious practices account for certain behavior patterns exhibited by some patients. The Catholic who refuses to go to surgery before receiving communion is not being uncooperative. Neither is the orthodox Jew who refuses to eat nonkosher food. The Jehovah's Witness who vehemently refuses a blood transfusion places his religious tenets above immediate health considerations. Should those with differing religious beliefs refuse to honor the convictions of such patients? Should we be furious that the operating room schedule is delayed, that the kitchen must make special dietary arrangements, or that the need for blood must be reconsidered? Do we have the right to add to the patient's discomfort by being angry and argumentative while trying to convince him to do what we want him to do? Showing respect for the religious beliefs of others, no matter how widely they vary from our own, helps one to make an honest assessment of the patient's behavior. He certainly is neither stubborn nor uncooperative if he tries, even in a time of stress, to adhere to the teachings of a lifetime.

The patient from a low socioeconomic group may view his placement in a single room as a luxury. He may not want to "bother" the staff and, therefore, gets out of bed to go to the bathroom even when on strict bed rest. At the other end of the scale, the patient from a high socioeconomic group may complain that the paint is chipped off the bed, or that the linen is not changed often enough. He may demand a great deal from the staff, even though he is permitted to be up and around ad libitum. Either patient may be thought of as a "problem" unless viewed in the context of his background. Acknowledgment by the staff of the first patient's need to be completely independent, and of the second one's need for a coterie of people to order about will help both patients understand their own behavior. Often, such a simple phrase as, "It must be difficult for you to have to depend on others for all your needs," or "It must be frustrating for you not to have people available to help you immediately" will enable the patient to think through his reaction to his present situation.

Often when a member of one of the medical disciplines becomes a patient, he presents many problems to the hospital staff. He tries to guess his diagnosis from tests being done. He may question the necessity or wisdom of medications or treatments ordered for him. He often will not ask questions about himself directly but rather will say, "This test is usually done for cancer, isn't it?" He interprets an evasive answer as an indication that he does indeed have cancer. In such an instance, it may be helpful for the nurse to say, "Yes, it may be done for cancer, but it is also used to confirm other diagnoses as well. Your doctor will tell you about the other conditions that he was considering when he ordered the test."

The health professional who has been involved with patients in the clinical situation may become anxious when methods other than those he is familiar with are used to carry out procedures. He may note that sterile equipment appears to have become contaminated, or that he would do things differently. If the staff can discuss these differences with him and offer a theoretical basis for the techniques being used, he will probably feel more at ease. His knowledge and experience may be broader than that of many of the staff. For example, if he is the medical director of the service, staff members may have to remind themselves that being a patient is as difficult for him as caring for him is for the staff. All his expertise will not make him less anxious than any other patient. Perhaps, knowing as much as he does may *increase* his anxiety. Air in the intravenous tubing, crooked needles, contaminated equipment all add to his stress, particularly as he tries to have the situation corrected without showing his distrust of the staff. His desire to be a "good" patient may increase his anxiety even further as he tries to reassure himself that others can be as knowledgeable as he is, and that his care will be as excellent as any that he would provide for one of his own patients. Considering these factors, it is not difficult to understand why he questions everyone and everything.

Nonprofessional hospital volunteers or their family members who are hospitalized frequently present problems in that they often have preconceived notions of what their care should include. They may misunderstand procedures or test results, but be unwilling to admit their lack of knowledge by asking questions. In addition, they may request special privileges because of their association with the hospital. They expect an acknowledgment of their services and may be upset if staff members do not recognize them as very important people.

Previous hospital experiences also modify patients' behavior. If this is yet another admission for the same condition, the patient may be very upset and discouraged, for it indicates that he is not improving. The patient with heart or kidney disease, or with diabetes, may feel that following the rigid limitations of diet does not make a difference, that he will be sick whether he follows or disregards the rules. He may be angry that he has deprived himself of foods that are forbidden but enjoyable, only to become ill anyway. Talking about his feelings will help because it gives him the chance to ventilate his anger as well as find out where he may have made mistakes. (Patients on a self-restricted diet have been known to scrupulously avoid sodium chloride while freely using monosodium glutamate, not realizing that the sodium is the harmful substance.) The approach might be, "How do you feel about being back in the hospital? Some people find it frustrating to stay on an unappealing diet and still become ill. Let's take a look at your food intake and see if you might have overlooked something that is responsible for your present difficulty."

The patients' previous hospital experiences may have involved the illness of family members or friends rather than themselves. They may remember these incidents pleasantly or apprehensively depending on the quality of the care they received and the outcome of the hospitalization. If a biopsy was performed, and a negative report received, they remember the hospital as a happy place. If, conversely, the report was positive, and the friend or relative later died, their memories of the hospital may be very distressing ones. When the patient is relatively well and comfortable, visitors tend not to notice hospital shortcomings. This is particularly true if staff members have been helpful to the patient. Conversely, staff members who may be short tempered or argumentative often cause visitors (as well as patients) to become hostile and angry. Individuals who enter a hospital after being involved in a pleasant or unpleasant previous experience, whether their own or someone else's, will have initial feelings that are colored by that experience.

Children are particularly influenced by how they were cared for during prior hospitalizations. They remember the attitudes of staff members in great detail, especially in relation to truthfulness. If children have been told that a procedure would be painless, and found the opposite to be true, they now anticipate that every procedure will be painful. Conversely, they place greater trust in the staff if, during previous hospitalization, they had been told exactly what to expect before a procedure was done. Being in the hospital is less frightening and less anxiety provoking when the child knows that health workers are reliable, supportive people who do not enjoy causing pain but are truthful about it when it is unavoidable. Memories of unhappy childhood hospitalizations continue to haunt some patients through the years, and resistance to later admissions may be based on those memories.

Some patients who are admitted to either a general or a psychiatric hospital have a long-standing history of abnormal behavior for which they have not been previously hospitalized, either because the symptoms were not severe enough or because the family insisted on keeping the patient at home. Some of these patients have created an unreal world to which they retreat so as to protect themselves against any feelings of anxiety produced by the real world that surrounds them. Their actions may be subject to orders from some invisible power in that secret world, their vision may be distorted, and their language may become unintelligible because of this power. The unreal world is, in a sense, the patient's protection against the unbearable feelings that he is experiencing in the real world. Some patients move back and forth between their two worlds, resorting to the unreal one only at times of great personal stress, and then they seem unable to see, hear, or feel anything going on around them.

Ujhely writes of *"sustaining the patient through the experience,"* an important concept in meeting the needs of *all* patients, but especially of those who lose contact with reality. Using this concept, the health worker must first become aware of the patient's *perception* of the current situation. How does what is happening appear to patients? Their perceptions may differ from those of others in similar situations because of their physical state (as when they have severe or constant pain), the culture in which they have lived (as the Amish farmer who regards the taking of x-rays as against the dictum of having "graven images"), or accumulated knowledge.

The second factor the worker needs to be aware of is the patients' *interpretation* of what is happening. They may be distorting what they have perceived because of their extreme anxiety, or inability to think things through properly (as the patient who refuses to have her chest shaved for a breast biopsy "because it will make hair grow on my chest later").

A third factor for the worker to note is the patients' *response,* which will depend on their capacity to cope with a given situation in light of their ability, background, and previously learned response in similar situations.

Having assessed the patients' perception, interpretation, and response, the worker can then move on to *sustain* patients. This is an all-encompassing term that indicates ways in which patients may be helped to cope with the situation now at hand. It calls for sensitivity on the part of the worker, the ability to let the patients' experience take precedence over the niceties of hospital care, accepting patients even when they are in their unreal world, and not forcing other standards of behavior on them until they are ready for change. It may take a long time before patients feel they are safe enough to change. This will usually happen as a result of their trusting those who care for them in ways that indicate sincere concern for them as human beings.

Travelbee notes the distorted perception of both the givers and receivers of care when the term *patient* is used. Individuals may easily be dehumanized when they are stereotyped and categorized according to a particular illness. Such thinking dulls the ability of the health worker to regard the patient as a person with unique qualifications, one who must be regarded in terms of background (ethnic, cultural, socioeconomic, etc.), physical status, home environment, and current problems.

Health workers can be of greatest help to those in their care when they are empathic and sympathetic, but not immobilized by either of these reactions. Patients sense that the worker understands them and wants to help. For some patients, the worker is the only individual in the world to whom they can tell all their worries, sorrows, and expectations. Their close emotional involvement with family members and friends may make such disclosures too painful. It is hoped that the worker is able to tolerate what is being said, and does not turn a confiding patient off with such trite phrases as "Don't worry," "Everything will be all right," and "Your family still loves you." If workers become involved (but not incapacitated by that involvement), they cannot help patients through their experience of illness, as well as help them learn how to deal with life more meaningfully when healthy.

Almost always, patients fear a hospital experience. They fear such unknown factors as the diagnosis, the treatment, the outcome, and the type of care they will receive. Some will conceal their feelings with a veneer of humor or boredom. Others will cling to hospital personnel, much as children do, seeking scraps of information about themselves. Occasionally patients will cry, a most upsetting spectacle for some health workers, who communicate their feeling by what they say and do. The pat answer, "There, there, don't cry," neither stops the crying nor helps the patient. Telling him to "pull yourself together" makes him feel that he is regarded as inadequate and that the worker is looking down on him. The patient needs to feel the strength and empathy of a worker who can stay with him, one who is not upset by the tears. Verbal communication helps to make the patient feel less guilty about his tears. "I realize how upset you are. Sometimes tears ease that feeling," implies that the worker believes the patient can mobilize untapped strengths within himself. This encourages his belief that the worker recognizes him as a person with assets still to be used. The feeling that someone else believes in him often furnishes the motivating force for the patient to find those strengths. Nonverbal communication is equally important. An arm around the patient's shoulder, a hand on his arm, or a gentle hand helping to wipe away the tears all indicate to the patient that there is acceptance of what might ordinarily be unacceptable. He can still retain his dignity, knowing that he is looked on as a very human being.

THE PATIENT IN CONTEXT OF WORLD EVENTS

Many areas of the world have been in turmoil during the past few years. Civil strife has resulted in displacement of populations, with families ripped apart by death or physical separation. In addition to the tragedies spawned by wars, there have been episodes of violence including bombings and other dastardly acts throughout the world. In the field of health care, illnesses thought to be conquered by modern treatments have once again taken hold. In addition, new organisms, or mutations of old ones, have resulted in virulent epidemics requiring new and even, in some instances, as yet undiscovered antibiotics or antiviral agents. Added to these problems have been international calamities, such as famine, drought, floods, fires, and other natural disasters.

In many cases, the physical conditions, horrible as they may have been, have been treatable. The more difficult problem for many has been the overwhelming aftermath of the emotional upheaval when children were left without parents, adults could not find loved ones, and homes disappeared from the face of the earth. People who had control of their lives were suddenly without their possessions or loved ones, and had little hope of regaining what they had lost. Is it any wonder that these victims have been overwhelmed? What can the health worker do to help those so affected?

It is impossible to guess how anyone will react to overwhelming tragedy. It is important for the caregiver to respect the approach initially chosen by the individual, regardless of how inappropriate it may seem to the onlooker. Intervention may have to await the building of a trusting relationship before the victim feels safe enough with the caregiver to attempt any changes. The professional needs to be patient, to allow the victim to determine the speed with which any therapeutic intervention can begin.

The problems that are seen today are not limited to any one country, not necessarily to even one section of that country. Often populations must be shifted from one geographical location to another because of the devastation of their homeland. In some instances, the receiving areas are unable to absorb those who arrive, having inadequate resources to feed or care for them properly. Medical care, including professional providers, may be lacking, although desperately needed. In some cases, there may be little, if any, understanding by the established inhabitants of the new setting concerning the culture of the refugees. If so, the refugees have to deal with culture shock, possibly an unfamiliar language, a lack of family or friends to act as a support system, and perhaps their own or a loved one's physical or emotional illness.

CULTURAL DIVERSITY

The United States Census Bureau has estimated that more than 135 million people, approximately 50% of the country's inhabitants, will be people of color by the year 2000. To add to the diversity, 32 million are likely to speak a language other than English at home. These numbers include health care workers as well as patients, and indicate the great need for understanding and tolerance among all peoples. This is unlikely to occur without education. With this in mind, some hospitals have already instituted programs to help their staff members appreciate the differences in cultures.

Beth Israel Medical Center is a large university-affiliated hospital located in the Lower East Side of New York City and is typical of a multicultural setting. Its population includes Whites, Native Americans, Asians, Hispanics, Blacks (native born as well as those born in Caribbean or other nations) and Hasidim (a religious Jewish sect). In 1991, a daylong program called "A Workplace of Difference" was made part of the orientation of every new employee. At this session, new workers discuss their own backgrounds, and are helped to examine the stereotypes they have accepted as well as their assumptions and perceptions that they hold about others. This is geared to increasing individual awareness of personal attitudes, and to stimulate a greater understanding of differences between themselves and others. At the end of the program, each employee is asked to create a personal contract to contribute to the healing environment at the Center.

This program introduces the staff to traditions of which they may be unaware, as well as solutions to problems that may arise. For example, Hasidic males are not permitted to touch females other than their own spouses. Therefore, husbands are not permitted to accept a child being given to them by a female nurse. Understanding the religious prohibition, the nurses now place the child on the bed or stretcher, enabling the father to pick up the child in pediatrics, the emergency room, delivery room, or elsewhere.

In the geographical area of the Center, there has been a large increase in the population of Asians and Pacific Islanders with different languages, dialects, and assumptions about health. To meet this challenge, a 10-month program was developed to provide those with previous health care experience in China to learn English as a second language. Nursing classes are also held, with a clinical practicum at Beth Israel. This program concludes with the LPN licensing examination. In this way, bilingual nurses are made available in a Center with a need for their services.

In other parts of the country, local needs are met by including transcultural training for nurses. This may include information about customs not usually familiar to Western health practitioners. For example, time may be described differently, as some cultures rely on social time (less punctual) rather than clock time. Other variations include the shunning of eye contact, feared by some as an unwanted intrusion that gives outsiders a view through the eyes into the soul. When this is understood as a cultural phenomenon, the avoidance of direct eye contact by some groups is no longer regarded as an unfriendly practice. Training programs such as these help staff members respect the diverse cultures in their communities, understanding differences rather than being angered by them.

Some immigrants have been treated by folk healers, herbalists, or spiritualists. These practitioners may use mercury, shark cartilage, pigeon blood, snake oil, or other substances in an effort to cure their patients. Other healers may resort to chants, drawing patterns in sand, voodoo, or Santeria (including animal sacrifices), with a blending of African and Catholic beliefs.

If the patients' beliefs are deeply rooted, they may not feel comfortable with, or have confidence in, the conventional practitioner of Western medicine. To counteract this, some practitioners with an understanding of the customs and practice of the healers, have been able to work with healers, combining folk and conventional practices. In doing this, they hope to gain the trust of the patients and convince them to accept the Western methods, while rejecting any folk treatments that may be injurious. If the folk methods are not harmful, the Western practitioner may let the patients continue using them, thus building trust between them.

Although the population of the United States has referred to itself as a "melting pot" through the years, the actual mixtures have not been very varied. In the past, most of the permanent inhabitants could trace their origins to European ancestry, with a minority having arrived from Africa, Asia, or South America. This has changed radically in the past few years, to the extent that many newer immigrants are from areas that are totally unfamiliar to those with whom they are trying to integrate. This is true also in some European, African, and Asian nations, as they receive settlers from other parts of the world.

Many of the new arrivals come from war-torn countries, or to escape terrorism, persecution, starvation, overcrowding, or natural disasters that have made life unbearable. In many instances, those in the receiving countries object strenuously to accepting those who may require financial assistance, or are unable to fit into the lifestyle of the community. Economic fears are also part of the problem when newcomers arrive. Will these immigrants take over jobs held by the original population? Will they overrun neighborhoods, so that the original population flees in fear or misunderstanding? And what if the new inhabitants require medical care?

When those of differing cultures require medical assistance, they may find themselves in a totally unfamiliar situation. They may be used to a different approach to illness, perhaps herbal remedies or acupuncture or other treatments with which local practitioners are unfamiliar. This is particularly true in psychiatry, where differences as experienced by the newcomers may lead to problems in diagnosis and treatment.

Some syndromes experienced by immigrants are unknown in the areas where they are now living. In other situations, the newcomers are unable to talk about their problems in words that can be understood by the health care provider. One reason that psychiatric diagnoses are affected by the cultural origin of the patient is that idioms rule the language needed for patients to understand and describe their experience. For example, *zar,* a syndrome known in North Africa and the Middle East, involves a belief of being possessed by a spirit. The patients react by shouting, laughing, perhaps banging their heads. As strange as the behavior is, it is not considered pathological in their native setting. Because it is not included in an official diagnostic system, treatment offered by practitioners unfamiliar with it, may be inappropriate.

Some disorders are actually included in an official diagnostic system, but may be totally outside the realm of understanding by those unfamiliar with it. One example of this is *taijin kyofusho,* recognized in Japan as an intense fear that one's body or its functions may displease, embarrass, or offend others. Conversely, anorexia nervosa, so familiar to health care workers in the United States, is considered absurd by most other cultures. This is especially true in areas of the world where shortages of food are an everyday occurrence. In those countries, self-starvation by choice is unfathomable.

2

Looking at the Health Worker

Health workers' observation and understanding of the patient are prime considerations in determining the care that is to be given. But unless the workers understand themselves, their perceptions of the patient may be incorrect. Workers, as well as the patient, bring to the bedside a value system that is based on socioeconomic, cultural, health, religious, educational, and work backgrounds. It is impossible for workers to make an insightful evaluation of the patient if they consider their own standards impeccable and use them as the basis for evaluating the patient. Even though the professionals' standards may be "perfect" within their own social group, they cannot expect to develop therapeutic relationships by applying their beliefs indiscriminately when evaluating the status and needs of patients.

Workers usually enter one of the health professions for special reasons. For many, the chance to help others is the prime consideration. For others, the stimulus may be provided by the availability and stability of job opportunities, the status of belonging to a respected profession, or even the prodding of parents, relatives, and teachers. Some are influenced by serious illnesses they have had as children, or books they have read about heroic medical achievements. And there are also those who can give no conscious reason for having chosen a career in one of the health services.

The health worker who has led a sheltered life, protected by environment and parents, may find it difficult to become attuned to the needs of others. Conversely, workers whose lives have been full of problems, and who have not had their own needs met, may find it equally difficult to hear a cry for help. It is not that these workers are unwilling to be helpful. Rather, they are unable to assess situations because their backgrounds are limited in scope and experience. When workers have lacked the opportunity to compare their own backgrounds with that of others, they may be unable to understand how changes in their rearing might have provided them with greater insight and empathy in their relationships with patients.

The workers reared in homes in which family members always subdued their emotions may be uncomfortable when faced with a highly charged situation. It is easier to become busy with other tasks than to face the obvious difficulty of entering a patient's room when anticipating a tirade. Workers may see no reason to accept abuse, particularly if they have always been kindly, "good" persons respected by others. They may regard the patient as nasty and ungrateful, and not think in terms of understanding the patient's unmet needs. The patient who cries, moans, screams at relatives and staff is looked upon as an unpleasant individual, one to be avoided if at all possible.

The reverse situation may occur when workers are confronted by the saccharin-sweet, quiet patient, who denies discomfort or illness even when obviously very uncomfortable or very ill. If workers have had a volatile family life, they may see this patient as a "delight," one who doesn't seem to have a care in the world and whose concerns are minor. Workers may spend a great deal of time socializing at the bedside but, again, never think in terms of what is behind the facade presented by the patient.

The worker who has been reared by people he considers "normal" will probably use them as the basis for his perception of normality in others. The authoritarian father, the dependent mother, the selfless sister, the strong brother may be acceptable to the worker, whereas the dependent father, the authoritarian mother, the selfish sister, and the weak brother are not. He does not look at the patient's situation and evaluate it for itself, but rather is judgmental in terms of his own upbringing.

Health workers must be aware of their own physical and emotional state when approaching a patient. Anger at a coworker, worry about an ill family member, or such physical illness as a cold or an arthritis attack may result in a preoccupied, angry, or pained facial expression that the patient may think reflects the workers' response to his actions. It is wiser for workers to postpone giving care—when this is feasible—or to explain to the patient that certain extenuating circumstances are causing their appearance of distress rather than to allow the patient to feel that his own actions are the cause. There are occasions when health care workers undergo personal crises that are overwhelming.

It may be difficult to muster the inner resources necessary to provide proper professional service to clients under these circumstances. At such times, the provider needs a strong support system, one that will allow ventilation without fear of judgmental reprisal. However, others may make themselves unavailable, fearful that they are intruding. This is particularly so if the worker in crisis is a colleague upon whom they have depended for help.

Where can the provider in crisis go for help? Obvious choices would be supervisors or other therapeutic professionals within or outside the work situation. For some, the need to ask for help, to share their own pain, is an unacceptable sign of weakness. As professionals, we need to accept the fact that we cannot always be in command of every aspect of our lives. There are occasions when we may feel as fragile as our clients, as impotent as they, as unable to recognize our options as those whom we may consider to be helpless. We may need the input of someone who is not emotionally involved in the problem, someone who can see beyond the immediate to the long-term aspects of the situation.

Often coworkers shy away from even mentioning the crisis. This may be regarded as callous indifference unless the provider understands the reluctance of others to interfere. There even may be some coworkers who are unaware that the provider is in a crisis situation. In a sense, this is equivalent to a "secret" in a family, where abnormal behavior or responses are noted, but the reason is hidden. How much better for all if the "secret" is aired in a discussion with coworkers, to whatever depth the provider feels appropriate, affording everyone the chance to offer support.

The provider in crisis may be overwhelmed by the illness or death of a loved one, a marital, social, or financial problem, or even a work situation that is formidable. Coworkers can show support just with an act of kindness, perhaps taking over tasks for which they are suited at work, visiting the ill person, providing a meal for other family members (particularly children), or just letting the person talk. The chance to describe what is happening to an interested listener is therapeutic. It does not imply a search for a solution, nor should the listener feel compelled to find one. There are times when a resolution is unattainable, but the warmth felt from those who have shown interest will be enough to get the provider back to a functioning state.

Because cultures differ widely, they affect the worker's approach to a patient. One who enters an old-fashioned Japanese home without removing his shoes is regarded as uncouth. Yet walking shoeless into an American mansion would be equally unacceptable. Recognizing, accepting, and acting within cultural determinants help prevent the worker from developing misconceptions of patient behavior, and thus help establish a therapeutic atmosphere. The patient who senses that the worker lacks respect for his values is unlikely to establish a feeling of rapport with the worker. For example, a physician who conducted a filmed psychiatric family therapy session in a Black patient's home, complained later that the family had not been amenable to therapy. He felt that they resented him because he was White, middle class, and Jewish. A review of the film supplied the real answer. The physician and his cotherapist had taken off their jackets and ties before being seated, and were blowing billows of cigar smoke through the well-kept living room. Meanwhile, the nonsmoking family stiffly maintained the formal appearance they normally exhibited in their most important room. The physician was unaware that his behavior, attire, and smoking were being regarded as signs of disrespect.

Religious beliefs that are different from those of the health worker are sometimes cited to explain one's inability to establish rapport with a patient, or as a reason for disliking or not understanding a patient. For example, staff members often show their anger at the "stupidity" of a severe cardiac patient who has refused to disavow religious scruples about birth control and who has become pregnant. The unkind remarks they make have their roots in religious bigotry. "Why not try self-control if you can't use birth control?" "Put a television set in your bedroom." "Don't you ever stop to think about the lack of natural supplies if the population continues to explode?" The patient may smile uncomfortably in her embarrassment, too upset to discuss her fear that she may not live long enough to raise her children and her even greater fear of perdition if she practices birth control.

The staff may also become furious with diabetic Jewish patients who insist on insulin that comes only from kosher animals. It becomes troublesome to exchange the medication on hand even when the other is easily accessible. The request ties in with the picture of "that demanding Jew," and does not consider his training regarding important religious observances.

The worker, too, may have to face expressions of intolerance. "I usually don't like Blacks, but you're different." Such a remark by a patient may make the worker wonder, "Why should I help nurse this person back to health?" The worker has to accept the statement as one born of ignorance and may safely counter it with, "Aren't all people different? Shouldn't each of us be judged for personal worth rather than race, creed, or color?" If the worker speaks calmly, and without rancor, the patient may recognize his prejudices and start to review them. If the worker becomes angry, and storms out of the room, the patient will likely become indignant at the action of "that arrogant, lazy, stupid worker. I was only paying him a compliment."

Health workers find themselves changing in the face of constant involvement with patients who are suffering. Some are frightened at the thought of developing a warm relationship with a patient, particularly one who may die, because of fear that the pain the workers will then go through will be too much to bear. To avoid that pain, they may remain detached, perhaps focusing on incidents in the relationship that can be regarded humorously but disregarding those that indicate the patient's suffering. To some, such a detached attitude is "professional." But is it? It is certainly not professional to avoid responding to the cry of the patient for a meaningful human relationship.

Assuming a facade of caring for only the specific "illness" of the patient may lead to feelings of guilt on the part of workers. Although the patient may have a diseased gallbladder, his entire being is not encompassed by that organ. In fact, that aspect of his being may be minor in comparison with his view of himself in relation to others. The health workers who have empathy, and listen to the patient's complaints or problems, no matter how unrelated to the present illness, can provide a great deal of support. If they do more than just empathize and become involved (again, we stress, not immobilized), they can help the patient adjust to his life situation or make some changes in his behavior that reflect new insights.

Some health workers have a compulsion to be the *total* suppliers of all care to the patient. This attitude is often born of an inner need to be in complete control at all times. It does not take the needs or desires of the patient or family into consideration. Workers who function on this level do not allow the patient to plan any part of his or her care—bathing, eating, sleeping, and recreational activities are all predetermined by the worker. For example, a mother "interferes" if she stays with her child; an adolescent is "disturbing to others" when quietly seated at a patient's bedside; anyone who receives special visiting privileges, because he cannot come during the designated hours is met with hostility, and the visit will be interrupted for checking the patient's temperature or blood pressure, or for giving special treatments; the patient with a chronic illness is discharged without the needed practice in self-care, and is made to feel that he cannot possibly make decisions or do things for himself.

At the other end of the continuum are workers anxious to relieve themselves of responsibility for the patient. Some nurses consider themselves fortunate to be assigned to the care of children whose mothers remain in the room almost around the clock. In one case, nurses would bring the bath supplies, linen, meals, and medications into the room, and say to the mother, "If you need anything, just call." They did not offer to care for the child, nor speak to the mother or child about their feelings or problems. They were happy not to watch the child going downhill. By keeping their distance they avoided any emotional involvement. They were unprepared for the mother's angry outburst when the child came nearer to death. "Of course I have to be here all the time! If I weren't, who would bathe, dress, and feed my child? No one takes any interest in us . . . no one cares." The nurses' own anxiety had been so high that they had failed to recognize the needs of the mother. It would have been far better if the mother had been relieved of responsibility for the child's nursing care but had been allowed to work along *with* the nurses if she so desired. The mother would have then felt more confidence in the availability and competence of nursing care, and the child would have had a chance to develop rapport with the nurses. Then both mother and child might have been able to express their worries to the nurses, thereby easing their tensions.

A patient who bears great responsibility for others (a sick spouse, elderly parents, young children) is usually greatly admired by the hospital staff because his anxiety is ostensibly centered not on himself, but on the welfare of others, a trait that inspires admiration as well as empathy. One patient was frantically worried about her blind diabetic husband, who in three sightless years had become totally dependent on her. "Who will take care of him if I die?" "What will happen if I have to stay in the hospital for a long time?" The staff looked upon this woman as being full of virtue, always extending herself in consideration of her husband. Their own standards for being a "good" wife blinded them to a major fact—the patient had needlessly relegated her husband to the role of helpless invalid, even unable to pour a cup of coffee for himself. He, in turn, felt emasculated, but blamed his resulting sexual impotence on his diabetes. (Although this disorder is frequently associated with impotence, the patient's emotional reaction to his feelings of helplessness was the much larger factor.) The patient was helped to find practical solutions for her worries. A worker at a local institution for the blind went to the patient's home and taught the husband the necessary elements of self-care. A college-aged son, still living at home, was happy to learn that he could help his father. Finally, the wife was able to speak to the hospital staff about her past hidden resentment at always having to be "the strong one." She also talked about her feelings of guilt when her husband developed the diabetic retinopathy that caused his blindness. "Maybe if I had been stricter about his diet, it wouldn't have happened." Had the staff not been so overly impressed initially by the patient's "goodness," she might have received the help she needed sooner.

At times, hospital workers may feel outranked by patients who are better educated than themselves and avoid any meaningful discussion with such patients not to reveal any missing aspects of their own education. The patient is then isolated, unable to have his needs met, simply because the insecurities of the workers make maintaining their own prestige more important than being involved in any exchange. For example, nurses may have been graduated from a diploma program, an associate degree program, or a baccalaureate program. Small wonder, then, that even experienced nurses who have had little advanced education shudder at the thought of caring for the nursing director who holds a doctoral degree. Yet, if staff members can look at the patient as a human being who has all the hopes, worries, loves, and disappointments that other people have, rather than as the holder of a prestigious degree, they may be able to overcome their anxiety and provide empathic care that is also technically superior.

As health workers gain experience, they have the opportunity to refine their techniques and become more effective. They learn to evaluate what they are doing and how they affect the patient. They will learn as much from their failures as from their successes but only if they can truthfully assess their own contribution to both. They should evaluate the image they have projected— have they been directorial, permissive, judgmental, hostile, seductive, or concerned? How have the patients reacted? Would another approach have been more therapeutic? Were the providers meeting the needs of patients, or were they forcing patients to satisfy the needs of the staff? Should the workers have called in consultants to advise them more often?

If the workers have the interests of the patient at heart, they will be aware of the roles of the other disciplines. Just as the physician asks the nurse to give the enema that he orders, so the nurse should feel free to call in the clinical nurse specialist, social worker, psychologist, physiotherapist, or home care expert. Each discipline has much to contribute to the patient's well-being, yet each has limitations. Working harmoniously as a team helps promote better care for the patient.

Because no one knows everything, it may be necessary to consult with others of one's own discipline to ensure the best possible patient care. The obstetrical patient with heart disease may be assigned to a bed in the maternity division of the hospital, but she and her husband may benefit from a cardiac teaching program given in the medical division. Being aware of available programs and liaison personnel increases the scope of the workers' proficiency. If they limit themselves to their own field and remain unaware of the possibilities of using help that can be given by personnel from other areas, they may also not become aware of the divergent needs of the patient. It is an unfortunate fact that when workers do not recognize their own limitations, they also are unable to see a need for outside consultation. Occasionally, workers who do know of other programs do not arrange for patient participation because they fear that the patient will think less of them for seeking outside assistance. In such a case, the worker needs help in defining priorities—which is more important: the needs of the patient or the worker's fear of a possible loss of status?

On occasion, the beliefs of the workers and those of the patient may clash, with tragic results. A patient who had experienced several severe postpartum depressions became pregnant, although she had used a contraceptive. The patient, her husband, and the physician agreed that termination of the pregnancy was the only solution. The patient was assigned to a room on the maternity floor near the nursery because the admitting officer could not "tie up a gynecology bed for this." A nurse told the patient, "I can't take care of you because abortion is against my religion." The anesthesiologist said, "I have to receive my fee in advance. You people leave the hospital very quickly." Although the patient was in therapy, she had to be rehospitalized for her severe depression and guilt after the procedure. Each staff member was either disinterested or unaware of how his negative statements would affect the patient.

In another case, a brilliant octogenarian who had been a practicing psychologist was losing her hearing, her sight, and her financial resources. She resented her dependence on others, and withdrew from any association with staff or other patients, whom she had difficulty in seeing and hearing. She looked forward to death and frequently discussed her positive feelings about euthanasia for those who no longer wish to live. Staff members became very uncomfortable when she talked about euthanasia, a concept unacceptable to them. They described the patient as "haughty. . . . She thinks she's better than any of us." They overtly rejected her, and repeatedly placed her in the position of having to ask for help. One night, she encased herself in a sheet, and set herself on fire with her cigarette lighter. Staff members rushed in, beat out the flames, resuscitated her heroically, and spent long months treating her burns. When she was well enough, she was transferred to a state mental institution. After all, her suicidal attempt was a sign that she was crazy, wasn't it? Not one staff member had seen the need for intervention during the time that the patient was talking about euthanasia and isolating herself from others. Instead, they looked upon her ideas and withdrawal as a hurtful, unacceptable rejection of themselves.

The health worker who can look on himself honestly, taking credit for his virtues and trying to improve his shortcomings, will be able to care for his patients more effectively. The worker whose insecurity is too great to let him evaluate his own abilities and actions truthfully will be so anxious to protect himself that he will not hear patients' cries for help.

Fear of the patient's behavior may also hinder the thinking and actions of the worker. Occasionally, patients become assaultive, either because of a basic psychotic condition or a precipitating factor such as an electrolyte imbalance. Several days after extensive intestinal surgery, a patient who had previously been quiet and who was later found to have such an imbalance started screaming that the patient across the room was going to kill her. In defense, she threw everything she could get her hands on toward the other patient. Fortunately, her aim was very poor, and there were no injuries. The nurses who were on duty ran to the other patient to protect her, and themselves, from the onslaught. Only one nurse was unafraid. She walked directly to the patient and in a calm voice said, "No one will hurt you. I am beside you and will see to that." Hearing this, the patient reached out and grasped the nurse's hand. Within a short while, she relaxed and fell asleep. Had the nurse not been able to approach her, the assaultive behavior probably would have continued and even increased.

Workers also become fearful when patients harm themselves as well as others. One psychotic patient would start her assaultive behavior in the day room. After shouting a long line of expletives, she would start throwing whatever was available, sending other patients, and often staff, running for help. As they disappeared, she would look for smouldering cigarette butts dropped by patients, and burn her arms or legs with them. One day a nurse who had noticed this pattern walked quickly to the patient when she started to curse aloud and calmly said, "I am not going to let you hurt yourself today." The patient screamed more foul language and reached for a nearby ash tray. The nurse quickly maneuvered it away, saying, "I am not going to let you throw things, either." The nurse then extinguished the cigarette butt, which the patient had thrown to the floor. At this, the patient screamed, "I hate you. I hate you, you no good—." She banged her fists on the wall and began to sob. The nurse stood nearby, not speaking or moving. Finally, the patient sat down on the couch, and the nurse sat near her. "I couldn't let you hurt yourself. I know how angry you feel, but there are other ways to get it out of your system." The patient did not seem to hear what was being said but continued to sit on the couch, staring ahead. After a long silence she whispered, "You're a nice lady." After this episode, she continued to exhibit assaultive behavior on occasion but never when that nurse was on duty.

This nurse, instead of being afraid of the patient's actions, tried to understand what those actions meant. Thus, she was able to empathize with the patient and help to calm her. Had the nurse become fearful, she might have tried to control the patient physically, an impossible task in view of the patient's greater strength and agility.

It may take time and experience for workers to overcome their apprehension about working with difficult patients. However, if they expend their energies toward understanding why the patient is behaving in an unacceptable manner, rather than concentrating on their own fears, they are more likely to be effective in the situation.

3

The Use of the Interview

An interview is a conversation on a professional level conducted by an individual educated in counseling techniques. Peplau notes that it has several purposes, including the *orientation* of the worker and the patient to each other, the *identification* of the patient's problems, and the *resolution* or institution of means to solve those problems. It differs from an ordinary conversation in that its function is not to provide socialization (except when that is a therapeutic goal), and it is usually planned for set times and places on a regularly scheduled appointment basis. The full time allotted for the appointment is kept by the worker whether or not the patient is present or responsive.

Orientation is the first step in establishing rapport with the patient. The worker greets the patient by name, and introduces himself by name and title. He then seats himself nearby, and tells the patient why he has come. "I understand that you are unhappy about your care," or "I have been called because you asked to speak to someone about your problems," or "How are things going?" The approach should be friendly but matter-of-fact, so that the patient does not feel as though he is going to be judged, as he might if the interviewer were to appear stern or threatening. If the person's anxiety level is high, he may not hear the introduction and will ask the interviewer to repeat his name, title, and the purpose of his visit. He may, in fact, request this information several times. "What did you say your name was again? . . . What do you do? . . . Why are you here?" If the worker realizes that anxiety and not inattentiveness is preventing the patient from hearing the answers, the situation will be more comfortable for all concerned. The worker should continue to repeat the answers in a friendly, matter-of-fact way, without showing any sign of annoyance.

Orientation may also focus upon the patient's stated desire for help. The fact that he recognizes his need for help is a step in the right direction, even though his perception of the actual problem may be distorted. The interview can then proceed to the next stage, that of identifying the problem.

Identification of the real problem is not always easy. The patient may focus on one symptom or event, and be unaware of what is really troubling him. It is up to the professional to listen carefully to what the patient is saying to discover the real problem. At times, the patient may shift the conversation to a different subject as the real difficulty starts to become apparent. He may become restless, say he is too tired to continue the interview, or develop a sudden pain that requires medication. These signs should alert the worker to the fact that the patient cannot tolerate further discussion along that line of inquiry. The patient may direct the conversation to safer subjects or remain silent, in which case the worker should just sit quietly until the end of the appointment. Before leaving, the worker should tell the patient the time and place for the next interview, and that he will be available should the patient need additional help.

Resolution of the problem often follows its identification. Once the patient has been able to recognize what is really at the core of his trouble, he can usually think it through and reach a solution that is satisfactory to *him*. This is not to say that it would be acceptable to another patient in a comparable situation. Nor is it necessarily the ideal solution in the eyes of the professional. The important factor is that it meets the needs of the patient. If it is unsuccessful when tried, the patient should be helped to think the problem through again and to find alternative solutions, one of which may be more helpful.

A nurse consultant was called to see a patient who suddenly began to cry hysterically four days after having had a complete hysterectomy. She greeted the patient by name, introduced herself, sat down so that she could be on eye level with the patient, and said, "Would you like to talk about why you are crying so uncontrollably?" The patient nodded "yes" and continued to sob. In an attempt to help identify the problem, the nurse then said, "Sometimes women worry about the effects of this type of operation. They're afraid that it may affect their femininity." The patient shook her head from side to side, still crying and blowing her nose.

Between sobs, the patient finally said, "I'm a very sexy woman, and I've been looking forward to this so that I won't have to be concerned about becoming pregnant, or be annoyed by menstrual periods. It's not that. I just don't understand why I can't stop crying. It's been going on for six hours. I'm exhausted, but I can't get myself to stop." More tears, more nose blowing, more convulsive sobs.

The nurse sat silently for a while, then said quietly, "Many people anticipate dying during surgery, and cry afterwards for the sheer relief of being alive and on the way to recovery."

At this, the patient suddenly stopped crying, broke into a broad smile, and blurted, "That's it—I'm alive and I'm so relieved, I'm really alive!" By identifying her problem she had resolved it, and her crying ceased.

A man who was scheduled for surgery to remove a cancer became depressed two days before surgery, refused to leave his bedside, and cried at intervals. Although his depression was understandable in light of the diagnosis, it seemed to be based on something more than that. The nurse consultant greeted him, introduced herself, and sat down near him. "The nurses tell me that you are very sad. Perhaps it would be helpful if you could share your feelings."

The patient's eyes filled with tears, and the nurse handed him a tissue. "I guess you must think I am not much of a man for crying." The nurse assured him that being a man was not at all dependent on whether or not one cried. "You know, I'm going to have a big operation, and the doctor says he can't tell how I'll be after it's over. I just don't know what to do."

The nurse said, "It's hard to face surgery when there are so many unfinished pieces of business to be completed." At this, the patient bowed his head and shoulders, and began to cry aloud.

"I've hurt so many people—everyone that I've loved. I lost my wife's money in the stock market, I stole from my best friend in business, and, worst of all, I've antagonized my daughter so that she refuses to see or speak to me. I'm no good to anyone, not even to myself."

The patient went into each of these reasons for his depressed state in great detail. Losing his wife's money and stealing from his business partner were rash acts in a desperate bid for needed cash; his fight with his daughter involved her new husband. The patient believed that it was unmanly to apologize and had, therefore, stopped communicating with his wife, his best friend, and his daughter. Now he needed to reopen those lines of communication to find inner peace. He finally decided that it was more important to ask each of them for forgiveness than to maintain his self-image of an unrelenting man. Although the reunions were tearful, they helped him resolve his inner conflicts. As soon as the stress of his emotional turmoil was relieved he was able to hold his head high again and face the surgery "like a man." His depression had lifted, and he became hopeful about the outcome of the operation.

During any interaction, the worker must listen attentively to what the patient doesn't say, as well as to what he says. Sometimes unspoken words are more revealing than those which are said aloud. One young patient discussed his work history in great detail, but skipped over a five-year span during which he had worked for his father. Toward the end of that time, the situation at work had become so distressing that the son could neither sleep nor eat, and finally had to be admitted to a mental institution for three months. Another patient did not mention or recall his daughter's serious bout with rheumatic fever years before, but ruminated at length about the car he had purchased just before she became ill. A young woman who told a nurse that she was afraid to go home because she might harm her children and herself was later unable to remember uttering that statement.

In some instances, communication is impeded because the patient speaks in a language of his own that is not understandable to anyone else. The interviewer should not permit such words and phrases to pass unchallenged because the patient may interpret this as a sign that he is being understood, or that the worker lacks real concern for him, or that he considers the patient "too crazy" to talk to. Pronouns may be misused (the patient may refer to himself as "he" rather than "I"), and neologisms (jargon coined by the patient) may hide the patient's thoughts. The worker can sometimes assess the meaning of confusing phrases by asking the patient to explain them. Unless both interviewer and patient have the same understanding of the patient's language, the patient's private world will remain impenetrable.

The patient who is totally mute is also communicating with the worker. His very silence becomes a challenge, because the worker must then try to unravel the mystery of this nonverbal communication. It may be difficult to tolerate the silence, to realize that it is part of the patient's illness. Spending time with the patient reassures him that he is a worthy person. Although silent, he realizes that he is communicating with you if you meet his physical needs by intuitively providing care that his body gestures suggest (offering him food if he seems hungry, a drink if his lips appear parched). In time, he may feel free enough to start communicating on a verbal level. However, coaxing him to do so before he is ready will increase his need to remain mute.

Listening to what a patient says during an interview involves more than just hearing the spoken words. The *content* of the discussion may only tangentially refer to the subject matter that the patient really wants to talk about. He may be fearful of his ability to deal with the matter once it is exposed, of being ridiculed, or of losing his status in the worker's eyes if the material is ludicrous or unsavory.

The worker must also be aware of the patient's mood during the interview. The patient may exhibit sadness, tearfulness, happiness, or anxiety that may be appropriate to the content of the interview. At other times, the affect (mood) may be totally out of context. The patient who smilingly tells the worker about a long series of disastrous happenings is reacting inappropriately.

As the interviewer listens to the content, his mind may rush ahead, trying to decide what is important, and what material has hidden meanings. The patient may begin to discuss his fight to get a hot cup of coffee with breakfast. The worker may sympathetically jump in to agree with the fact that coffee just never seems to arrive hot at the bedside. Actually, the patient's main concern was the fight, not the coffee. Each employee she asked had promised to bring in a fresh, hot cup of coffee, and each disappeared without doing so. If no one could meet that simple request, how could they be trusted to care for her following complicated abdominal surgery?

Sometimes a worker will sidetrack the patient when an item of common interest is brought up. The patient may start to discuss something that happened on a camping trip. The interviewer, also a camper, may say, "Oh, you enjoy camping, too. Where have you gone? What type of camper did you use?" The events that the patient wanted to bring up are lost in meaningless socialization.

Frequently, patients will direct personal questions at the interviewer, asking whether he is married, has children, lives nearby, and so on. If the worker feels comfortable in doing so, he may answer the questions briefly, without going into detail, and quickly switch the focus back to the patient. "I appreciate your interest in whether I am married. Is your basic concern whether a single person is capable of helping you solve your marital problems?" This brings up the fact that the worker understands that the patient is uneasy and has mixed feelings about talking and revealing himself. It also acknowledges the patient's curiosity about the worker's competence and knowledgeableness.

If the patient says, "Somehow, you remind me of my mother," the worker can use that by saying, "In what way?" or "Describe her to me." The patient can then proceed to discuss whatever he wishes because either phrase can refer to physical, emotional, vocational, educational, or other aspects of the patient's mother that are brought to mind.

The interviewer may find notes on the patient's chart that describe some behavior problem. Relatives or friends may also want to talk to the worker to share bits of information. Some workers like to read the chart and speak to others first, so as to have as much prior knowledge about the patient as is available. Other interviewers prefer to speak to the patient first, and not be "contaminated" by the reports and remarks of others. If the latter course is taken, the worker may seek other information later to get a more complete picture of the patient and to clarify what the patient has said.

A patient who was terminally ill with cancer and who suddenly became very depressed furnishes a case in point. Ostensibly, she was concerned about the fact that she would not be able to meet the expenses incurred by her illness. In a series of interviews, she brought up the changes that had occurred in her life since her husband's death several years earlier. She spoke of him in endearing terms, and told of how admired he was by everyone who knew him. Suddenly, her face reddened in anger. "Everyone, that is, but me! He never planned ahead for me. He spent everything he earned and didn't have much insurance. He changed jobs just two years before he died, and lost the pension and other benefits that he had accumulated. After he died, I had to go to work. I wasn't trained for anything and had to lie about my age and qualifications to get a job. It all worked out, but I hate him for putting me in such a position." She went on to tell of her difficulties in getting along with her daughter, and of her son's marital difficulties and divorce.

The notes on the chart indicated that the patient was always cooperative and pleasant, and that she stressed her desire to "not be a burden" to anyone. Although too weak to be out of bed without help, she went to the bathroom alone one night, fell and injured herself. She was very apologetic to all the staff members involved in getting her back to bed. The next day, a deep depression set in.

The daughter described her mother as "authoritarian." "She just won't let go. I'm almost 40 years old, and she still tells me how to dress, and how to live, and how to raise my two children. She's loved by everyone who knows her, but [and here she began to cry] I hate her. She has always made my brother the good one, and me the bad one. I won't have her in my home because she causes trouble between my husband and me. I can't help being angry with her, or feeling guilty about it later."

With all this information, the interviewer was able to help the patient look at her illness and its effects from a different angle. The worry about finances was only a ploy to disguise her anguish about losing control over herself and her daughter. Slowly, the patient was able to bring out her fear of becoming dependent upon others. The interviewer discussed this problem with the staff who responded by giving the patient as much latitude in determining her own care as possible. Medications for pain were adjusted in consultation with her. She wanted relief but did not want to be drowsy so much of the time. Smaller doses were given more frequently, until a happy medium was met. The patient was also urged to dictate her dietary preferences, and to decide upon times for her personal care. All of these steps contributed toward lessening her sense of dependency.

In further interviews, the worker discovered that the patient had always resented the close relationship between her husband and their daughter, and had remained aloof from her daughter because she sensed she would be rejected. Instead she developed close ties with her grandchildren, who loved her dearly. Gradually, as she explored her feelings, she lessened her attempts at control over her daughter, thus easing the strain between the two of them. Before she died, they were able to spend pleasant hours together, learning about each other, and gaining some of the closeness that each had wanted through the years.

To be effective, interviewers must remain nonjudgmental, regardless of what they are told. This was particularly true in the mother-daughter interviews cited earlier. If workers side with either protagonist, they are unlikely to help in the resolution of the patient's problems. By remaining outside the realm of the problem, workers are able to help the patient work toward a solution.

Once a counseling relationship has started, an inexperienced worker and the patient may find that they have developed a close personal relationship. This becomes a problem if the patient wants to continue meeting the worker socially after the therapeutic sessions have been terminated. One way to prevent this is to make it clear during the orientation phase that the worker will be available *until* the patient has determined ways to solve problems. As that time draws near, the worker should remind the patient of this. "I will be seeing you while you still need my help. After that point, arrangements can be made for you to receive help if you confront other problems that appear too difficult to manage alone."

4

Respecting Confidentiality

Patients reveal a great deal about themselves during the time they are involved in interviews. Feelings that they perhaps have not admitted even to themselves may suddenly come to the surface. They must be assured with certainty that anything they share with the interviewer will be held in confidence. This is imperative because confidentiality is a prime concern, particularly when the discussion involves action, thought, or feelings that might be embarrassing to the patient.

Information that the patient discloses must be regarded as privileged and must not be bantered about by hospital or agency personnel not directly involved in the patient's care. If the team approach is being used, every member of the team is obligated to respect totally and absolutely the information that is revealed by the worker in conferences. As a professional person, the worker's ethics should prevent him from divulging information about patients to neighbors, friends, or family, even though the patient is not known to them. In fact, discussion of confidential material is unethical even though the worker is away from the clinical setting, and feels certain that the patient is not identifiable.

Sometimes patients are so fearful of a breach of confidentiality that they will withhold pertinent information. In one instance, a White patient did not tell her physician that she had been having extramarital sexual relations with a supposedly sterile Chinese man. When her unknowing husband who believed he had impregnated his wife saw the oriental appearance of the newborn, he accused the hospital of switching babies. The wife was unwilling to divulge the truth about the baby's parentage until her husband initiated a lawsuit against the hospital. At that point, she told her husband the truth, asking him to drop the suit before the local newspapers printed the story. The marriage subsequently was terminated, with husband and wife each going into therapy.

What if the patient tells the interviewer that he is planning to commit suicide or a homicide? Can confidentiality be respected in such an instance? What will happen to the relationship if the interviewer shares such information with others?

The worker should never agree to meet demands of the patient before he knows what prompts them. If the patient says, "I'll tell you what I'm planning if you promise that you won't tell anyone," the worker should reply sincerely, "I can't help you fully unless I know what is really bothering you. I never make promises I can't keep. It wouldn't be fair to either of us. Furthermore, such a promise might make me incapable of giving you the kind of care and attention most beneficial to you."

When a patient discusses committing an act of violence, he is crying for help. He is afraid that he will not be able to control his impulses without outside assistance. The worker must then help him reach the point where he can discuss his intentions with his physician. The worker can support the patient and remain with him, but cannot accept the total responsibility for preventing an irresponsible action. He can say to the patient, "The fact that you are able to share this information indicates that you realize you need help. I am not in a position to offer all the assistance you need. Your doctor will be able to offer a wider range of suggestions than I. Until you speak with him, I shall try to help you in every way I can. It would be best if *you* speak to the doctor, rather than have me transmit your thoughts to him. How do you feel about this?"

Some workers find it difficult to respond in a professional manner if the patient rejects the suggestion that he confide in the doctor. If the worker himself has never been able to trust others, he may very well be adamant in his feeling that he should not disclose the patient's plans to anyone else. He reasons, "I wouldn't want anyone to interfere with my plans after I confide in him." His judgment is obviously impaired because of his feeling that what he would want for himself is best for the patient.

When the patient refuses to speak with the doctor, the interviewer should try to determine the reason. If the patient refuses to change his mind, the worker should state calmly and factually, "I guess I will have to speak to him, although it would be more meaningful if you did. It is important to me that you not be permitted to hurt yourself or others. The doctor can help in that effort."

The suicidal patient is often isolated and placed on certain precautions which may include locking the windows permanently, searching his belongings for dangerous implements, and keeping nurses at his bedside around the clock. One patient, in a riverside hospital, mulled over his rejections of various methods of committing suicide. "I'd jump out of the window, but I'm afraid of heights." "I'd jump into the river, but I can't swim." "I'd slash my wrists, but I can't stand the sight of blood." "I'd hang myself, but I can't stand anything tight around my neck." And so on, ad infinitum. It is important that staff members assigned to the patient share such information so that everyone can help protect the patient from himself.

Patients who are transferred from a psychiatric service to another area in a general hospital often worry about the reports that go with them. They should be assured that confidential information will not be placed on the chart, but that a note advising the staff of appropriate ways to care for them will be included.

Facts pertinent to the care and understanding of the patient may be shared with other staff members only if they understand and respect confidentiality. A patient's personal problems and motivations are not to be bandied about for the titillation of coworkers or friends. Health workers are legally responsible for confidentiality, and are liable for any unprofessional breach of that trust.

When a patient confides in the worker, the information must never be used to the worker's self-advantage. One worker became so interested in a patient's tales of her sexual prowess that he decided to test her skill for himself. The patient reported the seduction, noting that it was just one more affirmation of her belief that men were interested in her only for her body. Another worker became excessively attentive to a patient who told of his vast financial holdings. Her attention to this patient was noticed by the staff, and remarked upon by the patient who said, "She is probably after my money." Discussions with the worker revealed her plan to use the patient's acumen as a guide in her own financial dealings.

The staff must not use the patient's psychiatric status to intimidate him in any way. One health worker on a psychiatric unit told a patient that it didn't matter what the worker said to him, because "no one would believe a report from a nut." Fortunately, the patient did not allow himself to be intimidated, and reported the incident, which was then thoroughly investigated by the staff. Similar incidents were revealed by several other patients who had been afraid to say anything because they feared reprisals by the worker.

Often the change-of-shift report is a time when the staff gossip about the patient. This seems to relieve them of tensions accumulated during the tour of duty, but it is demeaning to the patient and prevents the formulation of more meaningful goals for his care. Noisy laughter and often total immersion of staff in stories about patients are sometimes overheard or observed by patients, who may then believe that their confidences are not kept. Although health workers are also human, they should not use staff conferences to denigrate patients who are, at the moment, less fortunate.

Telephones that workers use to discuss privileged information with the doctor or other professionals should be in a private area to prevent the conversation from being overheard. Oftentimes the health worker uses a telephone that is centrally located, with the result that any patient who is nearby hears what is being said. This may cause the patient who overhears to lose confidence in the staff's ability to maintain confidentiality. Once that happens, the patient is unlikely to confide in any staff member again.

The introduction of computers as a time-saving device for recording, retaining, and recalling information about patients has led to questions about the maintenance of confidentiality. Concerns that their histories will be shared with unqualified personnel may cause patients to withhold important material about present or past illnesses. The patient should be assured that information is available to the staff on levels that vary with their capabilities.

Certain computerized information, such as general care and dietary orders, can be made accessible to everyone providing care. This ensures continuity and accuracy. Information of a more sophisticated or personal level can be reached only by selected staff members in possession of computer "keys" that unlock further information. The more restricted the input, the fewer are the number of staff members having access to the "key" for that level of information.

A computer is only as helpful as the information fed into it. The ability to select pertinent, accurate, and important facts and incorporate them into the records in a concise way is a skill that can be an important factor in improving the quality of patient care.

ETHICAL CONSIDERATIONS AND CONFIDENTIALITY

There are ethical considerations that also arise in the sharing of information. Today, the field of genetics permits people to discover whether or not they bear genes that may lead to serious or even life-threatening disorders. For example, the genes for breast cancer are supplying clues for some families with a history of the disorder. However, it is not simply a case of finding one suspected gene. It is known that there are at least two, and possibly four or more genes, each with additional mutations possible, that enter into the preillness diagnosis. These same genes may also have a role in male breast cancer as well as cancer of the prostate, colon, pancreas, ovaries, or tumors of other organs. What will the knowledge do for the individual?

Although genetic tests would theoretically be helpful by giving advance knowledge to individuals who may develop a disease, that knowledge may be regarded as a death threat by patients in situations for which there is no known cure. Not only does the concern about the disease add to patients' distress, but side issues of confidentiality become paramount for some. If patients are known to have the possibility of developing a serious illness, they may lose their jobs as the employer fears that they will need time away for medical care and, therefore, be less productive. In addition, although federal legislation may change the possibility, individuals with genetic disorders may find themselves uninsurable. No wonder that those undergoing the expense of genetic tests need assurance that the results will be handled with total confidentiality.

Psychiatric professionals are necessary to help patients through the period of genetic testing. In many places, testing is not undertaken unless it is preceded by professional counseling. The field of genetic testing is so new that full implications are not always understood. Presently, patients who test negatively for the known breast cancer genes cannot be told that they will never develop the disease because the known genes are only involved in a small percentage of cases. Conversely, those with positive results may never suffer from the disease. In some instances, they may choose to undergo bilateral mastectomies as a preventive measure. This radical procedure should not be considered foolproof because it may reduce but not eliminate the risk.

It is important that counseling include discussion of available treatments for those who test positively. The importance of frequent testing to discover the disease at its inception should be stressed because cures are more likely to succeed with early detection and intervention. In addition, information on life style, including the latest knowledge on diet, and the effects of injurious substances should be offered. The patient may also seek information on whether or not to have children because there may be the possibility of passing mutant genes to the next generation. There may even be a question of whether to marry if there is too much danger in bearing children. Ethically, false reassurance should not be offered about the future. Certainly the need for counseling may be ongoing as the full implications of negative genetic information become known. Again, confidentiality is imperative as patients try to sort out the effects of their situation.

5

The Health Worker
in the Community

When the health worker is knowledgeable about the extent of mental illness in this country, he realizes also that an awareness of the factors in prevention must become part of every health worker's armamentarium. The institution of treatment after mental illness has taken hold is not enough. It is imperative for all health workers to recognize those situations that may give rise to causative factors and help the patient find options for their resolution.

As far back as 1964, Dr. Gerald Kaplan noted that prevention of mental illness can take place on three levels. On the *primary* level, the health worker tries to prevent or alleviate situations that may contribute to mental health problems. Perhaps this can be accomplished by efforts to change the home, community, or work environment, or by helping people to anticipate and handle crises that are of maturational or situational origin. On the *secondary* level, the health worker strives for recognition, diagnosis, and early treatment of problems. On the *tertiary* level, the worker tries to prevent a worsening of the illness, while working toward rehabilitation of the patient. At times, workers find themselves involved with a patient on all three levels at one time. For example, the patient's illness may have been recognized and treatment instituted. During the same period, his work situation may require intervention. Meanwhile, rehabilitation is started with vocational training geared toward placing the patient in a job that would create less tension for him or use his newly learned coping skills in his work setting.

Hospitalization for any mental illness should be for as short a time as possible. The patient should remain in the community whenever feasible, to prevent the additional problems that prolonged hospitalization often brings. Such problems often result from one's separation from home, friends, and work, and the development of a sense of hopelessness and a feeling of helplessness that comes from dependence on others for the gratification of every need and desire.

Who is available to help the patient with a problem? In a sense, everyone who has contact with another human being is a health worker. Neighbors, relatives, teachers, friends, shopkeepers, as well as social workers, nurses, psychologists, and physicians can recognize the beginnings of unhealthy behavior. Beauticians and bartenders are often privy to people's fears and anxieties long before any health professional is involved. It is the duty of the health worker to see that the public is made aware of community resources in the hope that they will be contacted if the need arises.

The public health nurse is in a unique position to uncover behavior patterns that indicate incipient psychiatric illness. Her excursions into homes permit her to see family exchanges that may be unhealthy. She may note that a certain member is the scapegoat for all family problems, or that another is the troublemaker, or that still another lashes out inappropriately in anger. The nurses may hear unrealistic expectations and note the patient's flights into unreality to escape the possibility of not meeting those expectations. Nurses may also become a link between school and home, informing teachers of an intolerable home situation that may result in poor school performance. If she enters the home with the idea of giving care for one specific condition, and does not note situations that may be contributing to mental health problems in the patient or other family members, she is not performing her function to the fullest extent possible.

The public health nurse may also be active in schools or other institutions. She may be present to conduct eye tests, but notice signs of other problems in the children being tested. A child may have a severe tic, lack control of bladder and bowel function, fall asleep in class, or show signs of drug abuse. If the nurse focuses all her energies on the eye tests, she will not be aware of these other signs of possible psychiatric problems.

Social workers also have the opportunity to note problems as they are presented in patients' homes or in institutions. Although workers may ostensibly be present to assess the need for public assistance, they may find a family in acute distress because of the illness of the breadwinner. The father may have become totally dependent, both physically and emotionally, on the mother. He may terrorize the children, or remain silent and withdrawn. The children may not understand what is happening, and attribute his illness and its effects to their own "badness" or "bad" thoughts. If the mother then tells them, "Be quiet, or you'll make daddy worse," they may be overwhelmed by the thought that their father's recovery rests on their ability to be quiet. Again, financial assistance may seem to be *the* problem to the social agency, while actually it is minor in terms of family mental health.

A child's schoolteacher may be the first to recognize physical or emotional problems. She notes that a child who has never spent much time in the bathroom suddenly starts to urinate frequently and is drinking copious amounts of fluid. The teacher may assume that the child is trying to avoid classwork, whereas the youngster may really be showing the first signs of diabetes. Another child may seem to doze off for a few seconds at a time, or be unaware of what is happening around him. He may be having petit mal episodes. Still another may find it difficult to concentrate on his studies, and may not be working up to his potential. The teacher may automatically label him as "lazy," or, conversely, she may investigate and find that certain definite factors are causing the child's behavior. Teachers can be excellent case finders, as the two following case reports indicate.

Eight-year-old Joey's teacher urged the child's mother to ask for help from a neighborhood mental health center because the boy had begun to wet himself frequently in class. The mother told the nurse at the center that the child had also recently become enuretic, and that she was disgusted with him. He was the second of five children, and had been born seven months after her husband committed suicide rather than wait for inevitable death from acute leukemia. She had not been able to care for Joey during his infancy, and had placed both Joey and his older brother in a series of foster homes for two years.

The mother regarded her husband's suicide as an insult to herself. If he had really loved her, he would have waited to see the outcome of her pregnancy. To help regain her sense of being desirable, she had entered into a series of romantic alliances that had resulted in three more children. The father of the youngest child wanted to marry her, but she felt his unstable work record was a drawback. He lived in the home sporadically, but would leave when he was out of work and unable to contribute financially.

Joey appeared to be very bright, and tested well on standard IQ tests. The mother wanted him to be the "best" student in his class, and envisioned him as going to college in the future. She placed great pressure on him to do his schoolwork, and forbade friendships with neighborhood youngsters, whom she considered beneath him both intellectually and socially. His only companion was the next younger brother, a year his junior.

Although the mother qualified for public assistance, she refused it as degrading. She held a full-time job and delegated household tasks to be completed by the three older children before she came home from work. (The two youngest were cared for by a neighbor.) None was allowed to leave the house or backyard after returning from school, or to invite playmates to the house because the mother looked upon other children as a possible contaminating source of bad habits, such as drug abuse or other antisocial behavior.

In describing his life, Joey said he didn't know how to make friends, and that he spent all his time studying. He looked sad as he described doing poorly in some subjects because he was afraid to ask the teacher for explanations. He wanted to join a Boy Scout troop, but his mother would not permit it when she was told she would have to be available for some activities. "It probably wouldn't have been any good anyway!" As for wetting, "I just get that feeling and then it happens . . . like I'm scared, and I don't know what to do . . . when the teacher calls on me, and I don't know the answer . . . when my mother yells at us, and says she hates us and she's leaving us forever."

Meetings with the mother revealed her erratic temper. She found that she could get the children to behave if she stormed out of the home in a rage, and did not come back for several hours. "I'm afraid I'll kill them when I get very angry." She had been unaware of their terror that she really would never come back. "I thought they knew I was kidding." As she talked with the nurse, she decided to try a new pattern of behavior. Instead of raging when angry, she would force herself to talk to the children about what made her angry, but would no longer threaten to leave home. The children learned to change their behavior when she would say, "I am getting furious." Joey in particular began to relax when the threat of desertion lessened.

The visiting nurse went to the school and spoke to the young, dynamic teacher who had made Joey her special project. The teacher was anxious to have him succeed, and recognized that he was hampered by insecurities. "I made him the monitor in charge of homework so that he would realize how much I think of him. He has to check everyone's notebook and report those who have not done their work." She was aware of his inability to make or maintain friendships, and asked the nurse for help in this area. The nurse helped her to understand Joey's role as homework monitor as seen by the other youngsters. Because many of them did not do their assignments, he was regarded as responsible for getting them into trouble. He was torn between his desire to stay on their good side and his responsibility to the teacher. She was concerned by the stress she had unwittingly caused with her well-intentioned appointment. She decided to talk with Joey, and offer him a choice of two other tasks instead—he could either become the monitor who distributes milk, or the one who controlled the window shades. He chose the latter since "some kids don't like milk, but everyone likes the sun out of his eyes."

The teacher also devised some games in which the children worked sequentially with different classmates in twosomes. Joey was thus able to widen his one-to-one contacts in the class. He befriended a new pupil who spoke only Spanish, and took great pride in being able to teach him some English. Although he did not form any close friendships with any of the other children, he began to feel more comfortable with them.

The mother discussed her expectations for Joey with the teacher and began to understand the pressure he was under to do both his schoolwork and household tasks. The teacher then realized that her own tactics in forcing him to produce were adding to the overwhelming pressure from home and decided to lessen her demands on him. "Even if he is bright enough to go on to college, they won't take him if he's still wetting himself!"

Joey's physical appearance changed as he felt less pressure. His shoulders were less stooped, and he smiled occasionally. His voice, which had been almost inaudible, became louder and firmer. He stopped wetting himself, both day and night. Although his mother still would not allow him any social contacts after school, he found it easier to be friendly with others at lunchtime and during recess periods.

The nurse at the mental health center met with Joey weekly during this time. At first, he sat on a chair several feet away, and kept his eyes averted. He would take a very large doll from the shelf, and talk to it. "You know you have to keep clean . . . I'm not going to wash your wet things. . . . What do you mean you were in trouble in school?" As time went on, he no longer needed the doll, and could speak directly about his troubles. On occasion, he would cuddle up to the nurse. From the beginning of their relationship Joey was told that the nurse "will only be able to see you for three months."

When he was reminded that the time for termination of his interviews was near, Joey silently walked to the window, shoulders dropping, hands in his pockets and, with his back to the nurse, quietly said, "I guess that's what always happens when you find a friend. They leave you."

"But Joey, the things we learned from each other will always remind us of each other. Even though we won't be together each week, we have had the chance to really know each other, and that was good."

"I guess so."

"Remember when we first met? I told you we would only be together for three months. There's nothing either of us can do about the short time."

Joey wet himself in school and during the night several times the next week. Both his mother and teacher had been warned of this possibility, and did not fuss about it. Joey asked that the last visit between himself and the nurse take place in school. There, he gave the nurse an ornament which he had made for her. He asked her to walk into the hall with him, and said, "Could you give me a kiss goodby, and then leave, fast, when I go back to the room? I don't want to say anything else." And so they parted. Joey's later history showed that he remained dry for the most part, and was more competent in school. Although he was more comfortable with others, he still avoided close friendships. It was hoped that as his mother would give him more freedom, this would change and he would find friendships that would last.

Ten-year-old Vivian had accused the school custodian of raping her. Physical examination determined that she had not been molested. The school principal was aware of the girl's seductive manner toward boys in her class, and suggested to the child's mother that she contact the neighborhood mental health center. After speaking with the mother, the nurse at the center determined that family therapy within the home would be most practical, since there were one older and three younger children to be cared for at home, making clinic visits on a regular basis unlikely.

The entire family looked forward to each session. The five children, mother and her boyfriend usually sat in a circle in the same order: 2-year-old, mother, 12-year-old, 4-year-old, 7-year-old, mother's boyfriend, patient, and the nurse. It soon became apparent that the patient was cut off every time she tried to speak. She was also blamed for all unpleasant family incidents. She initiated much dissension between the others, and was sexually provocative toward her mother's boyfriend.

Vivian's father had deserted his family after the last child was born. He was overwhelmed by his financial responsibility for five children. Although the boyfriend wanted to marry the mother, she refused, reasoning that by remaining unmarried she could continue to collect public assistance money.

As the oldest girl, Vivian was expected to help make beds, cook meals, and wash dishes, although not the pots. (The only other girl was the 2-year-old.) She resented this, along with the fact that she was not given "grown up" freedom consistent with her household responsibilities.

Although she was often placed in charge of the younger children while her mother visited friends, she was punished if she chastised them. She was ambivalent about being the mother-substitute. She enjoyed the sense of being trusted, but disliked the limitations placed on her. The others said she was "too bossy" while in charge. They would often think up ways to get her into trouble. The mother always said that she "knew" Vivian was the troublemaker, even without investigating. She hated doing housework and reasoned that it was "good experience" for Vivian to take over certain tasks, pointing out that she herself did the two most hated tasks—washing the pots and cleaning the bathroom.

The mother placed restrictions on all her children's friendships. If she knew and approved of the outsiders, they could be invited to visit. However, only the oldest boy was permitted to visit other friends. Vivian resented not being given the same amount of freedom.

As arguments took place during the family therapy sessions, the behavior of various members became apparent, and this was discussed. The other youngsters began to realize how they were goading Vivian until she would lose control and become dictatorial. The mother decided to stop relying on Vivian for the major portion of the household tasks. Vivian in turn reacted to the easing of the pressure by calming down and not ordering others about. The school principal noted less seductive behavior in school, and an improvement in her work.

At the last family session, Vivian insisted that her mother sit near the boyfriend. Vivian was permitted her full say when she talked and remained in good control of herself. Her mother agreed to let her visit two girl friends after school and praised her for her help that day.

In each of the cases cited, initiation of treatment was suggested by members of school staffs. It is unlikely that either patient would have received help without the referral. Early recognition of the problems allowed the needed intervention before unacceptable behavior patterns became too deeply ingrained.

Unfortunately, neither school had a school nurse attached to it. School nurses should be assigned to develop health programs that will benefit both the school population and their families. Even though teachers may notice abnormal behavior, they may be unable to get help for the child if the parent refuses to accept the recommendation. A school nurse could make a home visit and, because of her medical background, would be likely to recognize any unusual family patterns or problems which are contributing to the child's difficulty. Parents are more likely to accept her suggestion for seeking help, since she appears as an authority figure in the health field.

In many schools, the nurse is also responsible for individual health teaching and guidance. Information available to her about each child enables her to tailor programs to the needs of each. In a sense, she is the coordinator of health care for each child, collecting information from home, doctor, teacher, and community agencies that have contributed to the child's care. She sorts the information and shares appropriate sections with those who are involved with the child. She also makes referrals to mental health agencies if such care is required.

Community centers are another source of mental health referrals. Workers in charge of preschoolers can spot problems that may be due to retardation, lack of maturation, or environmental factors. Parents who are unaware of normal behavior patterns may either forgive or damn their children wrongfully. The normal "No" of the 2-year-old may be very threatening to the authoritarian parent, while the abnormal clinging of her 4-year-old may fill the need of an insecure mother. Group meetings for parents can be utilized for giving parents information about normal child development so they can become better prepared to deal with their children at all age levels.

In community centers that are available to school-age youngsters agency workers have an opportunity to note those who are overly aggressive and those who are loners, those who may be victims of child abuse, and those who are not reacting in an acceptable fashion. The perceptive worker can then refer these children to suitable helping agencies. Teenagers often present problems, particularly in the areas of acting-out with drugs or sex, that come under the scrutiny of the center's workers. "Rap" sessions often help these young people to look at their life styles critically and, for some, this may be sufficient to cause them to cease the pursuit of unacceptable or harmful behavior. Others may need more personalized professional help to solve their problems. Identity crises are common at this age, and it is invaluable for community centers to have workers present who are trained to recognize such problems.

Senior citizen clubs are another area in which community workers can be helpful in identifying the mental health needs of older people. Unless some social outlet is provided, older people tend to isolate themselves, and may not care for their personal hygiene, diet, medications, or financial affairs. They may begin to develop early signs of dementia, with the forgetfulness that may lead to dangerous situations (fires, flooding in the home, taking inadequate or overdoses of medication). The stimulation afforded by being engaged in activities with others is recognized as one way to lessen mental deterioration. This is an important consideration because the elderly are the fastest-growing segment of the population. It is estimated that there will be 100 million elderly (20% of the population) by 2050. As the elderly increase in number, concerns have been voiced that there will be a greater percentage of that group with emotional and physical problems. Much to the surprise of many gerontologists, the elderly seem to be holding up well, living longer, with less chronic disease or disabilities.

Data have been accumulated for over a decade through the National Long-Term Care Surveys that follow people enrolled in the Medicare program. One factor in the higher level of health status of the elderly seems to be increased education during their formative years, with resultant higher socioeconomic status. There also appears to be greater attention to better self-care, with less use of injurious substances as well as positive health procedures, such as regular exercise (including strength training and aerobics) and awareness of the need for regular physical checkups and adult immunizations. In addition, the elderly today seem less inclined to tolerate long-term disabilities, and seek surgery that includes cataract lens replacement, coronary angioplasty or bypass surgery, and even hip and knee replacements. They are also more aware of their nutritional needs, some relying on programs like Meals on Wheels to bring food to them if they are homebound.

One problem that has surfaced among the elderly has been alcoholism. For some, it is a continuation of a problem that was present before they became aged. Others blame the problem on isolation and boredom, ill health, retirement, loss of loved ones, and the presence of "happy hours" as a daily social event. There are an estimated 3 million Americans over the age of 60 with a drinking problem. Nurses may become aware of the problem as they screen or treat older patients. Although staff at the Center for Alcohol Studies at Rutgers University believe that the elderly can be discovered and treated successfully, many do not seek help because they see alcoholism as a sin rather than as a disease. Many do not want to join local groups of Alcoholics Anonymous because they are uncomfortable with the attitudes, language, and perhaps involvement with drugs found among the younger members. Older people with an alcohol problem tend to be more receptive to treatment, and are treated more successfully, when they are in a program with people of their own generation.

Crises in living occur when older people lose their mates, when friends die, and when they may be forced to move in with a child. There may be resentment at the loss of independence and unhappiness at being uprooted. Problems may arise as they have to revise schedules to fit those of their children. They may, in turn, sense the discomfort of children and grandchildren who loved them during short visits, but now find it hard to adjust to their permanent presence. Group sessions for these senior citizens may help ease their tensions. Sometimes members can arrange for joint living accommodations, thus providing themselves with compatible companions. Their families may also benefit from individual or group counseling available at the center or an associated agency.

The concerned health workers are also interested in efforts to improve community health care. Those efforts must extend beyond the individual to an involvement in society and active participation in change. They recognize community problems that may contribute to illness and work toward change. When individuals in the community become mentally ill, the worker is responsible for facilitating treatment before it becomes ingrained, and plans for long-range care and rehabilitation. To do this, workers must be familiar with local agencies and their referral systems. They should also be aware of any gaps in the provision of health services, and actively seek institution of missing services. They should be able to speak to community groups, coordinating their efforts with existing agencies, to make the community aware of its needs. Workers should be resource persons, able to help the community set priorities in meeting needs and to suggest ways that funds can be used most beneficially for the community at large.

In an effort to utilize mental health facilities to the utmost, some communities have implemented day hospitals and night hospitals along with the usual custodial residences and outpatient clinics. These provide necessary services for patients who do not require full-time hospitalization, yet are unready or unable to live at home. Some patients can work during the day, yet need the security of the hospital situation at night. Others are able to spend the night at home, but need the structured situation of the hospital during the day. Providing both types of facilities releases inservice beds without denying appropriate services for the patient who is preparing to return to the community. A full range of therapeutic programs is available in both day and night hospitals, including individual and group sessions, vocational, recreational, and rehabilitation activities. Patients continue to use these services until they are able to manage on their own. Frequently, they are given an emergency telephone number which they may call at any time in the event they need immediate help.

Some communities have set up crisis intervention centers, with telephones manned 24 hours a day by individuals trained in crisis techniques. Patients who call are usually given appointments to be seen within 24 hours at a nearby clinic. (If the situation is acute, the patient may be seen immediately.) After the initial consultation, the patient is given a follow-up appointment or is hospitalized if necessary. Many colleges have set up such centers on their campuses. They are frequently manned by nurses, psychologists, or social workers who are in graduate school. The calls they receive are often tied in with drug abuse, unwanted pregnancy, or poor interpersonal relationships. When threats of suicide are received, immediate preventive action is instituted. Appointments are made as necessary for follow-up care in the hospital or community.

Health workers who are assigned to the community find that their responsibilities go far beyond their job descriptions. Those involved with families in ghetto slums may find themselves battling with landlords and governmental agencies to secure housing that meets even minimal standards, sufficient food, proper clothing, and necessary health care for their patients. At first, much of their time may be spent in determining what the community *wants* as well as what it needs. The worker may have determined the needs accurately, but if those needs do not coincide with what the community wants, the worker's efforts will be met with resistance. The astute worker will recognize the demand for autonomy by the people. A community's intense desire to determine its own fate without outside direction must be respected if the worker is to gain the trust of its residents.

The community health worker soon finds that it is important for him to become a member of local committees. In so doing, he emphasizes his desire to be part of the community and to play a role in its betterment. It is equally important, however, that he approach his committee work as a part of the team, that he listen to others and not try to take over the leadership. He will need to determine where the real power of the community lies and what lines of communication he can use to reach that person. Sometimes seemingly powerful leaders are merely fronts for the quiet sideliners who wield the true power. Convincing the sideliners may be the most effective way of gaining the "leader's" support for needed programs to be backed by the community. It may also be necessary for the worker to inform the leaders that there are programs, agencies, and other resources available to the community if they desire to take advantage of them. Such information implies that the worker is sharing his knowledge, not trying to make decisions for the community.

Preventive psychiatry depends on the worker's competence in recognizing the interplay between the individual and his milieu. Workers must assess all aspects of the effects of the environment on the individual, determine the effect of these forces and the reaction to them. Unless the evaluation is complete and critical, important factors may be disregarded, and time wasted on trivia. To illustrate: Environmental catastrophes in various parts of the world have resulted in widespread evidence of emotional damage. Adults as well as children require guidance in calming their fears. They may complain of feeling weak and helpless and of an inability to sleep after the disaster, especially if it occurred in the middle of the night. Children suddenly orphaned have to deal not only with the grief of loss, but also with fears for their own futures. Mental health workers should encourage the victims to discuss their experiences rather than allow their anxieties to remain pent up.

Intervention must consider the physical effects of disaster, including displacement from homes, schools, and work areas. Arrangements for physical care may initially overshadow the need for psychological intervention but actually may be of lesser value when considering long-term needs. The new living arrangements may provide a higher standard of living than was present before the disaster, but the loss of loved ones may have a lifetime of negative repercussions.

6

Health Professionals in a Changing Workplace

The utilization of hospital beds is changing drastically under the leadership of managed care organizations. Throughout the country, the terms *restructuring, reengineering, redesigning, contracting,* and *downsizing* are being used. To the professionals working in the affected institutions, the words may be translated into "layoffs." Although more patients are being treated, shortened hospital stays reduce the need for beds. In addition, insurance companies, which pay most of the costs for hospitalized patients, often determine what hospitalizations are allowable, and the length of time that patients may remain. Many of the procedures formerly carried out within hospitals are now being performed on an ambulatory basis, or are judged to be unnecessary. Does this all mean that fewer nurses will be needed?

On the contrary, according to Margaret McClure, the vice-president of hospital operations and executive director of nursing at New York University (NYU) Medical Center in New York. Nurses who formerly practiced at the hospital bedside must now change their focus, so that they can be available to care for patients in other settings. Newer technology permits ambulatory care to be used for surgical procedures that formerly required in-hospital stays. For example, cataract surgery used to be performed in the hospital, with patients required to have their heads immobilized by sandbags to prevent movement for varying lengths of time after the surgery. Because most of the patients were elderly, many became confused and disoriented. Although their eyesight was helped by the surgery, the restraints were detrimental to their emotional status. Certainly today's outpatient cataract surgery is advantageous to the patient.

Using the cataract surgery as a model, the changes for the nursing staff should be examined. Under the old system, a bedside nurse admitted and educated the patient as to what could be expected. The operating room nurse had little, if any, actual nontechnical contact with the patient. Following the surgery, the recovery room nurse checked vital signs and determined when the patient was to be returned to the assigned floor. In some hospitals, the patient may have been returned to another room, and even assigned to another nurse, all adding to the possibility of disorientation while immobilized. The patient may have had brief contact with four nurses, probably none of whom had time to establish rapport or examine any but the physical problems presented by their patient.

Under the new ambulatory care, the nurse who carries out the initial intake has the opportunity to evaluate the relationship that exists between the patient and the person who accompanies him. The explanations and teaching will include both individuals, and will alert the nurse to the possibility of the need for home care on a professional level. The same nurse may remain with the patient through the surgery and after the procedure. Because the patient will return home within a few hours, there is less likelihood of a period of confusion or disorientation. The fact that the patient is not immobilized with sandbags to his head has not lessened the effectiveness of the surgery.

Patients were often kept in bed for long stays that were not only unnecessary, but often harmful. Another example of this was the treatment of postpartum patients in the 1940s. The newly delivered mother was kept in bed usually for a minimum of 7 days. She then "dangled" her feet over the side of the bed before she was allowed to stand up. As she left the bed, weakened by the prolonged bed rest, the mother often became light-headed and fainted. In addition, during the period of being bed-ridden, there were instances of thrombophlebitis, and even uterine infections, as circulation slowed down. Today, patients may deliver in hospitals, birthing centers, even at home, and be up and around within hours. The mothers under the newer program appear healthier and happier than those who were in bed for many days. The nurses fill a different role. One nurse may be with the woman during her labor, delivery and postpartum experience. She may help the woman establish lactation and educate the mother on how to care for the infant. She can also evaluate the response of the mother to the infant, and even help with the integration of the newborn into the family unit. The nurse then widens her role as she recognizes the importance of the mental health status of the family unit.

In past years, nurses became specialists, assigned only to specific aspects of the patient's care. In the case of the obstetrical patient, this fragmentation of care became noticeable as rooming-in became a hospital option. Could the nurses caring for the mother be expected to give proper care to the newborn? Programs were instituted so that nurses would feel competent to care for both. As nurses realized that they could expand their expertise, they became more amenable to being assigned to a wider variety of patients.

At the NYU Medical Center, emergency room nurses had the opportunity to practice in the intensive care unit (ICU). Reluctant at first, most later realized that the experience had been a good one, widening their area of expertise. In the same way, as nurses find their bedside hospital positions disappearing, the opportunities for expansion into other areas of care are growing. The operating room nurse will find her skills necessary in ambulatory settings, even in surgicenters located in physicians' offices.

Psychiatric nurses, too, will find the need for their skills in other settings. In past years, they were primarily assigned to psychiatric units, caring for patients already designated as having severe problems. In many instances, the nurses were limited to medicating patients or helping with treatments such as electrostimulative therapy. Today, those with advanced education in psychiatric nursing may find openings for their services in schools, senior centers, housing units, courts, jails, and above all, in homes. They may even become entrepreneurs, and enter into a private practice either alone or in conjunction with others.

Nurses can only move from one setting to another if they have the educational qualifications and experience. Moving out of hospitals requires nurses to be able to work on their own in a competent manner. Nurses will require more schooling to prepare for a more complicated case load. They will also need more experience after their graduation from a nursing school setting. At NYU, Dr. McClure has started a "nurse resident" program, analogous to a medical student's experience after graduation from medical school. The program is limited to 1 year, during which time the new nurses receive a detailed orientation, followed by an assignment to a preceptor who is an experienced practitioner. After the "residents" have been through the basic process, they are under the guidance of a mentor, who meets with them for follow-up at intervals. Although this is basically a teaching program, the residents are paid at about the starting salary of a newly appointed staff nurse.

As nurses enter this new era, their education will be a paramount issue.

Managed care companies prefer nurses who have been through a baccalaureate program and find even greater value in nurses with advanced degrees. For
this reason, Dr. McClure advises nursing schools to expand, rather than contract, and she encourages graduates to avail themselves of the chance to
become advanced nurse practitioners.

Nurses who choose to remain in hospitals will find their patients to be
much sicker because those less ill are more likely to be seen in ambulatory settings. Nurses will be used as case managers, acting as the patient's advocate.
Their essential task will be to see that the patient receives proper care from the
appropriate caregivers (physicians, physiotherapists, occupational therapists,
clinical specialists, psychiatric nurses, etc.). It is likely that the ICU as it is now
set up will be changed to include small units on each hospital floor, providing
for those requiring less complicated care. Patients who require more technological care will be placed in the acute ICU. The smaller unit, with its more
relaxed atmosphere, will provide nurses with more time to recognize the total
needs of patients, including the need for psychiatric intervention.

Those nurses who prefer not to be in the high tech environment will probably choose to work in an ambulatory care or community agency. Because
hospitals are discharging patients into long-term care facilities or even to their
own homes at a much earlier point in the recovery process, the nurses caring
for them must be of a high caliber. Their knowledge base must be such that
they can recognize the patients' needs and implement plans to meet those
needs before (or when) problems arise.

Managed care is seen as a way to keep costs down. However, there have
not been sufficient data collected to evaluate the worth of such care. In some
instances, managed care may have greater value in that there is more emphasis on preventive care. In fact, it is much more cost-effective to prevent illness
than to treat it. Early detection is important, but appears to be ignored if the
required tests are too expensive to be paid for by providers. For example,
mammography, which is essential for early detection of breast cancer, may be
paid for only once every 2 years by some insurance companies. And mental
health services to prevent more serious problems, have been excluded by
many insurers as too costly. Presently, this is being addressed by unions and
companies, showing that if the services are well regulated and appropriate, the
cost per insured member will not be that great. There may even be federal
legislation mandating the inclusion of mental health services. Returning the
patient to a productive life through early intervention is certainly less costly
than allowing deterioration of his mental health status to the point where
more intensive care, perhaps even hospitalization, is required.

7

Interactions of Nurses and Patients in Managed Care

There has been a long history of freedom of choice to determine the provider of care to the individual in the United States. During this period, patients have been free to pick and stay with the provider of choice. This has resulted in long-term relationships between the patient and practitioner, often carried on into the next generation. The practitioner knew not only the patient but often the entire family. A trusting relationship was established, with the caregiver responsible for supervising medical attention, and suggesting any needed specialists or treatments. If the provider was a family doctor, he may have done all examinations, immunizations, deliveries of babies, surgery as well as pediatric and geriatric care. He was often the family confidant and counselor as well.

As the practice of medicine became more technological and complex, there was more of a move to specialization. Patients found themselves shunted into medical offices that were unfamiliar to themselves or their families. Still, in most instances, they still had access to their original family doctors, who could then offer advice and reassurance. The "nurses" in those offices were often receptionists who may have been trained by the physician to do routine laboratory work. Those assistants usually were not permitted to offer advice, nor to overstep their limited knowledge base.

Once the costs of care became exorbitant, health care management corporations began to be looked on with favor. They offered consumers a way to receive health care at a lower price, but with restrictions that would make the offerings financially feasible. The structured "panels" of caregivers would accept patients for their practice, charge fees on a yearly basis, but restrict care to themselves or other practitioners on the same panel. As the process evolved, the original physician was regarded as the "gate keeper," who would decide when, if, and to whom patients could be referred. For many, mental health services were not included. Many consumers felt that they were not being consulted or provided for in an acceptable way under this program, but felt financially obliged to accept it.

At the same time, the economy of the country worsened, with a loss of jobs for many. That loss often resulted in the termination of health care insurance that could not be transferred to a future workplace. The employee was now left without a job, with the additional stress brought on by fear of what would happen if he or a family member became ill. In 1996, federal legislation prevented the nontransferability of health insurance. However, under most plans, the individual had little choice of caregiver. This has proved worrisome for many because it was often difficult to sever a long-term relationship with a trusted practitioner. Some health management firms now offer a greater variety of choices, even permitting the use of nonpanel practitioners (often at an additional fee) to their members.

Members who join managed care plans often look over the list of panel participants, choosing one that may list practitioners with whom they are familiar. If that is not possible, there is often a heightened feeling of anxiety as they try to choose the most suitable practitioners for their families and themselves. The health management organization (HMO) may realize the importance of well-educated nurse practitioners, who can be a supportive link for patients as they shift from individual practitioners to this new system. If workers do not appear to have the proper educational background, patients may distrust their judgment (often for good reason) and demand to see the nurse who is qualified to help them.

Nurses who work for HMOs are made aware of the cost factors of patient care. Prevention becomes an important way to manage the expense involved in care. Mental health has not received the attention that is necessary, with the fear that patients may overuse such services. Yet, if psychiatric nurses are used properly, the likelihood is that there will be substantial savings.

Another type of managed care program is offered by preferred provider organizations (PPOs), in which care is offered by participating primary care physicians and specialists. In this setting, enrollees usually are not required to have a referral before seeing any physician on the list. As with the HMOs, an additional fee is needed to see any nonparticipatory physician.

Patients need to be cautioned to read their insurance policies carefully so that they understand their coverage. Some organizations may not have specialists on their staffs who are capable of providing the latest in care for disorders that are uncommon yet will not pay for visits to specialists for care or treatments outside the plan. In some instances, it is wise for the patient to select a plan that has a specialist familiar with the specific problem or one that pays for care given by outsiders when their own staff cannot be of help. The patient's medical needs have to be balanced against the lower basic costs of enrollment in a PPO or HMO, with the understanding that the refusal to pay for specialized outside care may make the plan much more expensive if the enrollee has to pay for the additional care out of his own pocket.

Traditional insurance companies also keep costs down by limiting the care for which they are obligated to pay. In some instances, they will not provide coverage for any drug or treatment that they consider experimental. Among these are newer drugs for human immunodeficiency syndrome (HIV), or bone marrow or stem cell transplantation for breast cancer. The enrollee may choose to argue with the company, even starting litigation. If the patient wins, the company is then obligated to pay. The process may be so long that the patient may expire before it is settled. If so, the family will require support as they work through their anger.

Another way that health providers try to cut costs is through "downsizing," a newer way of stating that they are curtailing the size of the staff. Although lesser educated hospital nursing staffs have felt the brunt of these cuts, physicians (especially the specialists but including some primary caregivers) have been targeted in some institutions. Advanced practice nurses (APNs) have proved their worth in their ability to care for patients and are often used in their specialties, thereby preserving their jobs. By developing peer relationships with physicians, the APN can use skills in discharge planning and education of the patient and family to be certain that the patient will be safe after release from the hospital setting, and will receive the proper follow-up care. It is important for plans to be made so that earlier discharge will not result in readmission to the hospital for a preventable relapse. For proper evaluations to be made, accurate charting and record keeping are necessary as well as outcome studies that check on the status of patients not only at discharge but over a period of the time that it takes for full recovery.

Patients who require an initial hospital examination and evaluation by a designated health care practitioner were often seen by physicians in the past. In a bold move at Columbia University in New York, Mary O. Mundinger, Dr PH, and dean of the School of Nursing, was able to work out an agreement with two major managed care companies to recognize Columbia University faculty nurse practitioners as full primary care providers, with pay equivalent to that of the physicians. Patients will have the choice of receiving care from either a physician or APN as the primary care provider. This giant step by nurses is not meant to displace the role of the physicians, but rather to establish a stronger collaborative role as both professions work together to provide the best possible care for the patient while limiting duplication, and thereby lowering costs.

PART TWO

Approaches to Specific Psychiatric Disorders

In this section of the book, specific approaches to various psychiatric conditions are detailed. As far as possible, the individual chapters correlate with the titles found in the *Diagnostic and Statistical Manual of Mental Disorders* (4th ed.) to make it easier for the practitioner to complete forms required by insurance and other companies.

8

The Person With an Anxiety Disorder

The feelings of tension, uneasiness, nervousness, and apprehension that are created by stress, the source of which may or may not be known to the patient or worker, are called anxiety.

Anxiety is one of the most common problems the health worker encounters in patients, whether they be at home, in a hospital, or elsewhere. It may become apparent through physical or behavioral symptoms that make the management of the patient difficult. This is particularly true when the worker either does not see the relationship of the symptoms to the patient's anxiety or is unsure of how to handle the situation effectively. The worker himself may experience anxiety at such times.

Anxiety may occur on a continuum. Its start may be mild, with symptoms so innocuous that they are not recognized by the patient. Untreated, the symptoms may escalate to the point where the individual is immobilized, unable to function. Recognition of the signs and symptoms of early anxiety is the first step in teaching patients how to self-manage their problem. It may be difficult for them to become aware of the impending attack unless they have a basic knowledge of the initial behavior common to themselves. For example, tremors, rapid speech, wringing of the hands, excessive perspiration, repetitious questioning, complaints of palpitation or rapid breathing, diarrhea, a feeling of knots in the abdomen, inability to focus attention on any one thing for a period of time, difficulty in concentrating or sleeping, continuous forgetfulness, and frequent use of the call bell in the hospital are all signs of anxiety. Once patients are made aware of the early signs and symptoms of the disorder, they can learn techniques enabling them to keep their anxiety from progressing along the continuum to a more serious stage.

The first experience with anxiety may subside quickly, but may leave patients fearful of another attack. This anticipation may increase their vulnerability to the point where the physical symptoms, as described earlier, become somewhat debilitating. At first, individuals may not feel restricted, continuing fairly normally in social or work situations. However, as the disorder continues, they may begin to avoid situations that they anticipate will cause discomfort. They may have difficulty in concentrating, resulting in work-related as well as social problems. If the problem continues for more than 6 months, it is characterized as a *generalized anxiety disorder* (GAD). At this point, patients may realize the need for professional intervention.

Patients who seek help for their anxiety disorder are usually more aware of the physical symptoms than of the emotional components. Therefore, they may feel that the rapid heart rate, the excessive perspiration and palpitations are signs of an impending heart attack. This thought in itself may result in a state of panic, sufficient to bring them to a health professional, possibly in an emergency room. Being told that "nothing is wrong" will probably not end the attack. They may well counter with a tale of a friend who was also told nothing was wrong, only to die shortly after. It is more helpful to sit down with patients who are anxious, and review events that occurred before the attack started. By doing this, the target symptom may be elicited, making the episode understandable. At this point, the use of techniques to lessen the heightened state of anxiety will help patients associate their reactions with their emotional state.

Because early symptoms of GAD usually include rapid respiration, often to the point of hyperventilation, patients may complain of being out of breath or feeling light-headed. Implementing slow breathing at this point should lessen the effects of their rapid breathing. They should be instructed to breathe in slowly, counting to themselves to the number 2 as they inspire through the nose, and then, using the same slow count, expire through the mouth as they count to 4, using abdominal breath. They should continue this until their respiratory rate is under control. By using this technique, not only do they change the breathing pattern, but by concentrating on the counting, they interfere with their concentration on the topic that caused the anxiety. In some situations, using a paper bag (never plastic) over the nose and mouth accelerates the process because it increases the level of carbon dioxide that the patients breathe. (This simulates the use of a rebreathing machine.) It may be necessary for the professional to count aloud when starting this procedure, until patients are able to do it silently alone. In some instances, when a paper bag is unavailable, patients can be coached to cup their hands over nose and mouth while breathing to build up the carbon dioxide level.

Other relaxation techniques to lessen muscle tension are also helpful as symptoms begin. One such technique is to tense the entire body, and then visualize the body as becoming soft and pliable, relaxing each area until the whole body is relaxed. Remember that telling patients to relax is rarely helpful because they are often unaware of how tense they are. It is important to speak slowly and softly when giving the instructions, and, when possible, to lower the lights in the room, making the environment more conducive to relaxation.

Patients who recognize that they have the power to interfere with the progress of an anxiety attack can be taught to recognize their target symptoms as they occur. In this way, they can alter the progression of the disorder. In time, there can be an exploration of the basis for their feelings. Anxiety disorders may have occurred during childhood or adolescence, particularly if the patient is female, and may present a familial pattern. They may become aware that they always tend to anticipate disaster, worrying excessively about every possible future occurrence: Will they have enough money, pass a test, succeed at a business or household task, and be accepted socially? These worries may be accompanied by physical symptoms, such as muscle tension demonstrated by frequent urination or diarrhea, nausea or actual vomiting, tremors, and headaches. If these symptoms have escalated during previous episodes, patients may withdraw from their usual activities, fearful that any situation may bring on the discomfort that they dread. The earlier that patients learn to use self-management techniques, the less likely that their symptoms will escalate.

In instances in which early intervention is unsuccessful, or when the symptoms are deeply entrenched before the patient seeks professional help, the disorder may progress to the point where medications become necessary. Buspirone has proved useful for some patients. Other medications, such as benzodiazipines and antidepressants are also being evaluated for their effectiveness in patients with an anxiety disorder.

Despite outpatient therapy and medications, some patients require hospitalization as their disorder exacerbates. Hospitalization is a threatening situation that may cause patients to feel as though they are at the mercy of a vast impersonal institution. Their physical and mental health are now placed in the care of others whom they may never have met before. The stresses they face are many and real, and they react to them with symptoms of anxiety—sweaty hands, tremors, rapid pulse, dilated pupils, diarrhea, or urinary frequency. Palpitations, restlessness, and indigestion are not uncommon. Patients may be tearful for no apparent reason, and may complain about anything and everything. The workers' efforts to please them are to no avail. The patients may regard whatever is said as a personal attack, and be easily angered. Or, conversely, they may act as though they are at a hotel for a few days' rest, laughing and joking with such consistent cheeriness that the worker reviews the chart, wondering if indeed the patient is in the right place. Because hospital nurses work so closely with patients, they are usually the first to note changes in a patient's appearance, mood, and behavior. These changes may indicate that the patient is trying to relieve himself of inner feelings of tension which are mounting to the point of discomfort.

Some patients experience a severer form of anxiety that results in a panic attack. Typically, an initial panic attack is described as coming "out of the blue," without warning or discernable reason. Patients feel a sense of terror, believing that something horrible, over which they are powerless, is about to occur. They go on to develop physical symptoms that are uncontrollable, including a pounding heartbeat, chest pains, respiratory difficulties, a sense of unreality, and fear of losing control or of dying. The symptoms may last for seconds or minutes, gradually fading in about an hour. The fear that the feeling will recur is based on the fact that such attacks are unpredictable and overwhelming.

If panic attacks do recur, patients may develop *anticipatory fear,* awaiting further episodes. If a previous attack was connected to a particular activity, there may be avoidance of that activity. For example, if it occurred while in an elevator, patients have been known to climb innumerable flights of stairs rather than chance another attack in an elevator. Recurrence leads to a diagnosis of *panic disorder,* the repetition of which may seriously interfere with the patient's life. It is difficult for some patients to accept the fact that there is no physical basis for the intense feelings experienced during a panic attack. About a third of those who develop a panic disorder become agoraphobic, resulting in an intense fear of being any place where they cannot escape or receive immediate help. These patients may be unable to leave their homes at all or leave only in the company of a trusted individual.

According to studies at the National Institute of Mental Health, about 70% to 90% of those with a panic disorder are treatable. The first step is to have patients undergo a thorough medical examination, to rule out possible physical factors, including thyroid disorders, epilepsy, or cardiac arrhythmias, which are known to cause symptoms similar to panic disorder. If physical problems are ruled out, treatment may require the use of medications, including tricyclic antidepressants, high potency benzodiazepines, or monoamine oxidase inhibitors (MAOIs). In addition to the medication, *cognitive-behavioral therapy* is helpful. Using this form of therapy involves a search for the thoughts and feelings associated with the attacks, which often demonstrate a distortion in thinking that causes anxiety, with heightened feelings of an impending catastrophe. Patients can be taught to reduce their anxiety, and thus lower the incidence of panic attacks through the use of relaxation techniques as described earlier.

THE APPROACH TO THE PATIENT WITH AN ANXIETY DISORDER

Immediate Intervention by the Patient

Self-management techniques: Teach the patient to recognize the target symptom that initiates the feelings of anxiety (tremors, palpitations, rapid breathing, etc.). In that way, the learned abdominal breathing and relaxation techniques can be started immediately by the patient.

Professional Intervention

IMMEDIATE ACTION

Recognize the signs and symptoms of anxiety. The importance of making patients aware of the physical symptoms associated with anxiety cannot be stressed enough. As noted previously, those symptoms (tremors, rapid speech, palpitations, respiratory and gastrointestinal symptoms, etc.) can become the targets for intervening and teaching patients self-management techniques.

Do not make demands on the patient when his anxiety is high. Remember, he cannot cope with his situation as is, so one more stress may prove catastrophic.

When approaching the patient, speak slowly, briefly, and concretely. This increases the likelihood that the patient will grasp what you say. Do not use meaningless phrases such as: "Just relax." "Don't be nervous." "There's nothing to worry about." "Control yourself." "I think you like to worry; it gives you something to do." "Just pull yourself together." "Some people are just natural born worriers."

Employ measures to increase the patient's comfort. Warm milk in the evening; no blaring radios; warm bath or shower; eliminate glaring lights. Teach him techniques that include muscle relaxation and slow abdominal breathing; eliminate the use of caffeine or other stimulants.

Tell the patient you are concerned about him and his feelings. Let him know that by talking with him about those feelings and understanding them, you will be better able to help him. Give him the opportunity to talk by saying, "I wonder how things have been going with you in general?" or "It must be very difficult for you to be here, when your mind is on so many other things." The health worker who cheerfully grins and breezes into the room saying, "In a few hours time you'll be fine" or "Everyone gets better on my floor" is hardly credible. It is far better to acknowledge the difficult time the patient is experiencing.

INTERMEDIATE ACTION

Be understanding of the patient's feelings. Let him know that you recognize his present state. Tell him, "You must be very uncomfortable now. But, as your condition improves you will feel more at ease." Don't involve him in loud, noisy, or complicated activities. Start with individual brief encounters which are firm but supportive. When the patient is able to cooperate, direct his energy into some productive and meaningful activity.

Don't assume that the patient's anxieties are totally due to his mental illness. One sixty-year-old gentleman refused heart surgery, believing that he would die during the procedure. His fear was that his death would enable his son, whom he disliked, to complete his college education by collecting on a large insurance policy in which he had been designated as the beneficiary.

Tolerate the patient's tenseness. All too often health workers seem more anxious to reassure themselves than their patients. If you find your own anxiety level rising, arrange for frequent relief periods by other staff members. This helps the patient to feel that he is not alone and that others—as well as you—are concerned and interested. At the same time, you will be able to function more comfortably and therapeutically when with him.

Do make an attempt to understand what triggers your own anxiety. One staff member was immobilized when assigned to care for a patient receiving an additional course of radiation therapy. The worker's own medical history revealed a previous mastectomy followed by radiation therapy. The parallels between her own illness and that of the patient increased her anxiety about her own condition to the point where she could not function therapeutically.

Don't try to reassure the patient with empty explanations. "I'd be anxious too if my husband lost the bank book" or "Anyone would be anxious if they had parents like yours" are illustrative of statements that are usually ineffective because the patient doubts that anyone else would really have that same reaction. Additionally, if the patient thought he knew what was really causing his anxiety, he would have gained control of the situation long ago.

Offer any reasonable explanations or information to clear up the patient's misconceptions about his condition. For example, the patient may erroneously believe that staff members are avoiding telling him about test results because he definitely has an incurable disease. Tell him, "The laboratory tests and reports have not yet been completed. There is nothing on the chart that states a definite diagnosis. Neither the doctor nor I know whether you have this disease. I can understand how difficult it must be to worry about this alone." These statements allow the patient to save face regarding his behavior, and at the same time encourage the realization that some of his worries may be unfounded.

Do not be surprised if logic is useless. The patient may well see himself as physically ill, although this may not be so. This misconception can be corrected only at the rate tolerated by the individual. It is important to focus on the healthy and positive aspects of the way in which the patient functions rather than to try to convince him that nothing is physically wrong.

LONG-TERM ACTION

Do not dwell on what the patient is doing to relieve his tensions. He may be constantly calling for the nurse, persistently running up to the nurses' station, not taking medication, or otherwise ignoring the doctor's recommendations. Do not say, "Now, now, I expect much more from a person like you" or "You are acting like a 2-year-old. Now grow up." Such remarks only reveal your anger and inability to change the situation.

Do not become defensive when the patient complains. He may not like the hospital food, his nursing care, or even the placement of his bed. Instead, help him to talk about himself, to explain and describe to you what happened before he became upset.

Encourage the patient to verbalize his feelings about what he remembers that happened before he became anxious. If he doesn't remember, don't push. But every now and then gently lead him back to the subject. Soon he will remember situations and incidents that provoked his present responses and feelings. Help the patient to find healthier ways of responding to anxiety-provoking factors. If he does not want to talk to you at a given moment, he may vehemently maintain that nothing is the matter and that you should mind your own business. Do not react as though he is doing something terrible by not wanting to bare his soul to you. Remember, you are there to help the patient and to meet his needs, not the reverse. Therefore, do not reject the patient by going off in a huff because he has rejected you. Say, "I understand that you may not feel like talking now, so I will come back in an hour when you may feel differently." And then do that; keep your word and return. This demonstrates to the patient that you really do care, are reliable, and that he can trust you.

Don't offer suggestions as to the possible causes of the patient's anxiety. Anxiety attacks are often triggered by unconscious factors. You may inadvertently focus on such a factor and thus increase his anxiety. Don't assume that you know what is worrying the patient. Remember that there is no substitute for direct questions when trying to obtain information from the patient.

Do not expect the patient to change his behavior immediately. Remember that the method he has chosen to make himself comfortable may be one that he has used to relieve anxiety throughout his life.

FREQUENTLY PRESCRIBED PSYCHIATRIC DRUGS

Psychiatric drugs frequently prescribed for anxiety include the following:

Short-acting benzodiazepines: triazolam (Halcion), alprazolam (Xanax), lorazepam (Ativan)

Long-acting benzodiazepines: clonazepam (Klonopin), diazepam (Valium), clorazepate (Tranxene), chlordiazepoxide (Libritabs)
Propanediol compounds: meprobamate (Equanil, Miltown)
Diphenylmethane: hydroxyzine (Vistaril, Atarax)

9

The Person With a Depressive Disorder

Health workers are rightfully concerned about patients who show overt signs of depression. Patients who weep easily and frequently or express thoughts of dying present a problem to the staff. Before reaching this stage, they may have presented signs of mild depression that were not recognized as such— little interest in pleasure or daily activities, insomnia or hypersomnia, inability to concentrate, poor appetite, constipation, amenorrhea, impotence, or disinterest in sex. They may have appeared unkempt and unshaven, and gained or lost weight. They may have expressed thoughts of hopelessness, worthlessness, helplessness, and even hinted at the possibility of suicide. Most of these thoughts were related to a loss of self-esteem. Motor activity impairment, such as slowed speech and movement, may have also been noted.

Depression is rightfully monitored along a continuum. For some patients, the initial event may be an episode of seasonal affective disorder (SAD), beginning as the summer sun ebbs, and gray skies predominate. This disorder usually responds to a move to a sunnier area, or the use of electric lights that simulate the brightness of the sun. Mild depression may not even be recognized by family, friends, or the patient. It is only when more serious symptoms become apparent that notice is taken, and intervention is begun. The aim of treatment is to uncover the cause of the depression and to institute proper therapy.

Difficulty with memory may lead others to think that the patient is showing the first signs of dementia. This may change when the depression lifts under treatment. However, the major depressive episode may actually be the first sign of dementia and should be evaluated carefully. If the depression has escalated to a *major depressive disorder,* the situation requires immediate intervention, because up to 25% of those with this diagnosis will commit suicide. Patients who are older than 55 years of age are at even higher risk because their death rate is four times as high. If they have been admitted to nursing homes, they are even more likely to die during the year after admission.

Words used to describe depression may vary with cultures. Those with a Latino or Mediterranean background may talk of "nerves." Asians may speak of "imbalance." Middle Eastern peoples may refer to problems of the "heart," and some native Americans may describe themselves as "heartbroken." It is important to recognize the variations experienced by those of other cultures. Some may see themselves as being hexed or being visited by individuals who have died. At the same time, the statements should be viewed as part of an overall picture, possibly indicating a serious psychiatric rather than a cultural anomaly.

When a depression is recognized as such, the worker may want to intervene but sometimes hesitates for fear that this will cause the situation to worsen. It is unlikely that he would be the *cause* of any further deterioration, since the reasons for the depression are probably deeply rooted, and unrelated to his actions. Conversely, the fact that the professional shows interest, spends time with the patient, and listens to him is therapeutic in itself. It is important for the worker to let the patient decide how much, and when, he wishes to discuss any emotionally charged material.

Under certain circumstances, depression is a normal reaction. The individual who has lost a loved one, had a limb amputated, or been given a diagnosis of an incurable illness has the right to be depressed and to grieve. The patient will probably manifest decreased interest in his surroundings, boredom, and a tendency to ruminate about his loss. He cannot be expected to remain cheerful under such circumstances. As he adjusts to his new life situation, he comes to terms with himself, and the depression usually lifts. Health workers can help by listening to the patient as he talks, and by encouraging him to examine his feelings. This helps the patient free himself from his attachment to the lost object or individual and encourages him to seek new outlets.

The patient who cries, weeps, screams, or whines is expressing helplessness. His loss of control makes most staff members feel very uncomfortable. Yet tearfulness can be therapeutic in some situations. For example, a worker who remains with the patient and quietly says, "I understand how difficult this time is for you—crying sometimes helps when dealing with such situations," is letting the patient know that his crying is acceptable, and that he is not alone in his grief. Once the patient is able to control his tears, he should be encouraged to verbalize his feelings about the specific problems that caused his weeping. It is not uncommon to discover that factors, such as a lack of success in work, loneliness, concerns regarding physical appearance or the feeling of loss of masculinity or femininity have triggered the emotional reaction. Understanding the patient's perception of the circumstances increases the worker's ability to help him get his bearings and aid him in reorganizing his approach to life in a reasonably hopeful and realistic way.

The depression that is not based on external reality, or that becomes prolonged or incapacitating, requires a greater degree of intervention. For example, the worker would expect a patient to be relieved and happy when told, after a benign tumor has been removed, that no further treatment is needed. He would be concerned if the patient rejects this diagnosis, remains convinced that everyone is lying, and believes that he is going to die. At this point, the worker's efforts should be geared to helping the patient talk about his unhappiness. Possibly, as they talk, they will uncover the situation underlying the patient's unhappy outlook. It may be based on something too difficult for the patient to face. Then more realistic thinking can be stimulated. At the same time the worker can encourage the patient to accept the current situation by repeating the facts about his condition (i.e., blood work normal, pathology report normal, recovery progressing satisfactorily).

Severe depression requires ongoing support of the patient by all associated with him. The patient who is severely depressed has little desire or energy to do anything. Usually, he does not want to talk or participate in any activities because he thinks he cannot do them well and is fearful of exposing his weakness. Thus, his feelings of inadequacy and worthlessness increase. The worker, therefore, must assume the initiative in drawing the patient into conversation or activities. However, he should not expect the patient to be pleasant or grateful to him for this challenge to his behavior pattern. The patient may even express anger at the intervention. This, in effect, is a sign of improvement, for depression is largely the result of anger being turned inward upon oneself. Anger at another helps turn that feeling outward and is less destructive to the patient.

Depressed patients often need a tremendous amount of care, approval, and attention. No amount of support ever seems adequate. Their level of sensitivity is so great that a comment such as, "I'm unable to go to the gift shop for you now, but I will be free to do so later in the day" may be interpreted as a rejection. The patient's needs can never be completely satisfied; therefore, he always feels cheated, frustrated, and unloved.

Often the behavior of the depressed person is very infantile. Family, friends, and professionals may become exhausted and angry when their efforts fail to bring about improvement in his condition. It is not unusual for those who are involved with the patient to withdraw and say, "I give up. No matter what I do, it isn't enough." This further increases the patient's feelings of rejection and worthlessness.

The patient who is depressed usually gets an initial bonus of sympathy, attention, and pity. However, the price that is paid for this secondary gain is draining, considering the lengths to which the patient must often go, such as abusing drugs or alcohol, attempting or threatening suicide, or denying himself any pleasurable moments. He may go to extremes to become the center of attention. In one instance, a young man took an overdose of drugs because he felt overshadowed by his sister at a family dinner party.

Every depressed patient has feelings of futility. Whether the patient says so or not, he has very likely felt like killing himself at some point. Often the health worker picks up these feelings in the course of conversation, perhaps after he has noticed that the patient looks particularly upset, and comments on this. Common utterances of the depressed patient are: "I wish I were dead," "If I had a bottle of pills I would take them," "My family can use my insurance," "I'll show him," "He'll be sorry." Such statements should be taken seriously. The health worker should confront the patient by asking what plan or method he will use to carry out his threat. Thinking, "Oh, he's just saying that; he'll never really do it," is dangerous wishful thinking. It is an excuse one gives one's self when unable to face the possibility of a successful suicide attempt by the patient.

In one instance, a patient threatened to kill herself if the therapist went on a planned vacation. She rejected the offer of having another therapist take over during that time. Her primary therapist then suggested hospitalization during the period of the vacation. The patient declined that option, promising not to carry out any self-destructive actions during the therapist's absence. At this time, the therapist helped her explore the ways in which this experience differed from that of having been abandoned during childhood by her mother. Once the patient could differentiate between her feelings of being rejected because of the therapist going on vacation, and her memories of having been abandoned by her mother, she was able to sustain herself. She even called the substitute therapist once, to prove to herself that help was available if needed.

THE APPROACH TO THE PERSON WITH A DEPRESSIVE DISORDER

Immediate Intervention by the Patient

SELF-MANAGEMENT TECHNIQUES

Teach the patient to recognize the target symptoms that initiate the feelings of depression (overeating, refusal to eat, disinterest in pleasurable activities, unkempt appearance, etc.). Immediately start on routines that will have the patient involved in activities of daily living. Check on nutrition and hygiene, personal appearance.

Professional Intervention

Immediate Action

Initiate the approach. "You look unhappy today. Perhaps it will help if we talk about what's troubling you." Be alert to the suicide potential of patients who demonstrate lower levels of self-interest and who make suicidal statements.

Show concern for the patient, while letting him know that the staff will take over and protect him until he feels better. The worker can say, "I believe that you feel very unhappy now. People often feel that way when they are ill and need protection, temporarily, from themselves. The staff and I will not let you harm yourself, but will protect you until you have recovered." Proceed to take any precautions necessary.

Show the patient you care about him. Stay with him, accept his silences, and tolerate his tears. Be nonjudgmental. Accept him at his present level.

Pay attention to the patient's daily hygiene and nutrition. Offer assistance and direction when necessary. Keep him from appearing unkempt because he doesn't have the strength to brush his hair, shave, or change his clothes. Be patient and controlled with the patient when he behaves so helplessly. Be aware of your own frustration and avoid ignoring or rejecting him because this would only increase his feelings of worthlessness.

Contact supportive individual (therapist, friend, or family member) who can spend time with the person and evaluate the need for hospitalization.

Allow the patient plenty of time to react to your approach and to respond.

INTERMEDIATE ACTION

Tell the patient that you understand and recognize his feelings. Tell him you have known others who have felt the same way at times. You can say, "When a situation like this arises, people often feel helpless before they have had the opportunity to think it through."

Let the patient know that you feel he is worthy. Note his participation in activities. "You certainly are helping us by filing those cards." However, don't overdo the flattery, because excess praise often reinforces the patient's feelings that because he is really worthless you are trying to make him feel good.

Plan activities according to the patient's degree of depression and the place in which he is being treated. Active participation in sports, when feasible, is a helpful way of working out feelings of aggression. Tasks should be simple, and not require concentration; for example:

1. In the home: polishing furniture, folding laundry, scrubbing vegetables.
2. In the general hospital: setting up new charts, copying notices for the nursing staff, watering plants.
3. In the psychiatric hospital: recreational therapy (handicrafts, dancing, painting, poetry); occupational therapy (woodwork, sandpapering furniture, typing); classes in art or poetry. Individual and group therapy are also important factors in treatment.

Be constantly alert to any alteration in the patient's requests, affect, tone of voice, statements, or behaviors. Remember that a sudden positive mood change may be due to the belief that he can carry out a plan to destroy himself rather than an improvement in his mental state.

Although the patient's environment should be made as safe as possible, remember that restricting him severely may increase his belief that he is unacceptable, and foster impulsive negative behavior.

Check on the patient early in the morning because sleep disturbances may cause him to awaken early and increase his depression. The patient may be more vulnerable to suicidal thoughts and actions at that time.

LONG-TERM ACTION

Discourage the depressed patient from making major decisions. He may think of selling his house, making a new will, buying or selling stock, or obtaining a divorce. Get him to delay such actions.

Help the patient to reorganize his capabilities and attitudes in a hopeful realistic light as he improves. Offer him hope by communicating your belief that changes can be made and that alternative solutions for his problems can be found.

Do not tell the patient how improved he is because he may then feel obliged to make a suicidal gesture to prove that he is still very ill. Allow him to set his own pace and tell you when he is feeling better.

Make realistic plans for discharge. The patient may require time in a half-way facility before returning to his own residence. Is he ready for self-care? Does he need supervision? Are plans adequate for follow-up care, including appointments for individual or group therapy?

FREQUENTLY PRESCRIBED PSYCHIATRIC DRUGS

Psychiatric drugs frequently prescribed for depression include the following:

> Tricyclics: nortriptyline (Pamelor), desipramine (Norpramin), imipramine (Tofranil), amitriptyline (Elavil, Etrafon, Triavil), doxepin (Sinequan), maprotiline (Ludiomil), trazodone (Desyrel), amoxapine (Asendin)
> Monoamine oxidase inhibitors (MAOIs): phenelzine (Nardil), transcyclopromine (Parnate), isocarboxazide (Marplan)
> Selective serotonin reuptake inhibitors: fluoxetine (Prozac), sertraline (Zoloft), fluvoxamine (Luvox), paroxetine (Paxil)
> Other antidepressants: bupropion (Wellbutrin), venlafaxine (Effexor), nefazodone (Serzone)
> Mood stabilizer: lithium carbonate (Lithane, Lithonate, Eskalith)

The author refers the reader to Chapter 28 of this book for more on the topic of depression and its treatment.

10

The Person With Suicidal Ideation

The patient who is restless, paces, and is agitated presents symptoms that indicate the need for immediate intervention. He will often plead for help, saying, "I feel like jumping out of my skin" or "I feel like I'm going to explode." He should be closely watched to prevent any self-destructive actions. Medication is usually indicated to lessen his agitation.

The patient who contemplates suicide is desperate. His judgment and thinking are impaired because of his depressed emotional state. Therefore, every precaution should be taken to protect him from his inability to control himself. It goes without saying that the physicians and the oncoming shift must be alerted about the patient's statements and thoughts.

The actively suicidal patient may telephone others frequently to express his thoughts of dying. He may also write long rambling letters in which he threatens to end his life. He may make suicidal gestures, such as using a nail file to scratch his wrists superficially or swallowing an overdose of pills, perhaps asking for more water because they aren't going down right. He may repeatedly bang his head on a wall, or abuse alcohol before driving, to the point where he can become involved in a car accident. Most patients will talk openly about their disturbing thoughts and specific plans for suicide. However, there are those who do not, yet need to be evaluated seriously to assess the urgency of the situation. It is important to remember that most patients are ambivalent regarding their actions and usually can be persuaded that they have options other than death.

Suicidal communication is usually a request to be saved rather than a statement of action. However, there are higher suicide rates among those patients with a history of previous attempts or those who have a blood relative who has attempted or committed suicide. Other high-risk patients are those with a close friend who has attempted or committed suicide and those who have lost one or more significant persons in their lives and believe that suicide is a way to join those individuals. Suicide also appeals to patients who believe strongly that death is a pleasant sleep through which they will awaken in a better world and those who feel extremely guilty about past misdeeds and want to end the torture of self-reproach.

Predisposing factors may be traced back to the patient's childhood, when he developed a poor self-image as a result of overcritical parents or the loss of a very important and meaningful person. The feelings that disturbed him in those formative years may be reinforced by a recent crisis in his life, such as the death of a loved one, divorce, school or work failure, severe illness, leaving home for college or marriage, climacteric, or loss of a body part through surgery. The patient who has poor coping skills in dealing with stress is more likely to attempt suicide. He is, in essence, waving a red flag. It signifies, "Stop. Listen to me. I need help."

Health workers often become intensely anxious when hearing the suicidal patient's dialogue. For them, as for most people, self-destruction is contrary to everything they have learned about the sacredness of human life. In addition, they are often intensely involved in helping people fight life-threatening physical illnesses. They often have difficulty in understanding why a physically healthy individual deliberately attempts to end his life and may become angry, particularly when the patient's care necessitates attention that could be given to others who want to live. How often do health workers day, "He just wants attention, that's all"; "She'll do anything to get her own way"; or "How can she be unhappy with all that she has? It must be an act."

It is important to realize that suicidal patients can be intensely fearful of intimacy with others, yet at the same time are unable to tolerate the separation or rejection which they often invite by their behavior. When placed in a situation with increasing intimacy or when the possibility of separation or rejection exists, the patient may panic to the extent that his loss of self-control becomes apparent.

Health professionals must keep in mind that they are not omnipotent, and many times, despite all their hard work and therapeutic approaches, a patient will succeed in killing himself. At times like this, health professionals must support and help each other to work through their feelings, while at the same time searching for answers which may not be forthcoming. However, open discussion of this failure is important in preventing projection of blame on coworkers, supervisors, the physician, or the patient's significant others.

Suicidal patients *do* talk about their plans. The slightest hint must be taken seriously. Staff indifference or resistance to initiating therapeutic changes are detrimental to the patient's care. Extra staff members should be recruited from an on-call or per diem staff to relieve the regular staff of nonprofessional duties while they direct their energies to managing the patient. Strain and drain on the staff is intense, as the health professionals work closely together in a joint effort on a most complicated problem.

Not all suicidal behavior is overt. It may be hidden in such subtle ways as to be almost unrecognizable. Some patients appear to be very accident prone, falling down a flight of stairs or in front of a speeding car, later saying that they lost their balance. Others may "forget" to take life-sustaining medications or take double doses. Others indulge in activities which are medically unwise for them. Patients on dietary restrictions may go on a "binge," indulging in substances which are potentially harmful.

The health professional must evaluate the patient's potential for success in attempting suicide. Although women are more frequently involved in suicidal gestures, men are more likely to succeed, as are older or chronically ill patients. Those with specific plans, who have a lethal method available, should be taken very seriously. Patients who verbalize feelings of extreme helplessness, hopelessness, and guilt, particularly in the wake of a significant loss of a meaningful person or life style, are at great risk. In addition, if the patient lacks a support system of friends, relatives, or professionals, he is even more likely to choose suicide as his only solution.

A patient can be treated on an ambulatory basis if there are involved people in constant attendance willing to assume responsibility for him. In addition, the patient's main problem should not have a long-standing emotional basis. More than half of such suicidal patients in the emergency department at one hospital responded to techniques of immediate crisis intervention, returning for ongoing follow-up care. The therapy was reality based, exploring the alternatives which were available to the patient.

On the other hand, there are times when immediate hospitalization is needed to protect the patient from himself or to undo the damage brought about by self-inflicted actions. This is more frequently the case when the patient has been emotionally dysfunctional in the past and has deep-seated problems. The admission may be directly to an intensive care unit, where the stomach may have to be pumped to remove an overdose of drugs, or to an operating room to repair slash, stab, or gunshot wounds. The patient may be familiar to the staff from similar admissions in the past. If so, they may feel very hostile as he again diverts their time and energies from others who will appreciate their efforts. It is difficult to feel a deep commitment to saving someone who not only is ungrateful but even angry that he is still alive.

On admission a suicidal patient and his possessions must be thoroughly searched for anything which he may use to harm himself. He may have to give up his belt, razors, mirror, or any other sharp or breakable possessions. He may have to be observed when undressing and his belongings searched for harmful objects. One woman had hidden a lethal dose of medications in a vaginal tampon which no one thought to remove upon admission. She swallowed its contents during the night, nearly dying in the process. A man had taped a razor blade into the hem of a bathrobe and slashed his throat during the change of shifts when he knew the nurses were involved with sharing information. Still another managed to hide enough rope within a pajama leg to successfully hang himself on the unit's shower curtain rod. The patient may be very devious in trying to reach his goal!

Patients may be placed on suicidal precautions in any location—home, general or psychiatric hospital, or even a jail. The person assigned to his care must remain alert at all times to a sudden destructive action. One man who appeared to be improving was left alone while the worker spoke with the physician in the hallway. The patient took this opportunity to dash across the room, hurling himself through a closed window, landing on the ground four floors below. This particular incident should remind health care providers that patients who appear less depressed may be so only because they have formulated a plan for death which they believe will be successful. True improvement is often difficult to assess, but signs should include an increased sense of self-worth, a positive connection with significant others, and a sense that there is hope or options preferable to death. The staff should adopt the view that the patient has a treatable depressive illness and work cooperatively toward his improvement.

In 1994, more than 32,000 people were known to have committed suicide. It is suspected that the number was actually greater, but that the deaths were blamed on falls, automobile accidents, or overdoses of drugs or alcohol. Families may not divulge the truth because of legal, financial, emotional, or social reasons.

Is suicide linked to genetics? The rate is four times higher than average among close relatives, and six times higher among adopted children whose biological parent has killed himself. Identical twins of suicide victims are five times more likely than fraternal twins to commit suicide. The basic factor may be vulnerability to a psychiatric disorder, or to an inability to control impulses when under stress, or perhaps to a low level of serotonin or one of its metabolites. The imbalance of the brain chemicals may lead to a serious depression.

Suicide is now the eighth leading cause of death in the United States, involving 20% of the total population and 40% of those older than the age of 60. The rate increases with age, becoming three times higher in those older than 75, and six times higher for those older than 80. The highest rates are among the divorced and widowed, although those who have never married are twice as likely to commit suicide as those who are currently wed. The suicide rates among American descendants of emigrants tend to correlate with those in the country of origin, with the highest among those from German-speaking countries, Switzerland, Scandinavia, Eastern Europe, and Japan. Suicides are rare in Greece, Italy, and Spain.

In the United States, most suicides occur in the western states, and the lowest number in the northeastern area. At one time, 5% of all suicides were in the age group 15 to 24. That number has escalated to 20% of male suicides, and 14% of females. Suicides of those between 15 to 19 quadrupled between 1950 and 1988, and are now the most common reason for visits to hospital emergency rooms for those younger than 35 years of age. Accessibility to firearms in the home increases the risk of suicide nearly five times, particularly among adolescents and young adults. (In areas of strict gun control, other methods are used.) In addition, women who were sexually assaulted under the age of 16 are three to four times more likely to attempt suicide.

About 30% to 70% of people who commit suicide have a history of a major depression or bipolar disorder. Half of all suicides are the result of substance abuse, with the alcohol abuser three or four times more likely to kill himself than the average individual. Users of illicit drugs as well as tobacco smokers have high rates also, with narcotic addicts about five times as likely to commit suicide as the normal individual. Schizophrenic patients are at risk, particularly if they are abusing drugs or alcohol, and suffer from hallucinations or delusions. More than a third can be expected to attempt suicide, with 5% to 10% eventually succeeding.

Certain personality traits are more frequent among those who attempt suicide. They are more likely to be guilty of uncontrollable tempers, verbal or physical abuse, sexual violence, and other antisocial behavior. White murderers in the United States are 700 times more likely to kill themselves than the average person. Chronic physical illness in the elderly, particularly in men, is another risk factor. Despair, including a sense of hopelessness, is the most common motivator as well as a sign that the unsuccessful individual is likely to make another attempt in the future.

THE APPROACH TO THE PERSON WITH SUICIDAL IDEATION

Immediate Intervention by the Patient

SELF-MANAGEMENT TECHNIQUES

Make the patient aware of factors that can increase the risk of suicide. Health problems, family and marital issues, loss of job, loss of a significant other through desertion or divorce, or death, particularly if by suicide, or financial problems all create issues that may lead to the point of suicidal ideation.

Professional Intervention

IMMEDIATE ACTION

If the patient is at home, in school, or in the hospital, make others aware of the problem. The need for supportive and knowledgeable helpers helps prevent the isolation of the patient, and lessen the sense of helplessness and hopelessness. The environment must be made secure, with the removal of any objects that can be used lethally (guns, sharp instruments, ropes, razors, pills). Access to alcohol or poisons should be prevented.

INTERMEDIATE ACTION

Don't become a partner to the patient's actions by promising to keep his thoughts and actions secret. By sharing his plans with you, he is asking for professional intervention, even though he may deny that this is so. Tell the patient, "As a professional, I will never promise to keep such information secret, nor will I ever be a partner to your plans to take your own life."

Take the patient seriously. Ask him if you understand him correctly, repeating what he has said. Do not be judgmental. Rather, let the patient know that you are concerned about him, even though his behavior causes you some anxiety. Remember that inquiring about suicidal thoughts or plans is not the cause of action. The questions are a sign that you are interested and that you have the ability to handle a difficult subject. This will increase his confidence in you. Don't be misled by a negative response, since some patients believe it is useless to discuss their feelings because "nothing can help."

Long-Term Action

Evaluate the patient's ability to return home. If necessary, the patient may need time in a supervised environment, with adequate plans for follow-up care, including appointments for individual or group therapy, and adequate anti-depressant medication.

Determine whether the stresses of home, school, or work can be lessened sufficiently for the patient to return to the preillness environment. If not, help the patient select other options.

11

The Person With a Dependent Personality Disorder

Many patients diagnosed as having a dependent personality disorder may appear to have lost all sense of self-worth. Their diagnosis is one of the most frequently reported personality disorders treated by mental health providers. Incapacitated by illness, they have become unable to function effectively in any area of living. Some have lost jobs or been unable to maintain their former positions, and may have been replaced in their family or community roles. Constant worry about not being successful increases the fear of failure, and causes the person to avoid acceptance of any new responsibility or taking part in any new ventures. If the patient does not assert himself in social, sexual, or work areas, he avoids the possibility of further loss of approval.

The patient's dependency severely restricts his life. Often he is a prisoner in his own home, refusing to go anywhere unless accompanied by someone. Characteristically, he appears depressed, has a pessimistic attitude with little self-confidence, and exhibits anxiety in any situation where he feels alone or is away from a safe environment such as his home.

The individual with a dependent personality disorder tends to be submissive and clinging, and lives with the fear that he will be abandoned. He reacts to this fear by becoming increasingly submissive, and does everything within his power to appease those on whom he depends. If he loses the person on whom he relies for nurturance, he is likely to seek a replacement to supply the care and sustenance that he craves.

Dependency is related to a combination of early life experiences, anticipation of future events, and present circumstances. The health worker needs to evaluate factors in the patient's environment that may be influencing his behavior. For instance, a 45-year-old woman, reluctant to separate from her college-bound daughter, concealed her feelings by developing physical symptoms that left her bedridden and helpless. This resulted in a cancellation of the daughter's plans to live at school. Each time the youngster attempted to leave home, the mother's symptoms escalated markedly. This changed only after the mother was actively engaged in long-term therapy.

Well-meaning attempts by the health worker to encourage the patients to help themselves are often resisted. Activities are shunned. The patients cannot even take care of their own daily routines. They never seem to be capable of making a decision without repeatedly seeking the advice of others. They deny any responsibility for their situation, and blame all their difficulties on other people or factors beyond their control. This behavior is reminiscent of that exhibited by a small child. In essence, the patient *has* regressed emotionally to his childhood years and is using old patterns of behavior in seeking gratification for his physical and emotional needs. It is as though he is saying, "Take care of me because you can see I just can't do it myself."

The patient's dependency, his inability to do for himself, to make such simple decisions as what to wear, what to do right now, what to order from the menu, what to read, or how to take the next step, tend to evoke feelings of deep sympathy. The worker feels inclined to do for the patient what he is unable to do for himself. This may satisfy the worker's desire to be helpful and needed, but increases the patient's helplessness by reinforcing his dependence on others. Through all this, the worker may even neglect other patients who, on first impression, seem to need him less. Those others may then harbor ill feelings against the worker and even greater resentment against the patient who is taking up so much time.

Dependent patients avoid taking responsibility for themselves or others. In that way, they cannot make mistakes and thus are protected from being blamed by others. They withdraw from the world around them; friendships are lost, and family relationships are barely sustained.

Over a period of time, patients who exhibit an excessive need for care by others may evoke anger and a sense of frustration in those very people to whom they cling. Eventually, there may be resentment at the patients' inability or unwillingness to take responsibility for their own decision making. Their inaction may be perceived as a barrier to gaining insight into their basic difficulties.

When outsiders begin to feel the weight of the patient's dependency, assume that the patient just cannot be helped or does not appreciate all the efforts in his behalf, they may begin to ignore him. This justifies the patient's self-evaluation of being an unworthy and unlikable person. He says, to himself, "Why try when no one really cares?" Dependency is a defense used by patients who generally feel that they have no worth. Unfortunately, the clinging behavior does not solve problems but instead prevents meaningful interaction with others from occurring. It also stifles any growth toward a healthier behavior pattern as responsibility for major life decisions is delegated to others.

APPROACH TO THE PATIENT WITH A DEPENDENT PERSONALITY DISORDER

Immediate Intervention by the Patient

SELF-MANAGEMENT TECHNIQUES

Teach the patient to recognize the target symptom that initiates the feeling of dependency (inability to make a decision, continually asking others what they would do in his place). Encourage him to immediately choose from his options and institute his choice.

Professional Intervention

IMMEDIATE ACTION

Use a kind but firm approach to reach the patient whose fears have immobilized him. A gentle but positive tone of voice and short, clear sentences will let the patient know that the worker recognizes his feelings of dependency, but does not feel the situation is hopeless. The worker can say, "You feel as though you are not able to care for yourself at this time. That will change as you begin to feel better." This implies that the situation is temporary, and leaves the future open for improvement. The dependent patient needs patience and support while he learns to care for himself. The worker should focus on such simple tasks as grooming, care of one's room, and selection of food at meal-time.

Deal with the present when you talk with the patient. Focusing on the here and now counteracts his feelings of dependency that arise from his inability to make decisions.

INTERMEDIATE ACTION

Direct the patient's attention to his small gains or successes in activities instead of stressing his shortcomings. This increases his sense of accomplishment and, at the same time, supports his positive feelings about himself. For example, the worker can say, "Today you were able to finish making your bed and attend a group meeting."

Encourage a positive relationship with the patient so that he will enter into a discussion about himself. Clues to the patient's dependency may appear as he talks of events in his childhood. Frequently the history reveals the presence of a parent who stifled any initiative or outward expression of feelings.

Allow plenty of time for the patient to complete a task. Help him see that errors are correctable and need not be dwelt on. The dependent patient's fear of making mistakes usually goes back to his childhood handling by critical parents. Such a patient has learned to avoid criticism by giving up in the face of difficulty. Stress the importance of the "doing" rather than perfection.

Help the patient to experience success in a trying situation. Point out his positive efforts toward self-help (e.g., his ability to remain with the group for a full hour, to talk with the therapist, or to relate to other people at mealtime), and his improved appearance.

LONG-TERM ACTION

Enlist the patient's cooperation in planning his treatment, self-care, and therapeutic activities. This will increase his sense of control, and strengthen his defenses. If the patient functioned at all before his illness, direct his attention to those areas and stress his accomplishments—working at a job, cleaning the house, preparing meals, doing volunteer work, driving a car, and meeting social obligations.

Encourage any attempt by the patient to assume responsibility for himself or others (e.g., setting up the room for a planned activity, erasing the blackboard, baking a cake, stamping charts). If his efforts are unsuccessful, point out how they can be used as learning experiences rather than viewed as areas of failure.

12

The Person With a Brief Psychotic Disorder

Patients who meet this classification suffer from delusions and/or hallucinations. They may be incoherent, grossly disorganized, or even exhibit catatonic behavior for at least a day but no longer than a month. An example of this would be a patient who is hallucinating. Hallucinations are episodes in which the patient hears, sees, smells, tastes, or feels what does not exist in reality. In other words, his perceptions do not have any outside stimulus but come from inside himself.

Hallucinations may be associated with many conditions including surgery, disturbances in the body's electrolyte balance, head trauma, brain tumor, respiratory conditions, severe psychic stress (psychosis), a drug reaction, and alcoholism. Another cause may be prolonged isolation, during which the patient suffers from lack of stimulation to his sensory motor system.

The workers can pick up obvious clues that reveal the patient is hallucinating. They may notice the patient staring into space intently and paying no attention to the immediate environment or to any activity occurring nearby. The workers' attempts at communication are rebuffed. The patient may appear terribly frightened and report that snakes or devils or saints are surrounding him, or that a deceased parent or child had been with him. (If these episodes are common to his culture, he may seem untroubled. At this point, it is important to determine whether the experience is actually related to his culture, or whether it is due to a psychosis because the latter requires immediate intervention.) If the patient indeed suffers from a brief psychotic disorder, he may appear preoccupied and seem out of touch with his environment including the activities of daily living and prescribed treatment. These nonexistent images demand all of his attention. Workers do not know what the patient "sees" unless they ask. This should be done in a tone of voice that is of sufficient volume and clarity to catch or hold the patient's attention. For example, a staff member may say, "Mr. Simpson, I am Mrs. Best. What are you looking at?" or "Tell me, what do you see now?" It is important to use the patient's name in addressing him because most patients will respond to their names. In addition, this identification helps the patient remember who he is, even if he has forgotten who or where he is. The identification of the worker helps the patient reenter reality with a minimum of embarrassment. A patient may readily respond to such intervention with, "My aunt was here"; "Daggers are pointing at me"; or "The rocks are ready to roll down the mountain." If so, the worker can deal with the patient's experience, and at the same time can state that he himself has not seen or heard what the patient is describing.

Generally, it is not useful to question the reality of a hallucinating experience too soon because such a challenge may increase the anxiety to the point of making the patient unreachable. This may then result in denial of what is happening. For example, one patient was observed talking to "the nice little bugs" and was counting. "One, two, three." When asked about this, she denied the entire experience, even though she appeared bewildered as to where she was and what was happening to her.

Health workers can show their appreciation of the patient's reluctance to share an experience and of the patient's anxiety when the issue is pursued, by saying, "Sometimes people have the unique experience of thinking they see objects or people, or that they hear sounds. This is usually just a part of the person's illness and disappears gradually as improvement continues." Such a statement offers reassurance while letting the patient know that the worker understands and is concerned.

In certain instances, usually when the patient is quite ill, staff members may be incorrectly identified as the patient's beloved mother, old friend, teacher, aunt, or sister. At other times, the worker or any one else in the area may be seen as a hated, mean, hostile person who is out to "get" the patient. Voices, smells, or sounds may heighten the patient's misidentification. An 18-year-old psychotic girl responded to the health worker's voice by referring to him as her "teacher" and said, "You always loved me. I love you. You taught me photography. Can I go to school now?" She then accused the doctor, who smoked, of being her "rotten father." "You always tell me you hate me and that I'm bad and nothing but trouble. Don't touch me."

It is easy to discover the patient who is having auditory hallucinations, for he will be observed talking with an unseen entity to whom he is attentive and responsive as though listening for answers. The ongoing conversation may last for seconds, minutes, or longer. On occasion, the quietly attentive worker may find himself involved in the hallucinatory experience. For example, the patient may turn to him and say, "Hear how he talks to me. He said he is going to kill me. You heard him." Again, the worker makes clear to the patient that the voice has not been audible to others.

Auditory and visual hallucinations may occur together. One middle-aged woman insisted that the problem that most interfered with her life was not the fact that she lived with her mother, with whom she had shared the care of an aged grandmother for the past seventeen years, but rather that she was involved in continual conversations with different men who she said appeared on the walls of her room and exhausted her to the point that she was no longer able to eat or sleep. She said they had even pursued her to the hospital, where they continued to insist that she talk with them. The patient admitted that she knew others did not see or hear these men, but that they still bothered her terribly. Obviously, these hallucinations were filling a void that she had felt keenly during her many years of loneliness.

On admission, the patient usually responds honestly to routine questions as to whether hearing voices or seeing things have been a problem. Sometimes the worker has been informed of the problem beforehand by a relative who has accompanied the patient. If so, he can state openly, "Your mother mentioned that the voices you hear interfere with your ability to concentrate at home or at work and with your ability to get along with people. Is this so?" This gives the patient an opportunity to talk about the problem further. If he has already denied having hallucinations, the relative's report can be used to probe the subject but this must be done gently so that the patient doesn't feel threatened.

Workers should report the hallucinations, with descriptive details, to other involved staff members, noting any events that may be contributing factors. Sharing this information helps to uncover the basis for the hallucinations. Discussion of how you managed the patient successfully encourages consistent treatment. It also helps to lessen the anxiety of workers who fear being with a patient whose behavior is "crazy."

As the worker pursues the details of the patient's hallucinatory experience, he must remain aware that the patient is convinced of the reality of the experience. Because of this, the more information the worker has about the experience, the more effective and clearly defined his interaction will be. He must discover what the voices tell the patient, what the visions are, and what may precipitate the experience and/or influence its frequency. If the health provider is present at the start of a hallucinatory episode, it may be possible to help the patient become aware of the target symptom. In one instance, the patient was observed staring at bubbles rising in a glass of soda. The worker said, "It almost seems that those bubbles are trying to convey a message rather than just coming to the top of the fluid." The patient appeared startled as his very thoughts were verbalized. He was able to agree, stating that he realized he was watching a normal process. This initial attention to a target symptom provided a breakthrough, helping the patient to reality test other hallucinations as they occurred.

THE APPROACH TO THE PATIENT WITH A BRIEF PSYCHOTIC DISORDER

Immediate Intervention by the Patient

SELF-MANAGEMENT TECHNIQUES

Teach the patient to recognize the target symptom that initiates a hallucinatory experience (visual, olfactory, or auditory sensation not perceived by anyone else). Immediately start to reality test by concentrating on a real experience, such as a person in the room, an odor of food that is cooking, or the sound of music on the radio, with verification of its real existence from a nearby person.

Professional Intervention

IMMEDIATE ACTION

If you suspect that a patient is hallucinating, use open-ended questions that require more than a "yes" or "no" answer. For example, "What did you decide to do this afternoon?" may elicit a response such as, "I'm going with this policeman to court." This is more informative about the patient's state than asking, "Are you all right?" to which the patient can respond. "Yes." In this instance, there was no policeman, nor was the patient going to court.

As you approach the patient, state who you are and what your role is. Follow the introduction with an open-ended statement such as "Tell me about your day today" or "What's happening today?" Sit next to the patient, or walk along beside him. Your availability will make him feel your interest, warmth, genuine concern, and desire to talk with him. Spending time with the patient will enable you to assess more easily what is really happening. Reply to his lucid comments about his surroundings, his clothes, or his family. These are real. Be kind but firm when you refer to what the patient states he alone has seen or heard. Always let him know—outright or by implication—that you believe what he states but, for example, that you do not hear the voice he speaks of. This can be implied by asking, "Is the voice you hear male or female?" "Does the vision you see remind you of anyone or anything from your past?" Arguing with the patient and trying to convince him that his perception is unreal is futile. It only increases his anxiety and his use of denial, which stifles further communication. Ask the patient to describe his experience. "What do the voices say?" "What do you see?" "What is your reaction to what you smell?"

Maintain adequate protection and surveillance for the patient. This is a must for one who is frightened and/or appears to be responding to commands that he may think are telling him to run, jump, or hurt himself or others. The patient may have to be moved to a padded room on a closed unit so that he will not harm himself or others. A nurse may have to remain with him for extended periods of time in order to help him cope with his experience and interrupt it, if possible. Keep the patient's environment familiar whenever feasible, so that he does not have to readjust to the physical setup. Don't allow him to be flooded with visitors and well-meaning friends. Too much stimulation may increase his confusion.

Always try to use a verbal response. Arm gestures, finger-shaking, showing approval or disapproval by head movements or grimacing are ambiguous and may intensify the patient's hallucination. Use clear, uncomplicated responses when answering his questions. Try to orient him to time, place, and activities each time you approach him.

INTERMEDIATE ACTION

Try to get the patient to focus his interest on what is real or happening at the moment. "What kinds of flowers are in that vase?" "Who brought them to you?" "What is the book on your table about?" "What kinds of stories do you enjoy reading?" "What activities do you like?" "At what time was your dressing changed today?" "What kind of a day are you having today?" Always present reality when responding to an hallucinating patient. For example, "You say bats are flying. I do not see any. You are safe."

LONG-TERM ACTION

As the patient begins to improve, include him in group activities in which only a few members participate. The focus should be on "doing," as in occupational therapy—painting, sanding, woodworking, making ceramic objects, or sewing, for example. Encourage the patient to go on outside walks when this is possible and to participate in dancing, exercise classes, bingo, card playing, games, baking, or other available activities. Your joining in these activities will encourage the patient to accept them as valuable. Activities keep the patient focused on reality, reduce his level of tension, provide satisfaction and gratification, and expose him to interactions with others. When the patient is able, group or individual discussions that focus on preparing him for living in the community should be stressed. Discussions may center on such items as transportation, selection of proper clothing, obtaining a job or gaining admission to a school, budgeting, or improving existing skills. Encourage the patient to participate in his own care to the degree that he is able. Help him with what he is unable to do.

Always treat the patient with consideration, respect, and a concerned attitude. A warm human response will have a substantial beneficial effect, even though the patient may appear to be unaware of what is happening at the moment.

If you are present as a hallucinatory episode begins, give the patient an adequate explanation for what is happening, and help him understand any misinterpretation. For example, the patient may complain of a foul odor in an odor-free room. The worker may notice that the patient is concentrating on flowers that are withering and comment, "Flowers often develop bad odors as they die. What experience have you had with that happening?" In one case, the patient related the odor to the flowers in the funeral home when her father died. That association enabled her to work through her unresolved feelings of loss that had been present since his death many months before.

FREQUENTLY PRESCRIBED PSYCHIATRIC DRUGS

Psychiatric drugs frequently prescribed for psychosis include the following:

Phenothiazines: chlorpromazine (Thorazine), promazine (Sparine), fluphenazine (Prolixin), thioridazine (Mellaril), mesoridazine (Serentil), trifluoperazine (Stelazine), perphenazine (Trilafon), haloperidol (Haldol), loxapine (Loxapac)

Neuroleptics: clozapine (Clozaril), risperidone (Risperdal), olanzapine (Zyprexal)

13

The Person With an Oppositional Defiant Disorder

Some patients display tremendous negativism while under psychiatric treatment. They are defiant, disobeying any rules that are in place, regardless of the setting. This behavior pattern has probably existed for many years, perhaps throughout childhood, adolescence, and into adulthood. They are argumentative, and go out of their way to annoy and antagonize others. At the same time, they are easily hurt by the actions of others, blaming outsiders for their own shortcomings. They often appear angry, and may invoke actions that are spiteful and vindictive. Their actions and attitudes impair their relationships with others as well as their effectiveness in social, school, or work situations. If they are in the hospital, they have difficulty in relating to staff members. They reject any overtures by the health workers, refusing to admit that those approaches are offered to be helpful.

The patient says over and over again: "No"; "I don't want to"; "Not now"; "What for?"; and "It's dumb." He refuses whatever staff members may offer, whether it is a back rub, a walk, or a drink of juice, regardless of its attractiveness. He usually does not take part in scheduled activities. When he does attend he does not participate but complains throughout that the therapy is useless. He may then say that he is sitting in only because he has been coerced into it, or because he wants to please his family, or that attending is the road that leads to discharge because his cooperation will be noted in the nurses' reports. All efforts to talk with the patient are futile. The worker becomes aware of doing all the talking when with the patient in order to keep up the facade of a conversation. The patient shows little response. When he anticipates that the worker is on the verge of saying something to him or coming his way to make a request, he may protest animatedly either in gestures or speech. In other words, the patient shuts the staff out by closing the door on any help that is offered. He does not see that it is his behavior that prevents others from working with him. His misinterpretation gives rise to an inner feeling that nothing will ever help—that he can never recover.

No one wants to feel rejected, refused, shut out, hurt. Yet this is just how the rejecting patient anticipates he will feel if he becomes involved. To prevent this, he avoids *any* involvement. He scorns help, avoids interaction, says: "No; leave me alone"; "Please go away"; "I don't want to"; "That's that, I've had it"; "Please stop bothering me"; "I don't need your help"; or "You're a big pest." What the worker must understand is that these patients have usually had more than their share of rejection. They feel worthless and are asking for proof of staff interest in them.

Some have experienced the early loss of one or both parents and were consequently shuffled from home to home. Some were given up for adoption. Regardless of the quality of love and care provided by the adoptive parents, some adoptees never overcome the sense of having been rejected by the biological parents, and see themselves as unlovable: "If my 'real' mother didn't love me enough to keep me, no one else will." Others come from broken homes in which neither parent wanted them, or were so busy with social or work activities aimed at achieving status and position for themselves that they did not realize that more than food and clothing are needed for the healthy emotional growth of children. In some instances, parents may have been cold, stern people who never gave their affection freely; if love was given, it was offered as though it were a chore or an obligation. A patient with an oppositional defiant disorder may have been hospitalized during his early life because of physical illness, abandonment, or unacceptable behavior. As a result, he may have experienced actual physical and emotional isolation from any kind of familiar environment or close relationships.

The feeling of being unwanted and unloved may be deeply rooted or the patient's early history may reveal no actual episode of rejection. Sometimes there is a symbolic episode which has been misinterpreted by the patient as a rejection. In one case, a 20-year-old girl spoke of her resentment when her younger sister was born almost 15 years before. She interpreted the birth as a sign that her parents no longer loved or wanted her, that they were rejecting her and attempting to replace her. In another case, a 30-year-old female who had received financial help from her sister-in-law expressed profound feelings of rejection when the same sister-in-law also provided help to another family member. It takes a long time for the patient who believes he has been rejected to place trust in others or to feel even a little bit good about himself. The initial effort often has to be made by the worker, in order to make the patient realize that at least one person thinks he has worth. One negativistic patient repeatedly refused to come out of her room, eat with others, or talk with anyone. Her response to the nurse's concern was, "Who would be interested in me? I've never amounted to anything and never will." She appeared stunned when the nurse proceeded to bring two lunch trays into the room, and sat down to eat with her. However, this initiated a meaningful relationship between them.

Sometimes a person is promised something that he really counts on and if the promise is not fulfilled, he interprets this as a rejection of himself, even though the explanation offered refutes the thought. One extreme example of this occurred when a patient's husband, having promised to take her on a trip after he retired, died suddenly three days before his retirement, thereby making it impossible to fulfill his promise. The patient felt that if her husband had really loved her he would have lived to make the trip. His delaying it until his retirement, and its cancellation by his sudden death was proof to her that he never really loved her.

Consider the obviously handicapped person who finds that he is repeatedly turned away when he applies for admission to schools or for job employment. He may very well attribute his inability to be successful to his personal appearance, even though this may not be entirely true. Young adults who have severe acne, stutter, or are unduly obese may anticipate being shunned and rejected by others. The rejected individual finally makes up his mind (unconsciously, of course) never to expose himself to that possibility again. It is too painful to have to cope with the feeling of rejection. In his mind, it would be better to push others away, prevent experiences—in essence, avoid life—before he suffers more hurts. The patient loses all his confidence in others and cannot believe that anyone really is sincerely interested in him as he is now, or ever could be in the future. Furthermore, he will not give you, the health professional, family, or friends, the chance. Why should he, when people have always failed him before? When you approach him, he says that you are staying with him because it's your job and you're getting paid, or because your superior has told you to do so. Your motives are always questioned. He projects onto you what he really feels about himself. One young woman said,

"You don't really care; no one ever has." Another said, "Why bother with me? There are others you could have fun with." Both individuals saw themselves as unlovable, unacceptable, worthless people, not significant enough to be given genuine affection. The worker was therefore seen as uncaring, and perhaps playing with the person's feelings to amuse himself.

It is not uncommon for these patients to be extremely sensitive, to make gross misinterpretations, and to attach personal meaning to everyday occurrences. A patient who was last on the list of those scheduled for electrostimulative therapy interpreted this as meaning that the doctor thought the least of her. One patient resented a lack of individual attention from the doctor following his participation in a course for family physicians. This was interpreted as a slight because the patient felt that the doctor was pleasant at first only to use him as a guinea pig, but now had abandoned him. In another instance, an unanticipated change in the scheduled time for a group meeting precipitated a strong reaction in which one patient accused the nurse of deliberately trying to "get rid of" her. Scheduled vacations or sudden absence of personnel often create crises as the patients feel they are being deserted.

At times, the professional worker becomes annoyed, irritated, frustrated, and plain tired. He may have spent an inordinate amount of time with one patient, been as therapeutic as ever, and yet was totally unappreciated. Increasingly, the patient's behavior and attitude irritate him. He begins to ask himself, "Why bother?" It is much easier and more satisfying to work with someone who appreciates staff efforts, or at least responds a little. So, the next time he goes around the unit, he inadvertently passes the patient's room. He forgets to ask him to come to the group sessions, does not remind him that the barber is on the unit, and neglects to include him in patient outings. After all, the worker knows ahead of time that the patient's response will be an unequivocal "no," and he doesn't appreciate feeling rejected time and time again, either. His pride in himself is shaken, he begins to doubt his professional skills, and his self-confidence decreases. If the worker could magnify his own experience a hundred times, he might have some concept of how desperately the patient fears rejection. He needs to understand that the patient is not rejecting him personally, but is very fearful of any experience or interaction that may lead to an arousal of his feeling of being unwanted. It is important to remember that the patient has not developed the ability to sustain normal give-and-take in everyday relationships. When he cannot have what he wants when he wants it, he feels that others disapprove of him, cannot love him, and are trying to hurt and reject him.

THE APPROACH TO THE PATIENT WITH AN OPPOSITIONAL DEFIANT DISORDER

Immediate Intervention by the Patient

SELF-MANAGEMENT TECHNIQUES

Teach the patient to recognize the target symptom that initiates the need to respond negatively. Is it the tone of voice used by the individual, perhaps reminding him of someone in his past? Is it the content of the offer? (One patient was furious when the offer of orange juice was made. "And that, after I said I was allergic to oranges.")

Professional Intervention

IMMEDIATE ACTION

Recognize the negativism as part of the illness. Do not retaliate by pointing out his unkempt appearance, or other negative features.

Recognize how you feel when the patient rejects you. Do not demand reasons or explanations for his rejecting behavior. Be nonjudgmental.

Offer a professional relationship. Tell the patient, "I have come to accompany you on the walk" or "I have come to eat dinner with you." If he questions your motives, reply, "I wouldn't have come in the first place if I really didn't want to."

Always keep the patient informed of any changes in the schedule, forthcoming events, or procedures. Avoid promising what you cannot deliver.

If the patient will not talk with you, spend at least 15 minutes just sitting quietly and being with him. Keep the immediate environment low pressured. Do not push the patient to do more than he can; be content with small gains at first. For example, if a patient refuses to go on a walk with the group, you can suggest that he sit alone with one of the health workers on the patio or in the day room. Do not push him to talk if he is obviously uncomfortable. Tell him, "When you feel more comfortable we will talk together again," and do so. When he can tolerate it, encourage the patient to express his feelings in a verbal manner. At the same time, indicate to him that you accept his expressions of his feelings even though you do not always agree with them. This will make him realize that you are not suggesting that he imitate your behavior.

INTERMEDIATE ACTION

Don't try to interpret the patient's behavior to him. This may increase his anxiety, and possibly interfere with the start of any therapeutic relationship. The patient needs to feel wanted before he can tolerate any threats. Allow sufficient time for progress, even though it may be slow and uneven. Be consistent in your approach. Several attempts, spaced at intervals throughout the day, will remind the patient that you are really interested and will also inject some doubt into his belief that no one cares.

LONG-TERM ACTION

Cultivate feelings of trust. This can be done by using nonthreatening activities in which the patient can achieve some degree of positive feeling (e.g., exercise class, body movement to music group, walks, ball games, shuffle board, bingo, helping with cleanup). Include the patient in all activities. Even though he is reluctant to participate at first, offer him the opportunity to change his mind. Avoid using empty phrases (e.g., "Your skin really isn't that bad" or "I'm sure everyone really loves you"). Instead, offer validation of the patient's feelings with constructive measures he can employ or the opportunity to explore his difficulty. State, "Your skin condition must be distressing. Perhaps with medication, treatment, and less tension it will improve."

14

The Person With a Conduct Disorder

As noted in the previous chapter, individuals with an oppositional defiant disorder are difficult but not physically abusive. Conversely, those who suffer from a conduct disorder are unable to restrain themselves when angry, and repeatedly violate others by harming them physically or damaging their property. They also ignore rules, and tend to bully others, threatening them or even hurting them by using a weapon or assaulting them. The destruction or theft of another's property is a common feature of this disorder as is physical cruelty including rape or homicide. Lying is a common component as well as theft (snatching purses, car or home break-ins, shoplifting, or forgery) and conning people into giving them whatever they want at the moment. People with this diagnosis may exhibit extreme hostility to everyone with whom they come into contact.

It is usually easy to recognize the person with a conduct disorder. His angry tone of voice and facial expression are apparent to everyone. Others readily observe that the hospitalized patient is often sarcastic, offers unwarranted criticism in the face of adequate staff performance, condemns his surroundings, is uncooperative no matter how simple the task, and is argumentative with little or no provocation. Obvious overt manifestations of his anger may include throwing magazines or pillows across the room, smashing glass, or kicking a chair. The person appears to be easily upset, and anything or everything may become a focus for his faultfinding. He does not want to be bothered in any way and may be actually insulting to those who try to approach him. His choice of language may be colorful and/or vulgar. Covert hostility should be suspected when the person is excessively polite, yet manages to convey his constant dissatisfaction with everyone and everything.

When confronted with his behavior, the hostile person may act as if he does not know what on earth you are talking about. Some people will offer elaborate explanations for their reactions to justify them. These supposedly acceptable reasons for behavior given to himself are called rationalizations. Sometimes the individual will tell the nurse about problems that are unrelated to what really bothers him. This is because the subject is too painful to deal with at the moment. He may be unaware or only partially aware of what is upsetting him. Again, if this glimpse of insight is painful, the person may deny his anger vehemently and refuse to talk at all. Instead, he displaces his anger onto other people (nurse, aide, social worker, or doctor), or whoever is working with him and trying to help. Denial and displacement are often observed when he suffers a loss (real or imagined) and feels unloved, rejected, and uncared for.

The person with a conduct disorder arouses fear and anxiety in those around him, particularly if he is assaultive. One practical reason why others keep away from him is that his behavior and responses are unpredictable. Fear of being physically hurt leads others to avoid the particularly angry person.

Sometimes there is no forewarning that the individual is becoming angry and unable to control his actions. Several aspects of his behavior, however, may indicate the possibility of approaching trouble; for example, a rising pitch of the voice and cutting comments—"You think you know it all"; "Well, if it isn't the big wheel herself." The person may also angrily refuse to accept medication or treatment, show clenched fists or slap one clenched fist into an open hand as if into a baseball glove. Often he will complain about his living quarters, kick the bases of the furniture, forcefully dump utensils into the waste basket, or just throw things onto the floor. He may walk in and out of rooms, or up and down the hall in brisk fashion, his glance darting to and fro, but particularly toward the exit door. He may ask a question, such as: "Are the windows breakable here?" or make such statements as: "I'll get even with him if that's the last thing I do," or "I'd burn the place down if I had a match." He may also say things, such as: "They think I'm stupid; well, we'll see about that"; or "If she thinks she's going to run my life, she's dead wrong."

Another excuse for avoiding the angry person is that most people do not like their services to go unappreciated. Because some health workers interpret a patient's hostility as a personal affront to themselves, they tend to walk away from the angry individual. This may occur when workers' own feelings get in the way of their dealing effectively with the patient.

Many people are not in the habit of dealing with their own anger or that of others. They keep angry feelings to themselves, sometimes accumulating them for so long that a depression results. In effect, depression is anger turned inwardly on oneself. When these feelings are finally allowed to come out, they may be directed against the dog, cat, spouse, a parent, or sibling—"safe" individuals who will not retaliate and with whom they feel secure. Some people express anger only when with a group of people, so that a response is unlikely. One family stated that their daughter (the patient) always waited for family gatherings to express her feelings that "all people are rotten. No one cares about me. Everyone is a piece of garbage." Some people displace their anger onto an authority figure and, fearing repercussions, avoid verbalizing or acting out their anger directly. Instead, they may "gripe" to a peer. The assassination of a public figure is sometimes blamed on this type of displacement.

Among the many reasons a person may have for being angry is the disability created by his current affliction or the threat it has brought to his job or economic status. He may be angry because he has received inaccurate information from professionals in the past, and may complain that he is being hospitalized unjustly and against his will. Past relationships or occurrences at home or at work that have disappointed him may have never been resolved. He may feel anger at having to experience this problem which he never asked for in the first place! Those old angry feelings are now displaced onto people in his new situation, which somehow seems similar to the previous situation. Therefore, certain aspects of unresolved conflicts of the past are reactivated.

The patient's hostility impairs his relationship with others. People turn away in a rejecting manner. This serves as further proof to the person that the world is mean and uncaring, increasing his anger. For some, being the butt of negative reactions is somehow better than the isolation of no reaction at all. Yet it is not uncommon for individuals to hide their hostility from health care providers for fear that care will be withdrawn if anger or displeasure is expressed.

The hostility may be an outgrowth of childish feelings or jealousy, reminiscent of his not wanting to share a parent. This becomes evident as health workers become very involved with administering medications or assisting another person. The patient, unable to tolerate the workers' involvement with others, may act out in a hostile way, in order to get attention focused on himself.

Young adults often become hostile as a result of disillusionment brought about by what they regard as unfair treatment by adults who promised otherwise. They also show hostility when they see flaws in the character of a cherished role model or when they face the inequities and social injustices of the world.

THE APPROACH TO THE PATIENT WITH A CONDUCT DISORDER

Immediate Intervention by the Patient

SELF-MANAGEMENT TECHNIQUES

Teach the patient to recognize the target symptom that initiates the need to respond abusively and to recognize the body tension that accompanies his hostility (clenched fists, tight facial muscles, or squinting eyes). Teach him to convert that energy into an acceptable act, such as punching a bed pillow to control the desire to assault another person.

Professional Intervention

IMMEDIATE ACTION

Get help immediately if it becomes necessary to disarm or subdue a patient. (Incidentally, if you fear talking with such a person alone, always have an assistant with you.) A controlling environment often helps the person to control himself. Inform him that you understand he cannot control his actions at this time; therefore, you are helping him to do so. Don't humiliate him while restraining him or giving intramuscular injections of medications to diffuse his assaultive actions and help him regain self-control. Offer the patient the opportunity of cooperating with you for his benefit. State, "You need this injection. I have to administer this to you even if you do not recognize the need for it. It will be much more helpful if you cooperate with me while I give it to you."

Avoid excessive smiling and ingratiating remarks. The danger here is that the person may interpret such behavior as insincere and feel that he is being laughed at.

Keep the tone of your voice low and well controlled. React to what the patient says with an honest, open, concerned attitude. You must convince him that you care and want very much to understand his problem.

Remember not to take the person's criticism personally. This will help you not to become defensive. Quietly answer any tirade by offering an explanation for your functions or the hospital or health care agency's routines. The idea is to acknowledge that you recognize his anger but doubt that it has a direct relationship to you. Then stay with him for a few minutes, demonstrating ease and control in the situation. This allows the person to feel increasingly comfortable with you and tells him that you are really sincere in wanting to assist him.

INTERMEDIATE ACTION

Let the patient set his own pace. Asking questions too soon or giving advice at the beginning of the relationship is premature. Instead, be available at definite short intervals to talk with the patient.

Reassure the individual that you are interested in his situation. If he screams, "I'm going to kill myself," try to discover what reasons he has for doing so. This lets him know that you are not afraid to discuss the possibility that he may harm himself. Try to have him tell you what it is that he thinks is making him so angry. This allows you to work with him to find other less drastic ways to relieve his uncomfortable impulses and thus lessen his need to hurt himself or others.

LONG-TERM ACTION

Allow the patient an opportunity to talk with you and express himself, without having his feelings hurt. You can do this by saying, "You seem to feel as though someone has disappointed you"; "You sound as if you are upset about having to be monitored by others"; or "You seem to be saying that I have done you an injustice. I can understand that it is difficult for you to be in this situation. I am wondering how you are dealing with it." Remember, allow the patient to save face. Do not use expressions that shame him or show your annoyance, for example, "We don't act that way here"; "That's immature"; "No wonder people avoid you, the way you behave." Such statements are not helpful and prevent further positive interaction.

Listen to what the person has to say. It is essential that you be absolutely honest in your responses. Stick to the reality of the situation. For example, if the patient yells, "You can't get anyone in this damn place to help you. I rang hours ago," reply, "Although it is only 10 minutes since you asked for help, I know it seems longer to you. I'm sorry that all of us were too busy to come immediately. But now that I am here, may I help you?"

Try to channel destructive energy into constructive areas. Exercise (e.g., shuffle-board and walks); simple work tasks (e.g., sanding furniture, stamping envelopes, and ripping up discarded paper); and sports (e.g., punchball, volleyball, and kickball) all give an outlet for such energy and reduce the possibility of its use against himself or others.

Above all, do not place your need for acceptance above the needs of the person you are trying to help.

15

The Person With a Paranoid Personality Disorder

People who are overly suspicious of the provider's actions or overly distrustful of his intentions, and who question every pill, sheet, towel, or glass of water that is brought to him or her are described as being "paranoid." Some degree of paranoia is usually present in most people. There are those who function well in most areas, yet exhibit some suspiciousness when they are involved with others either at work or in social situations. However, when paranoid behavior is carried to an extreme, it becomes trying to the health care provider and makes working with the individual difficult. The professional will frequently encounter this problem on the psychiatric unit. In other locations, the patient's paranoia may not be recognized as the primary reason for his problems. His suspiciousness and distrustful behavior is often attributed to physical discomfort, an unpleasant previous experience, or dislike for a particular health care worker. The stressful situation of hospitalization, with its many unfamiliar and unknown qualities, may indeed heighten the paranoid characteristics that have always been present in subtler forms. It is not uncommon to find out that in the past the paranoid patient was known as an overly cautious person.

There is usually some acceptable explanation for the patient's way of seeing or judging events. Attempts to determine what is real and what is an erroneous interpretation often just bog the staff down in a fruitless and frustrating endeavor. What is important is that the person's emphasis on these upsetting thoughts, and his inability to move from them prevent him from accepting treatment, being helped, or even functioning rationally in his everyday living.

When approached, the paranoid person is suspicious of what is said and why it is being said. He questions everyone's motives. He appears very tense and often has a suspecting, angry gleam in his eyes. He does not trust his family or friends, and certainly not the health care workers, whom he has neither seen nor met before. He feels that each worker is out to "get" him, and that his treatment is of the worst kind. He suspects that the water has either been tampered with or poisoned; the medication will "burn out his insides," or is being used to control his mind; and that the food has been harmfully prepared. He is suspicious of anything that requires explanation. He may go on to complain that the room is "bugged," that the telephone on the desk conceals a tape recorder, and that there are plenty of spies around, all plotting against him. He feels that evidence is being collected to be used against him and that the nurses' notes and charts are definite proof of this. Often, he relates that other people in his life (mailman, coworker, instructor) are conspiring against him because they are threatened by his special qualities. He insists that anyone who differs from him is wrong, and that only *he* sees things correctly. Frequently the paranoid person has strong inferiority feelings, and belittles others in an attempt to defend himself against these feelings.

The paranoid person feels unloved and unaccepted, and believes that almost everyone has let him down, has been unsupportive, and has rejected him. He assumes that others are jealous of him, and want to see him fail. He is angry at this world with all its injustices; this world which has misused him and has striven to treat him unfairly. In his eyes, everything bad that happens to him is unrelated to his own actions, but is the fault of others. He attributes to others the power of reading his mind, and accuses them of conjuring up devious ways to take over his life. He also believes in magical qualities, perhaps voicing great faith in extrasensory perception, mental telepathy, consciousness raising through the use of drugs and séances.

The paranoid person often distorts what is going on in order to have events fit in with his scheme of things. He is frequently fixated on a particular idea, and cannot accept the truth even when it is proven factually. He is usually argumentative, and may be easily provoked to violence. His anger may be stimulated by a staff member's pleasant smile which was intended to enhance friendship and communication. He interprets the smile as an indication that he is being laughed or sneered at, or that a plan is being contrived to cheat him or make him appear foolish. He is also extremely sensitive to anything that he may interpret as a slight. Even innocuous actions may be misinterpreted as when others talk to someone else before addressing him or interrupt a conversation with him to answer the telephone. Trivialities are not trivial to him; they are usually blown up out of all proportion. His resultant behavior is usually so offensive and disturbing to others that they attempt to avoid all contact with him, and, unfortunately, this increases his feelings of personal rejection.

Working with such a person presents special difficulties even when carrying out regular procedures that most individuals accept calmly, agreeably, and as a matter of course. For example, if a routine chest x-ray is needed, he may be leery of it or may adamantly refuse it, saying, "I know what it really is used for." A request for a urine specimen may be met with, "You really think you have me fooled, don't you?" Because he believes people are trying to "put him away for good," he will balk at signing routine consent forms for treatment and medication. He will read and reread the form, replying, "I am not signing without my lawyer." If his admission to a hospital is voluntary, the patient will doubt it. If it is not voluntary, he will indicate that the circumstances under which he has been admitted are proof of evil doings.

The paranoid person is acutely uncomfortable and is trying to cope with many painful feelings and problems that he cannot presently face. He handles this by projecting his distrust onto others. He will completely avoid recognizing his own feelings by stating that he feels the opposite. At times, he will be overtly belligerent. His illness prevents him from being able to comprehend the meaning of his behavior.

THE APPROACH TO THE PATIENT WITH A PARANOID PERSONALITY DISORDER

Immediate Intervention by the Patient

SELF-MANAGEMENT TECHNIQUES

Teach the individual to recognize any increase in suspicions or distrust that decrease his ability to function normally.

Allow the individual to inspect his environment. Let him explore the room, closet, bath, drawers, behind drapes, particularly if he feels someone has "bugged," wired, or tampered with anything in any way, even though it may be his own room at home.

Professional Intervention

IMMEDIATE ACTION

Look directly at the person. He perceives this as a sign of your concern for him. It also implies that you are comfortable in the situation when you return his gaze. If the person is severely paranoid, and is considered harmful to himself or others, he may have to be hospitalized against his will. Legal procedures must always be followed carefully in such a situation.

Establish your role as a professional person. Stress that because he has not known you before this, you can understand his hesitancy in trusting you. However, reaffirm that your interest in him is a professional one. Paranoid patients are difficult because of their reluctance to accept treatment and their lack of motivation.

Be aware of your own behavior. The paranoid individual watches your every move—when you giggle, cover your mouth with your hand, motion to another health care provider, or whisper in a secretive manner. Do not respond when your self-esteem is challenged with angry remarks. Be tolerant of any accusations he makes about you. Do not humiliate him with your reply but introduce reality whenever possible. Supporting the person's right to have an opinion that differs from yours encourages his sense of identity.

Recognize the patient's fear that he is not being treated fairly. Say, "This situation must be very difficult for you," or "I can imagine how upset you must feel." As health care workers develop a relationship with the patient, they may suggest that even if the patient finds it impossible to disregard his paranoid ideas, he can at least give some thought to workers' views of his situation. Say, "I accept your belief that your boss is cheating you. Even so, I'm glad you stopped threatening him and writing obscene letters. I believe that eventually you'll accept our perception that your boss has been very honest and above board with you."

Recognize the person's false belief system situation in establishing your approach. Tell him, "It sounds as though you feel that you were forced to come here"; or "It must be particularly difficult to feel that you were not properly informed about what to expect here"; or "You seem to be upset about the circumstances that led to your being here."

Try to enlist the person's cooperation in his treatment program. Give him adequate and intelligent explanations for all plans, procedures, and therapies. Truthfulness, consistency, reliability, firmness, acceptance, and understanding are imperative in establishing trust.

If you approach the person with medication, walk into the room surely, calmly, and firmly. First tell him with conviction and not as if you are anticipating difficulty, "This medication is to be taken now." If the patient asks about the effects of the pill, you can say, "It will help you to relax." If the medication is likely to cause any uncomfortable after-effects, tell the patient, "After a while your mouth may become dry." This will help him realize that you are not deceiving him. If the patient refuses the medication, calmly state, "We don't believe in coercion, but sometimes a person needs help to help himself. If you are unable to take this medication by yourself, I will help you take each dose until you can take it alone." Then give the medication without delay and with adequate assistance from others.

INTERMEDIATE ACTION

Do not react negatively when the person expresses extreme suspicion or distrust. He is sensitive to rejection, and has feelings of inadequacy and worthlessness when you question his beliefs. Be prepared for changes in his behavior when he encounters situations that kindle these feelings.

Encourage the person to talk to you and the physician. Tell him, "By talking, you will be able to be helped, and thus cut down on your time in treatment."

Do not humor the person when he makes irrational or outrageous demands. Instead say, "I am interested in your request to watch the preparation of your food for every meal and snack. However, that is not possible. I am certain, though, that there is no support for your belief that poison is being added to your particular portions."

Limit your interpretations of the person's words or actions. Do not confront him with his pathology; this is too threatening to his self-esteem. Instead, when he continues to verbalize paranoid beliefs, say, "Your involvement in discussing your treatment must mean you think you can be helped in some way." The person may ask difficult but real questions at the time of admission or during a hospitalization. "Am I wrong to think that?" or "Is it crazy to believe this?" or "Isn't it possible that what I say is true and that my husband is the crazy one?" You may explain, "Anyone may misinterpret events at one time or another"; or "The answer to right and wrong is not so easily determined. What is right for one may be wrong for another, or vice versa in a different time or place. Deciding what is right or wrong is something that you have to discover for yourself. It may take time." Then reassure the person that he will have the help of the doctors and the staff, who will relate to him with honest concern for his benefit. If he accuses you of playing tricks on him, or of having special reasons for saying and doing what is part of your job, explore his previous reactions with him. Say, "I wonder if anyone ever played such a trick on you." Avoid directing jokes or funny remarks to this person. He interprets them as an attempt to make him look foolish.

Be aware of your reaction to the patient. Always be courteous, relaxed, and honest. A trusting relationship will help the person see the situation more realistically.

LONG-TERM ACTION

Work with the person on any problems that he acknowledges. He often believes he is not sick at all and, therefore, needs no help. Do not provoke him or argue with him about his false beliefs. Instead, reaffirm correct ideas even if they are not complimentary to you. If the patient says, "You are a big one, aren't you?" and you are, reply, "Yes, I am very heavy." False illusions and beliefs (delusions) serve a purpose. They help explain fears, unfulfilled expectations, and diminished hopes. Let the person know that his false beliefs interfere with healthy functioning. When he tells you a bizarre tale and demands a response, reply, "I accept what you say, but I cannot find any evidence that supports your belief that someone is trying to kill you."

Let the person know you realize that he does not like to have any limitations placed on him. If he is on an open psychiatric unit, point out its minor limitations but stress as well the wider range of freedom that contrasts with that on the closed unit. Stimulate his motivation by giving him special responsibilities and by allowing him choices in such areas as group or occupational therapy, but also set limits. Do not allow him to harass or threaten others whom he distrusts, or be destructive to his environment; it is in no way helpful to the person.

16

The Person With an Obsessive-Compulsive Disorder (OCD)

When a person dwells so tenaciously on an idea or thought that he is unable to think of anything else, he is said to have an *obsession*. For example, a person may concentrate on the unwelcome and upsetting idea that he has cancer. Then, despite all medical evidence to the contrary, and a diagnosis of sound physical health, he continues to be plagued by the same thought. As a result, his ability to focus on such simple everyday functions as eating, drinking, sleeping, or dressing is impaired.

A *compulsion* is the persistent urge to carry out a repetitious action. In other words, the person must continuously perform the action to manage his anxiety. One patient kept washing and rewashing his clothes. Another kept returning to her room to count all her belongings and make sure they were all in a certain place, arranged in a special way. Still another patient took hours dressing in the morning because of a compulsion to wash her hands repeatedly. Such ritualistic behavior acts as a form of self-punishment and atonement and thus serves to undo any misdeeds the person thinks he has committed.

Although obsessions and compulsions may occur independently of each other, they commonly are seen together. When a patient has an obsessive-compulsive reaction, he experiences recurrences of a repetitious thought, as well as the need to perform a repetitive action. One obsessive lady came to all group meetings with pencil and paper. She took notes of everything said, and anything that happened. She also made lists of everything and anything that came into her head. She involved herself in compiling trivia in order to avoid discussing anything that pertained to her situation, problem, and feelings.

The obsessive-compulsive person tries to hide or prevent demonstration of his feelings. He fears losing control. He strives for order, structure, and a sense of sureness. The individual usually appears neat and fastidious. He cannot tolerate spontaneity or unscheduled activities. Requests or changes create a problem because they intrude into his orderliness. The health care provider can expect an angry outburst accompanied by much resistance if he informs the patient of recently ordered tests, introduces a new activity, or brings in an unexpected visitor. A person with OCD may even become upset if the furniture in his room or home is rearranged.

Unrealistic goals are often set by the person with this disorder. Attempting to reach and maintain these goals causes much stress. One woman could not leave her home unless it was absolutely clean, with the beds made, laundry done, even the silver polished daily. As a result, morning appointments caused such a high level of anxiety that she would become immobilized.

Recurrent thoughts that are baseless, yet continue to plague the individual are recognized as a product of his own mind. The person realizes that the process is coming from himself and is not the result of an outside force. However, he finds himself unable to stop the thoughts from starting. To reduce his distress, he may perform a specific action each time the obsessive thought occurs. By doing this, he believes that he is preventing a catastrophe from occurring. It is not important to him that his action is unrelated to the event that he is trying to obliterate. All that matters is that his action lessens his anxiety.

The obsessive behavior takes over to the extent that the individual's normal routines are ignored. If accompanied by a compulsive reaction, many hours may be used, preventing him from carrying out the necessary activities of daily living. As the situation continues, he feels increased anxiety and is no longer able to function normally. He is overwhelmed by the need to continue the excessive and unreasonable rituals. For example, he may fear that he will contract a terrible disease if he touches a doorknob or shakes hands with someone at work. To counter that possibility, he may wash his hands repeatedly, perhaps to the point where his skin becomes irritated. Still, he is unable to stop the ritual. In another case, there may be an unrealistic fear of being trapped in a store, even though the closing time is several hours away. To counteract the fear, the individual may check his watch every few minutes.

This time-consuming activity results in a failure to complete any necessary purchase.

In general, the most common obsessions center on fears of contamination (touching dirty objects or people), recurrent thoughts about actions that have been taken or forgotten (locking doors or windows, taking prescribed medications), keeping things in a specific order (obvious distress if there is a disturbance of clothing stored in discrete piles within a drawer), with additional obsessions centered on the possibility of aggressive actions or of thoughts related to sexual matters. The compulsions, also repetitive, are the actions used to relieve the anxiety caused by the obsessions. Washing hands, checking for the completion of tasks (checking and rechecking whether doors have been locked), and using prayers or specific actions to block out thoughts of unacceptable acts are common methods used in reaction to the obsessive behaviors.

Is all obsessive-compulsive behavior abnormal? Certainly not! We all know individuals who demonstrate some degree of this behavior. It is the degree of the behavior rather than the behavior itself which determines its abnormality. Sometimes it is helpful. For instance, in order to get through school or some long and intensive training, one usually establishes certain habits. The room may have to be quiet, or very well lit, or there may have to be certain pencils available before one is able to buckle down. Take, for example, a nurse whose job requires her to be an expert in operating room technique, or one who must carry out isolation technique on a communicable disease unit, or one whose responsibility involves the preparation and administration of exact medications at different precise times. In each of the above situations, the exactness and repetitiveness of the behavior are helpful in achieving constructive goals.

However, when one's thoughts and behavior interfere with, prevent, or obstruct functioning so that one is immobilized and unable to participate in his ordinary life, hospitalization may become necessary. The difficulties in working with such a person become apparent quickly. He repeats the same absurd idea or irrational thought over and over. No matter how others try, they are unable to get the individual to respond to simple reasoning.

Cognitive-behavioral therapy has been used successfully in treating OCD. The person is helped to separate the response from the initial intrusive thought. For example, he may be plagued by thoughts that he has forgotten to shut down his computer. Usually he would return frequently during the next few hours to check on its status. As part of his therapy, he is coached to go to another room after turning it off and to wait for increasingly longer spans before going back to see if it has been left on. In time, the need to check should be obliterated. For some, medications may have to be incorporated into the treatment. Between 40% to 50% of OCD patients will improve significantly within 12 weeks when involved in a combination of psychotherapy and drug treatment.

THE APPROACH TO THE PATIENT WITH AN OBSSESSIVE-COMPULSIVE DISORDER

Immediate Intervention by the Patient

SELF-MANAGEMENT TECHNIQUES

Teach the individual to recognize the recurrent thoughts that initiate his compulsive actions. Have him delay the compulsive response by increasing amounts of time.

Professional Intervention

IMMEDIATE ACTION

Do not confront the individual with what he says or does. Instead, encourage him to elaborate and discuss his feelings further. Allow him to repeat himself over and over again because this helps him clarify his feelings. Help him to identify his feelings by saying, "You seem to feel unhappy"; "You appear to feel upset"; or "You seem to feel angry." Comment on his facial expressions, grimaces, or downcast eyes. The patient usually feels more than he reveals.

Don't be judgmental or verbalize your disapproval of the person's behavior. Because you recognize that his obsessive thoughts and compulsive behavior are a way of managing his anxiety, do not interrupt or attempt to change his activity. This will only increase his anxiety. Help him to channel his energy into satisfying activities. The use of nonverbal activities is better for reducing anxiety than verbal activities. Group activities involving dance, exercise, yoga, bicycle riding, playing shuffleboard, jogging in place, or walking out of doors are all helpful.

INTERMEDIATE ACTION

Do not pressure the person. Allow him plenty of time to eat, dress, take his medications, and report for activities. Do not hurry him. Do not ask him, "What shall we do?" or "Do you want to do something now?" because such questions pressure him into decision making. Do not insist that he maintain a strict schedule. If he could control himself and his activities, he would.

Help the person develop confidence in his own choices. Encourage him to find answers for himself. If he says, "It's up to you to talk to me about my problems," the health worker can respond, "What specific problems would you like to work on today?"

Reassure the individual of your interest in him. Let him know that you desire to work with him in an effort to help him. Maintain this interest by staying with him at several intervals during your time with him.

LONG-TERM ACTION

Help maintain the person's physical condition if necessary. Limits must be strictly and consistently enforced to prevent malnutrition, fatigue, and lack of cleanliness.

As the individual learns about his feelings and becomes more comfortable with them, he will be able to channel the discomfort they arouse more effectively. Trying to argue him out of his obsessive-compulsive behavior or influence him with logical reasoning is to no avail because his problem has an emotional basis and cannot be solved by merely forcing changes in his behavior.

FREQUENTLY PRESCRIBED PSYCHIATRIC DRUGS

Psychiatric drugs frequently prescribed for obsessive-compulsive disorder include the following:

Tricyclic antidepressant: clomipramine (Anafranil)
Selective serotonin reuptake inhibitors: fluvoxamine (Luvox), fluoxetine (Prozac)

17

The Person With a Borderline Personality Disorder

People with a borderline personality disorder demonstrate a wide range of behaviors, which can cause havoc by totally disrupting their environment. They exhibit little tolerance for anxiety and frustration, a weak capacity for controlling impulses, and a limited ability to consider others. They focus on self-indulgence, feeling they are entitled to whatever they want when they want it. Their moods are unstable. Their interpersonal relationships are poor, with much ambivalence and vacillation. They have difficulty in tolerating being alone and often suffer from chronic boredom. They have a problem in integrating good and bad aspects of their personalities, demonstrating poor judgment and difficulty in separating reality from unreality. They may make suicidal gestures.

These individuals are best kept out of a long-term hospital situation. However, because of masochistic features and suicidal gestures, it frequently becomes necessary to provide the patient with a safe environment on a short-time basis until he regains control. The staff will generally feel the intensity of the patient's chaotic behavior during the hospitalization. The result of this attention seeking, demanding, and narcissistic behavior is to seriously disrupt the unit activities and has a negative effect on other patients.

The borderline patient has serious personality problems, with patterns of behavior that are self-destructive and long lasting. During any period of stress, the patient will view his relationships as all perfect or all negative (splitting). This has a disturbing effect on those relationships as the patient has difficulty distinguishing between what is real and what is unreal. The patient can be impulsive and may suddenly create a chaotic atmosphere in the workplace, at home, or in the hospital. For example, here may have been a recent warm, trusting relationship with another person considered to be "wonderful" by the patient. Suddenly the patient's perception of the valued person changes, with the blame always placed on actions by that other individual. The sudden turnabout is difficult for those who are involved, often raising their stress to high levels. In a hospital situation, staff members need special training to develop the skill, endurance, and psychiatric sophistication needed to help these patients.

The person may exhibit a grandiosity in which he presents himself as a "perfect" person who is the victim of others' ungratefulness. There is an amazing belief that the world should or will soon wake up and recognize his goodness. Insight is absent or extremely short-lived because he is unable to cope with the anxiety created by the need to be regarded as perfect. One patient wondered why her boyfriend left her after she repeatedly threw things at him and impulsively hit him. "After all, I was only trying to test his love for me," she explained. She firmly believed that "If he really loved me he would love me no matter what I did."

If the person with a borderline personality disorder is encountered on medical-surgical units, the health worker should present the need for new tests by using a paradoxical approach. For instance, if a barium enema has been ordered, it is unwise to say, "A barium enema has been scheduled for you today, and it is important." This patient is likely to respond, "Oh yeah, who says so?" and an outburst will likely ensue. However, if the health worker approaches the patient with, "I have unpleasant news and I don't know how to break it to you. A barium enema has been scheduled and the test is uncomfortable, embarrassing, and can be difficult. I don't know how you're going to get through it," the patient is likely to respond by saying, "Oh, it can't be that bad. You are a worrier. I've had that test before." The borderline patient likes to be the controller and demonstrate his power, regardless of the situation.

Borderline patients receiving psychotherapy on an outpatient basis are usually unresponsive to the therapeutic commitment, seeking help only in times of acute stress. Even then, the patient's goal is usually to manipulate the therapist in order to obtain gratification of unmet infantile needs. One patient came to six sessions hoping to convince the therapist that his wife was a terrible person. The patient refused to address his own role in their turbulent relationship and avoided any focus on his feelings. The therapist asked whether he thought that throwing his wife's bedding out of the window, and destroying her bed as well as the Father's Day present she had purchased, might have provoked her into leaving him. The patient responded, "Oh, that was just a joke. I thought it would be fun to do it to her before she did it to me." He subsequently denied that the incident had occurred. This same patient idealized his mother while he referred to his wife as "scum" (devaluation).

Those with a borderline personality disorder usually display an inability to control their feelings and are very vulnerable. Their childhood histories reveal unresponsive social and family interactions that have not provided them with the opportunity to learn how to trust their own emotional responses. They try to determine how they should react by picking up signals from those with whom they are interacting. They regulate their own behavior through angry outbursts, or by suicidal thoughts or attempts. Their suicide rates are highest when they also suffer from a major depression and/or alcoholism.

The reaction of borderline patients to drug treatment is controversial because they tend to have strong responses to placebos. Within a short while, they tend to complain of side effects, in line with their hypochondriacal tendencies. They may discontinue the drugs on their own, or refuse to take the prescribed amount, never reaching a therapeutic level. Conversely, they may take an accidental or deliberate overdose. Low doses of neuroleptics have been found valuable to control these patients' symptoms. Other useful drugs have been fluoxetine (Prozac) or selective serotonin reuptake inhibitors, to treat associated depression, suicidal thoughts, and impulsive aggression.

The health worker may react strongly and negatively to the defenses of the borderline patient, labeling him as manipulative, angry, faking, and bad. Once the worker recognizes his feelings toward the patient, his own tensions and frustration are likely to decrease. A consistent approach in which the responsibilities of the patient and health worker are firmly defined is essential.

THE APPROACH TO THE PATIENT WITH A BORDERLINE PERSONALITY DISORDER

Immediate Intervention by the Patient

SELF-MANAGEMENT TECHNIQUES

Teach the patient to recognize the initiation of his chaotic or self-destructive behavior when responding to his disappointment in what he perceives as negative changes in the behavior of others. Help him realize that few individuals are totally good and without any faults, and should be evaluated realistically.

Professional Intervention

IMMEDIATE ACTION

Do recognize your own feelings and reactions to the patient. Focus on helping the patient acknowledge his own feelings and accept responsibility for his own actions.

A mutual agreement is generally helpful in delineating what is acceptable behavior at home or in the community or before an admission to the hospital unit. The patient needs to be involved in planning his therapeutic program.

INTERMEDIATE ACTION

Avoid interpretations that diminish the individual's self-esteem and increase his feelings of inferiority.

Set realistic limits and be consistent in enforcing them. If the individual is destructive, say, "Stop breaking the chair. You appear to be upset. Let's talk about what led to this feeling."

If destructive behavior continues, be consistent and decisive. Seclusion and medication can be utilized to help the patient regain self-control. (They should never be used in response to the worker's fear of being hurt or in reaction to anger at the person.)

If the person projects his hostile feelings onto you, don't personalize his attack. Recognize his defense and respond to the feeling (i.e., patient: "Your stupidity is obvious. I thought people with low IQ's weren't allowed into professional schools." Worker: "You sound furious with me. What's the anger all about?").

Utilize a neutral approach to patients who tell you that you are a great professional or those who confront you with, "How did you ever get a license?" Respond with, "You feel things are going well (badly) today? Let's talk about it."

Use a paradoxical approach when making requests of these patients (i.e., "Mr. S., I know this will be difficult for you and I won't blame you if you want to leave the hospital, but we are transferring you to the coronary care unit because of changes on your electrocardiogram").

LONG-TERM ACTION

Health workers need to be in agreement regarding interventions. Consistency in setting limits is essential to avoid manipulation of the staff by the patient.

Recognize that your own intense feelings stirred up by the patient's actions (guilt, love, rage, disappointment) might well be an indication that the patient has a borderline personality disorder. Realize that borderline patients usually reach a state of equilibrium when they come into their thirties. Most marry, have children, and are able to hold jobs. Work meets their need for contact with others, and gives them a sense of satisfaction. Their personal lives may continue to be unsatisfactory, with high rates of divorce and a lack of closeness to their children.

Help the individual focus on constructive ways to obtain satisfaction, rather than acting out in a destructive way.

Do not blame yourself if the patient fails to change.

18

The Person With a Manic Episode

Manic behavior is characterized by generalized physical and emotional over-activity and results from a disturbance in mood (affect). Mania may be thought of as an attempt to avoid or deny depression. Often an unhappy occurrence is cited by family members as having preceded the manic episode. For example, one individual was upset when the therapeutic community in which she was living informed her that she was to be trained for new responsibilities. The person exhibited manic behavior two weeks later. The psychiatric interview revealed the patient's feeling that she would be unable to learn the necessary new skills. She totally lacked any confidence in her ability to cope with the new situation.

The manic person appears elated, is constantly active and talkative, and may be quite boisterous. His behavior is not related to what is happening around him. He has little patience for anything and is easily distracted from what he tries to do. His attention can be directed to anything but is just as easily lost. In the space of a few minutes, he covers numerous subjects, and goes from one to the other for no apparent reason. He is constantly involved in some activity, but accomplishes very little. Sometimes he is so talkative and speaks so rapidly that his speech is not entirely clear to the listener. Depending on the degree of his manic behavior, he may or may not be confused. If he is not confused, and his illness is mild, he usually does not believe he is emotionally ill or that he requires psychiatric intervention.

Individuals in moderate to severe manic states may yell, become argumentative and unreasonably demanding. They may also become abusive and resort
to pushing, shoving or hitting. Logic is usually absent. Often the patient is
grandiose, believing that he is a millionaire or a public official with untold
power, or that he is capable of carrying out business deals that are actually
impossible.

The manic person thrives on love, affection, and attention. Generally
speaking, he is likable because of his responsiveness and outgoing qualities.
He is amusing and full of fun. He may speak in rhymes and make puns. He
talks up and tells jokes and anecdotes. When he talks he rambles on with little
connection between thoughts, and there is little validity or rationality to what
he is saying. Sometimes he will go to ridiculous lengths to prove a point. He
may name-drop, cite events that never took place, and fabricate people and
circumstances. It is not unusual to find that the manic patient may be uncertain about the identity of strangers. He may greet visitors or even strangers as
though they are his close friends.

The manic person is an eager participant in all activities. He is always ready
to go and has a quick remark or witty reply on hand. He is the life of any
community meeting, jumping up without any apparent provocation to dance,
sing, or give a speech on any subject that comes to his mind. He appears to
have few inhibitions. If allowed, he will take over and monopolize every activity. One he gets started, it is very difficult to interrupt his behavior since he is
completely unaware of what he is doing and has usually captivated everyone's
attention. But, after a while his very behavior turns people off and they seek
to avoid him. What at first seemed cute and humorous becomes irritating and
threatening when one realizes that the individual really cannot control his
actions. In a hospital or other psychiatric setting, other patients are, themselves, striving to control their behavior. They may fear losing whatever control they may have achieved. What is more, their confidence in the staff's
ability to provide limits and appropriate intervention measures may be seriously undermined. If some staff members harbor secret wishes that they
themselves could be just a little less inhibited, they may even go along with
the fun—until it becomes impossible for them to handle it.

The worker may become so entertained by the patient's behavior and
amusing tales that he forgets why the patient needs care and supervision.
Usually it was this very behavior that caused chaos at home, at work, and in
relationships. There is also a tendency to overlook therapeutic approaches to
the person because he appears to be in such "good spirits" and can "do so

much so quickly for himself." One may even get caught up in some of his ambitious schemes, which may range from grandiose land deals or stock ventures to promises of large contributions to the hospital.

A 42-year-old man was admitted to the psychiatric unit of a hospital with a diagnosis of mania. Before his illness, he was considered a good husband and provider, friendly and outgoing. In the hospital he was very active, flitting from patient to staff member, asking numerous questions, but never waiting for a reply. Out of the side of his mouth he interjected his talks with imitations of Donald Duck or Bugs Bunny. He walked around the unit whistling, joking, hopping, and skipping. He indulged in anything that caught his fancy. He ate all the food in the unit refrigerator, kept long lists of notes, and wrote numerous letters to friends encouraging their cooperation in his wild escapades and plans. At one unit meeting he pounced into the middle of the group and began to sing and dance. He then became erotic, displaying himself and making lewd remarks, upsetting those nearby. He reacted to direction with an angry outburst and stamped out of the room. He then quickly made light of the entire matter and returned to his previous jovial demeanor.

Another manic patient bombarded everyone in the unit with a stream of long words used in a fast, witty manner. No matter what anyone said, he had a reply that directed attention back to himself, even if it meant introducing a subject other than the one under discussion. He constantly reminded others that his major problem was how to spend his recently acquired $30,000 annual raise. He ate triple helpings at mealtime and yet lost weight. He talked incessantly, kept copious notes, walked around with a pencil behind his ear and holding a clipboard, as if he were involved in an important urgent undertaking. He frequently contradicted himself, but attached little importance to this when it was brought to his attention. He informed the staff that the physician was planning special treatments particularly for him. When the staff checked on this they found it to be untrue. At one large group meeting, other patients told him to give someone else a chance to express an opinion, and the patient left the meeting, saying that he had to go to the bathroom. Instead, he proceeded to make several telephone calls. He returned at the end of the meeting, and immediately began to talk about his sexual escapades in an exotic country.

Both of the preceding patients benefited from the structured program within the hospital unit. Their overactivity lessened as they regained control.

THE APPROACH TO THE PATIENT
WITH A MANIC EPISODE

Immediate Intervention by the Patient

SELF-MANAGEMENT TECHNIQUES

Teach the person to recognize the target symptoms that initiate the feelings of the manic behavior: overactivity, increased speed of speech and actions, darting from activity to activity without any completion, grandiosity (including financial or political schemes).

Professional Intervention

IMMEDIATE ACTION

Try to protect the person from undesirable effects of his behavior. Be aware that he is easily distracted and may need assistance in the activities of daily living. He may need supervision to ensure an adequate food intake and to help him relax. It is important to reduce such exciting external stimuli as loud sounds, bright lights, flurries of activity.

In the hospital setting, staff members must be available to the patient at all times. They should be supportive in a quiet, calm, understanding manner. A consistent approach from the staff is vital so that the patient can begin to formulate realistic expectations concerning reactions to his actions. Spend frequent, short periods with him even if you feel nothing therapeutic is occurring. Your presence is supportive and demonstrates acceptance of him. *Reduce all stimuli.* Keep environment quiet. Play soft, slow music, read nonexciting short articles with an attempt to concentrate on the content. Watch food intake with an increase in calories to offset the energy used in manic activities. Stay away from caffeine (coffee, tea, cola drinks, and chocolate).

INTERMEDIATE ACTION

Help the person to rid himself of pressure when he is in an excited state. Divert his attention with repetitive tasks—for example, tearing foam rubber in occupational therapy, sanding wood, or assembling charts.

Help the person modify his behavior along lines that are socially acceptable. Be alert for sudden mood swings from exhilaration to anger. When the person is behaving in a manner that may prove embarrassing to him, isolate him until he is able to control himself. Set reasonable limits for him. As the person gains ground (becomes healthier) and is able to relate his difficulties, let him know that his joyous mood and joking behavior do not appear to be in keeping with the sad story he is telling.

Keep the person out of group therapy at the beginning of his treatment. His talkativeness and rapid sequence of ideas is disruptive. He may be hurtful to others by citing their shortcomings and, in so doing, prevent others from looking at their own behavior or problems.

LONG-TERM ACTION

Be aware of yourself. Do not encourage or react to the person's risqué remarks, coarse jokes, boisterousness, or pranks because you are having a good time or would like to indulge in similar activity.

Do not take offense, argue, or react negatively when the person becomes angry, argues, or makes unkind, cutting remarks. Instead, say to him, "You must be feeling uncomfortable. Tell me what happened." Then stay with him and provide a calm atmosphere for talking.

Do not encourage or respond to erotic or lewd behavior. Effect a therapeutic atmosphere by redirecting the patient, in a firm but kind manner, to socially acceptable activity. Tell the patient, "I will help you put your clothes on. Then you and I will be able to go for a walk on the grounds."

Provide the person with privacy during interviews. Because he is covering up much unhappiness, do not be surprised if he cries. Provide warmth, understanding, and acceptance.

19

The Person With a Phobia

The person with a phobia is overwhelmingly and uncontrollably fearful when anticipating usual life situations. His reaction is out of proportion to the event and usually causes him to be extremely self-conscious. His complaints include physical symptoms, such as weakness, faintness, blushing, and tachycardia. These may increase markedly when he is confronted with an unfamiliar or even more threatening situation. He has a heightened level of anxiety, low self-esteem, and a fear of being laughed at or humiliated by others. Hypochondriasis is not uncommon. The patient has a fear of not being perfect and avoids activities that he thinks may lead him to fail, even if the "failure" only occurs in his own head. Above all, he is concerned with dying, and with separation from people and places that are comfortable for him.

The person with a phobia tries to avoid situations likely to increase his symptoms. For example, a 25-year-old woman discontinued her schooling, stating that she was not interested in the subject matter. In fact, she dropped out because she anticipated experiencing unpleasant physical sensations if she were called on to answer questions during class. In another situation, a 45-year-old woman avoided all shopping trips after experiencing a panic attack while in a department store.

It is not unusual for the individual to develop agoraphobia (fear of open places) in an effort to avoid panic attacks. He increasingly curtails his activities until he virtually becomes a prisoner in his own home. Needless to say, family and social lives are disrupted as the individual refuses to go out, even to attend a movie, a wedding, a ride in a car, or a much needed family vacation.

Much of the agoraphobic person's fear is due to separation anxiety, as he avoids leaving the place (home) or people (mother) that are involved with his abnormal and inappropriate level of dependency. In some instances, sexual fears may play a part in agoraphobia. The thought that he may be attracted to, or active in, sexual activity may be so frightening that it is safer to remain at home. In some instances, the person may find comfort in taking something from home with him. This may be a family picture, a book, or a scarf belonging to a significant other, much as a child uses a transitional object, until his ability to separate without anxiety is strengthened.

Agoraphobic individuals are encouraged to go outside in the company of a therapist or a family member. On successive days they are encouraged to walk a few steps from the doorway, gradually increasing their distance from the door with the help of the accompanying person. The goal is to have them eventually walk out alone, acknowledging but not giving in to any fear that occurs.

The phobic person may be severely depressed and may demonstrate hopeless and helpless qualities, tending to perceive the world as a hostile place. In working with this individual, the health worker needs to develop skills in responding to the patient's endless questioning, such as "What happens if I get nervous? . . . if I faint? . . . if I get sick on vacation?" These questions reveal the patient's underlying fear of losing control when away from his familiar home setting. Additionally, there is the fear that others will be aware of his phobic state.

The phobic person often has a history of experiencing humiliation during childhood. One 22-year-old woman revealed that at the age of 6 she had accidentally lost control of her bladder while in school and that the entire class laughed at her wet clothes. Other individuals seem predisposed to phobic attacks when in situations that stir up feelings similar to those that occurred during childhood episodes of separating from home or mother.

Staff members or significant others may become frustrated and feel angry when the phobic patient refuses to go out on walks or attend group therapy sessions because it appears as though "he could if he wanted to." Some may even view these patients as obstinate and manipulative. It is important for them to understand that the patient has erected these barriers to protect himself against his phobic episodes and what he perceives as "death." Additionally, health care workers need to be aware that alcohol or other drug abuse may occur if the person, in his desperate struggle to alleviate his symptoms, turns to chemicals for relief.

Patients often tell the health worker that they believe and/or fear that they are going "crazy." Once the person begins to recognize that his symptoms are due to his phobia and that he can be helped, he feels encouraged and often begins to feel relief. He needs help in accepting the fact that some level of anxiety is normal, even helpful, in everyday living, that anxiety will not kill him, and that his anxiety about the *possibility* of having an attack may actually precipitate an attack.

Although some people suffering from phobias are treated only with anxiolytics and antidepressant medication, most will require a combination of pharmacotherapy to alleviate or control attacks, psychotherapy to resolve the psychological aspects of the problem, and behavioral therapy to sensitize them to situations likely to provoke phobic responses.

Phobic individuals should be encouraged to participate in the areas that frighten them. For example, those who are claustrophobic (fear of enclosed places), and therefore avoid riding in elevators, are sensitized by first looking at pictures of people in elevators. They can then talk about the fear the pictures provoke. The next step in the process might be to spend time with the health worker near an elevator, talking about the feelings that are evoked as people enter, ride, and leave the elevator. Once comfortable with that level of anxiety, the patient can be helped to enter and leave the open elevator with the health worker. As the anxiety lessens (and it may take many such entries and exits before that happens), the patient is helped to stay in the elevator with the care provider while the door is closed and then quickly opened. This is repeated, lengthening the interval that the door is kept closed. The time schedule varies with the patient, with the goal being to have him conquer his anxiety and the resultant phobic reaction.

THE APPROACH TO THE PATIENT WITH PHOBIA

Immediate Intervention by the Patient

SELF-MANAGEMENT TECHNIQUES

Help the patient to acknowledge the occurrence and to remain as calm as possible while confronting it. The use of relaxation techniques (see p. 63) may lessen the anxiety symptoms that occur in reaction to confronting the situation.

Professional Intervention

IMMEDIATE ACTION

Encourage the individual to make eye contact and talk with others. This not only reinforces socialization skills but also lessens his concentration on his shortcomings, thereby building self-confidence.

Interrupt negative obsessing and anticipation of events by concentrating on the here and now.

INTERMEDIATE ACTION

Help the person change his maladaptive thinking. Gently challenge his belief that it is unacceptable to appear nervous or that he will be rejected by others for appearing anxious.

Support the person as he learns to tolerate his distress. Often he believes he should be anxiety free, never encountering any uncomfortable moments, regardless of the circumstances. Focus on the irrationality of this belief. Reassure him that "although you feel uncomfortable, the discomfort will be short-lived and will not be a danger to your life." Additionally, help the individual to realize that many dysphoric feelings are normal reactions to life crises.

Enlist the person's participation in understanding himself. Help him look at his self-destructive patterns by confronting him with statements, such as, "you seem determined to view yourself as inept. What positive thoughts can you substitute that would help you in this situation?" When the patient begins his self-blame cycle, help him refocus by concentrating on the event rather than his feelings.

LONG-TERM ACTION

Develop a behavior program whereby the patient builds confidence in his ability to carry out feared activities. Tell the patient, "The more you practice, the easier it will be."

Encourage the individual to separate his self-worth from behavioral tasks or outcomes.

Help the person experience and accept small successes in an effort to improve self-esteem.

20

The Person With a Somatoform Disorder

Sometimes, when a person's anxiety is so great that he cannot handle it effectively, he displaces it onto parts of his body where it is felt as actual physical discomfort. One specific area of the body or several areas may be involved.

Perhaps the simplest illustration of a physical symptom caused by psychological factors is the tension headache. Commonly, one develops pain in the forehead, temples, and/or back of the neck and shoulders, which he associates with fatigue, tension, or worry. Characteristically, the pain is described as tightness, or "like a tight band." This feeling results from muscle contraction, which is the physical expression of emotional tension. The pain may be severe but can often be relieved by a mild analgesic. Eventually, the headache disappears without one ever really thinking through the reasons or events that precipitated it. One hospitalized patient's severe headaches occurred during the morning hours, when the house physicians made their rounds. He was sure that he would be told his condition was deteriorating and that he would have to extend his stay in the hospital. The anticipation of such a finding had the physiological effect of producing severe tension headaches.

Physiological responses that are a reaction to a current situation are easily identifiable. Some individuals, on observing others with more severe degrees of illness than they themselves have, are apt to identify and imagine that they have the same difficulties. They feel pains and discomforts in specific areas of the body, although no organic disturbance can be found. Later, when reassured that they do not have the more serious disease, the aches and pains disappear.

When an illness is diagnosed as psychosomatic in origin, the intimation is that the person is reacting to earlier events that caused unconscious stress, and for which he is now showing physical symptoms. One woman complained of frequent migraine headaches over a period of five years. She was often so irritable that she lost various jobs and social relationships. Medication to relive the throbbing helped, but not for long. Finally, she was referred for psychiatric care after a thorough neurological examination in the general hospital revealed no physical abnormality. When she was informed that no organic pathology for her headaches existed, she became upset and her complaints intensified as proof that she was being truthful. After many interviews, she was finally able to talk about a long-standing marital problem. Her husband had been seeing another woman for several years and while she didn't want him to leave, she could not tolerate the situation as it existed. She expressed her humiliation, resentment, and rage not only toward her husband but toward herself. Until this time, she had not recognized that the conflict of intense hostility toward her husband, and her strong need and dependence on him, was being expressed in the form of a migraine headache. The patient was able to accept this interpretation more readily when told by the physician that the stress of her situation actually was causing the physiological changes that made her head throb.

A young college student was admitted to the hospital with severe headaches and tingling sensations in the arms and legs. She explained that these symptoms had existed for over a year, but now she felt they prevented her from continuing in school. The pain was intolerable. She had sought several medical opinions, but no organic reason for her discomfort had been uncovered. She was not hospitalized on the psychiatric unit but was seen in the general hospital for daily psychiatric interviews. During these interviews, the patient disclosed fear of being away at college, loneliness, inability to have meaningful friendships, lack of a boyfriend, and difficulty in achieving excellent grades. Initially, she was made aware of the tensions and anxieties that brought about the physiological changes which produced her symptoms. Because many tests were done, she felt that her symptoms were also important in themselves. As she expressed her feelings and attitudes toward the difficulties she was encountering, she revealed a deep underlying resentment toward an older brother. He was a very successful student; had an outgoing personality; and was, she felt, favored by their parents. Her inability to do as well in her studies as he did made her feel like a failure. Not being as popular as he was made her feel worthless. Her being away at school (despite the fact that this was her choice), while her brother was now at home, was interpreted as proof that her parents loved her brother more each day while rejecting her.

At this point, the patient was not aware that her symptoms were helping her to obtain attention from her parents and brother. At the same time, she had an acceptable reason for not doing as well as she thought she ought to in her work. Many weeks passed before she began to see that there was no reason for her to compete with her brother—that she was seen and liked by others for herself alone. Then she began to realize that she had to acknowledge and build her own strengths and work toward realistic, achievable goals instead of unobtainable ones. The expression of her feelings, and the acceptance of them, along with a great deal of staff support for the patient as she was, evoked a gradual subsidence of her symptoms.

The person with a somatic complaint dwells on the ailment or discomfort and repeatedly reports his symptoms to whomever is available. He seems to fear that unless he does so, no one will really believe him. He is concerned that if no real physical pathology is found, he will be labeled "crazy." As a result, some individuals will go to great lengths to prove how incapacitated or uncomfortable they are—they moan and groan loudly, voice constant complaints, and request medication before the last dose has even begun to take effect. Citation of any improvement results in denial and is interpreted by the person as a great injustice to him. He may even feel that those caring for him are trying to rob him of something quite precious and resolves that he is not going to give up without a big battle. In a sense, he is justified in feeling this way, especially if he does not have anything better with which to replace his physical symptoms.

Usually, those with somatic complaints do not have demonstrable pathology; but some do, and then the physical sickness is actually triggered by emotional factors. This relationship has long been recognized. Just think of how the heart increases in rate and pounds in the chest when one experiences intense excitement such as meeting a lover or being in an automobile accident. Think of the intensity of gastrointestinal symptoms (nausea or diarrhea) that may occur when one anticipates taking an examination, giving a speech, or going to the analyst's office—all events that produce anxiety. The symptom manifested is the escape valve that relieves unbearable anxiety.

In the general hospital, the nurse cares for patients with ulcerative colitis, cardiac problems, asthma, obesity, and hypertension. Although there is usually no doubt that actual physical changes which have adverse effects do exist in these patients, it is believed that emotional factors play a significant role in the course, and perhaps in the cause, of their physical illnesses. Flare-ups are common during periods of emotional stress. The patient will usually indicate that he feels "nervous" and "tense." However, he attributes the upset to his physical illness. One patient who survived several life-threatening bouts of ileitis told the staff that she would force herself to have an attack in order to get her husband to meet her demands. Occasionally, talking with the patient about how feelings and emotions cause illness can be therapeutic. But any long-term improvement in the condition demands long-term treatment. Recognition of this will decrease the feeling of ineptness one may experience when working with these patients, and increase one's tolerance and patience in a frustrating situation.

A patient with an acute illness such as myocardial infarction, cerebrovascular accident, or who has undergone gallbladder surgery has already sustained a jolt to his physical system and experienced much fear and anxiety. If his personality structure before illness was defective, the illness may be used manipulatively to escape difficult and unpleasant situations in the future. Thus, he may voice many complaints that are unrelated to the primary illness. This becomes especially apparent during convalescence, when the patient finds it threatening to recover completely. It is more satisfying to him to continue deriving the secondary gains that the illness has provided. These gains are seen in terms of extra attention, pity, a dependency relationship, and even disability insurance payments. An example of how this latter gain may be utilized was seen in the patient who was admitted to the hospital for long-standing neck pain. To offset the pain, he kept his head bent toward one side. For years, this prevented him from working. He sought treatment only when his disability payments were discontinued. But by this time his neck muscles on one side had become permanently shortened, and his condition was not amenable to treatment.

The patient admitted to a psychiatric unit for treatment of a psychically influenced somatic illness is incapacitated to the extent that his symptoms interfere with effective functioning. He hopes that psychiatric treatment will assist in alleviating his physical condition, which has been caused or intensified by tensions. He is told that if he can learn to deal with the emotional aspects of his life, his symptoms will decrease appreciably. This is often a difficult concept for the patient to accept. Thus, it is up to the staff to help him gain confidence and obtain some satisfaction in life that will replace his need for the symptom. This is no easy task. But the discomfort, unhappiness, and incapacity created by the patient's situation, plus his willingness to accept voluntary hospitalization, means that he recognizes the burden of his present predicament. He would like to make some changes, if only he could do so and at the same time save face.

An example of such a dichotomy is furnished by a young woman who was hospitalized because of severe anorexia. She had lost much weight, and her physical strength was deteriorating. Her behavior was related to deep hostility toward her mother, and was expressed by rejecting the food her mother prepared. This maladaptive pattern was corrected after much perseverance by the staff in trying to help the patient to see herself as worthy and meaningful, not just as an object who would not eat. No attempt was made to interpret the unconscious factors. The patient began to see how detrimental her behavior was to herself, and also that change was possible. As her good qualities were reinforced, her self-esteem improved, and successful treatment became possible.

In another case, a young woman in her twenties was admitted to the psychiatric unit because of a severe depression. She had made a suicidal attempt that was precipitated by a broken engagement. After admission, she developed pain in her legs and groin. She was unable to ambulate or stand erect. This persisted for 2 weeks, during which time a medical workup was completed in an effort to discover the source of her pain. Results of all tests were negative. She refused to discuss her engagement or other aspects of her personal life, and clung adamantly to her physical incapacity. In the course of many interviews, she revealed guilt regarding her sexual activity with the boyfriend and an incestuous relationship with an uncle when she was quite young. At this point, her physical complaints were explained to her as manifestations of the great anxiety she was experiencing regarding her sexual experiences. Her disappointment over the broken engagement and her embarrassment at telling family and friends revived the original repressed guilt related to her uncle. She unconsciously sought to avoid these aspects of her life which presented problems, and punished herself by developing symptoms in the body areas associated with sexual activity.

The patient cannot voluntarily control the symptom that develops in response to the stress of an earlier event. This is important for staff to keep in mind, as there is a tendency to regard the patient as being able to recover if only he would put his mind to it. This, of course, is not the case, as the patient is not able to view his condition with his conscious mind. The need for effective treatment and a supportive approach is intensified when the worker realizes that physiological symptoms which continue over long periods of time may result in unalterable body deformities.

THE APPROACH TO THE PATIENT WITH A SOMATOFORM DISORDER

Immediate Intervention by the Patient

SELF-MANAGEMENT TECHNIQUES

Help the person to become aware of the circumstances that occurred before his physical symptoms began, even though he cannot see a connection between the two events. Encourage him to discuss this with the health professional.

Professional Intervention

IMMEDIATE ACTION

Evaluate the person's complaint of physical pain. Do not be judgmental, even though the complaint does not appear to be valid. Inquire what was taking place when the person first noticed the pain, and when and where it began. Express your willingness to understand what he is experiencing, without suggesting that it may be unreal. Remember that the person's physical symptoms and his emotional problems influence each other. It may well be a sign of improvement if the person's rash gets better or his diarrhea decreases.

Let the person talk about the physical aspects of his illness first. This will give you an understanding of his feelings about illness, its cause, prognosis, and the limits it imposes. Try to discover which family members react to his illness, and how. Listen to what he has to say about how his life is affected or influenced, for better or worse, by the problem. Never underestimate the reasons why a person clings to his symptoms. The illness may be less of a problem for him than having to face his other difficulties. Discourage him from searching for shortcuts, such as a new pill or a different medical regime, because they are unlikely to have any lasting effect on his symptoms.

INTERMEDIATE ACTION

Tell the person that it must be very depressing to suffer as he does. He may then validate the existence of depression. It is difficult for most patients to admit that their pain is a result of a preceding depression. They prefer to believe the reverse, that the pain causes the depression. The individual with psychosomatic complaints has an absence of any organic findings. He often feels frustrated as his multitude of somatic complaints result in negative findings, baffling the health professionals. Those with chronic complaints seek a reaction and a loving response from those involved in his care in the same way that a sick child seeks love from a parent. Unfortunately, their repetitive complaints drive away the people they need most. At the same time, the painful disorder satisfies an unconscious need for punishment.

Encourage the person to talk about things that have increased or decreased his aches and pains. Then help him to see that sometimes an upsetting telephone call can create a nervous reaction, resulting in diarrhea, headache, or other symptoms. Ask the person, "What would you do if you were well?" Perhaps plans should be changed if the patient's illness is a way of avoiding his work, forthcoming marriage, moving to another state, engaging in sex, and so on.

Avoid giving well-meant but meaningless advice. Although you can suggest that some emotional problem may be increasing the physical discomfort, avoid confrontation. Asking the person what emotionally upsetting incident was going on when his pain first started is too direct a confrontation for the individual's defenses to handle and might prove disastrous. Stay away from such meaningless recommendations as, "Just learn to take things easy," "Relax," or "Don't be such a worrier." These suggestions accomplish nothing. Instead say, "I noticed you became upset when your mother visited you," or "I noticed you seemed upset when you didn't receive any mail this morning." This allows the patient to comment on real situations or problems that might be bothering him.

LONG-TERM ACTION

Never reject, avoid, ignore or humiliate a person because he has "no right" or "no cause to be sick." Never say, "The pains are all in your head." Accept him as he is and communicate the attitude that there is a reason for an illness. Say, "The staff will help you during your illness by working with you to understand yourself better."

Do not increase the person's anxiety by telling him what seems obvious to you. If you say to the asthmatic, "Oh, I bet your hatred for your dead father is behind all this," you may well precipitate an attack. Do not attach a label to the patient or shake him off with an abrupt, "There is not one thing wrong with you. You're a perfectly healthy specimen." Patients who have somatic complaints use them for a purpose, whether to communicate with others or to protect themselves from unconscious fears. Encourage the person to talk about times when the symptoms appeared. Tune in to periods in his history of loss, loneliness, disappointments, and dependency.

Encourage the person to find small satisfactions and experience small achievements. This may allow him to feel secure enough to begin giving up his somatic complaints.

21

The Person With a Psychiatric Emergency

The health worker will often become involved in an emergency psychiatric situation. Such emergencies occur when an individual (or several individuals) experiences so much anxiety that his thinking, actions, and total organization become seriously affected, and he cannot assume any responsibility for himself. He usually arrives at a hospital unit accompanied by friends or relatives, but occasionally may come to the hospital unaccompanied.

Usually everyone in the situation is under a great deal of stress and appears very anxious. Often the patient cannot communicate adequately, coherently, or effectively. He is unable to state just what is bothering or troubling him. All that comes across is that he expects you to do something to make everything all right again. He may even cry out, "Just help me." He seems to expect a magic, instant solution that will resolve all his problems without the necessity of his revealing anything. Of course this is not possible. At this point, the health worker must talk with the accompanying friends or relatives to obtain some understanding of what may have happened that led to the patient's present state. At the same time, if the patient cannot control his emotions effectively the health worker may need to provide some effective restraints.

Health workers who interview the patient and/or accompanying relatives or friends need to assess and explore the situation without becoming unduly upset. They must be calm. If they become anxious they will not be able to perform effectively and competently. It is imperative that they impress others with their command of themselves, demonstrating control of what is occurring in the immediate situation.

There should be professionals who have been trained to treat patients with psychiatric emergencies available to health personnel working in emergency room settings. In addition, emergency room staff should receive specific help with their own reactions to offset their anxiety. Often the workers have to deal with a multitude of emotional problems shown by patients brought in by police, social workers, or friends. It is unfortunate that some health professionals in emergency rooms do not recognize the importance of their roles in saving the life of a psychiatric patient. Their help is as necessary to the emotionally distressed person as it is to the patient with a medical problem.

Psychiatric emergencies require immediate attention. It is important to focus on the behavior of the patient, as well as what caused it. A patient may have been exhibiting destructive behavior without receiving any medical attention. However, as soon as his behavior affects someone else, the family is likely to respond. For example, one man had been abusing medication for a long time, but it was not until he threw a lamp at his mother that the family dragged him to the emergency room for help. Conversely, a patient in the emergency room may seem very subdued; yet the police may report that just a few moments earlier, he attacked an innocent pedestrian.

Every health worker should be aware of the patient's physiological condition. It is not unusual to find that a brain tumor will reflect itself in a patient's unusual behavior. It goes without saying that every patient should be evaluated by a knowledgeable professional.

Initially, the health worker should give the patient the opportunity to talk and tell about the events that made him feel he needed help. Often the patient will relate that "it was all too much," or that he felt he "couldn't continue like this any longer."

The health professional should inquire how the patient arrived at his present state and whether he thinks the problem is an emotional one. If the answer is affirmative, the patient should be asked what makes him think so. This gets the psychiatric nature of the difficulty out in the open and clears the way for the patient to relate some of his unpleasant thoughts and feelings. Often he declares that he is unable to function because he cries all the time, as did a 60-year-old man following his retirement. More often he will reveal suicidal thoughts and fear of losing all self-control because he has engaged in impulsive acts in which he threatened, hit, or struck out at himself or others. Many patients will say quite openly, "I can't think straight"; "I just can't get myself together"; "I feel like I'm falling apart"; "I can't remember the simplest things, and I forget what I'm doing when I'm in the midst of it"; or "I know it's in my head because I'm so miserable and don't know why."

If possible, it is most helpful for the health worker to obtain information about some of the occurrences that preceded the illness It is not uncommon for the person involved in an emergency situation to be in a very depressed state. The depression can be the result of the loss of a parent, sibling, lover, or even a pet for whom his attachment was very strong. He may feel completely lost now that his loved one is gone. A very dependent person may feel that he can no longer continue living without the support of this most important individual. One such case involved a single girl whose closest girlfriend became engaged and planned to marry soon, leaving her alone.

Incidents in which a person loses self-esteem and confidence to the extent that he feels demeaned can also precipitate a severe depressive reaction. Such situations may include not being chosen for a much desired promotion, losing a job, being asked to leave school, or ending a relationship with a significant other. The patient may relate that he feels totally hopeless and that he is contemplating suicide. By the time the health worker on the unit sees the patient, a suicide attempt may have been made in the hope of ending his severe emotional tensions.

Another type of emergency situation involves the patient who is overwhelmed with anxious feelings that make him unable to control his impulses. For example, a man leaving on a vacation with his wife became fearful that he would strangle her when they were alone together. A mother feared she might do harm to her children. A student found his learning ability impaired and feared he would fail all his courses and be dismissed from the university. A woman was deserted by her husband, and became frantic at the prospect of managing herself and her children alone and of being regarded as a failure. A man became overwhelmed with guilt and anxiety at the prospect of taking care of his ill wife; he felt that he would not be able to cope with the situation.

A current situation may also arouse fears which may not be recognized by the person involved. All he knows is that he is distressed and has uncomfortable feelings which may be incapacitating. A somatic reaction may occur, and affect him in such a manner that he is unable to walk, he faints or falls, or is unable to use an arm, to swallow, or to speak. It is not unusual to see an upset, bewildered family following the health aide who is wheeling such a patient into the psychiatric unit for admission.

The health worker who admits the emergency patient to the hospital can assume that the patient, whether or not he accepts the idea, realizes he needs help. This is definitely so in a voluntary general hospital. The patient may be fearful of what will happen, particularly if he has had an unpleasant prior hospitalization or in any way identifies hospitalization with mistreatment. He looks to the worker as one who will help take care of him and provide relief for his distress. Some of his anticipations are valid, while others are based only on his deep, unconscious needs. The valid expectations can be immediately acted upon by the health worker. But those which are products of unrealistic wishful thinking may be impossible and may never materialize. The worker can reassure the patient about what is realistically available, thereby reducing the patient's anxiety and lessening his depression. Although immediate solutions to problems may not be possible, the health team must stress that while he is in the hospital, the patient will be helped to understand himself. The hope is that he will eventually become strong enough to make his own decisions and to cope with the reality of difficult and unpleasant situations. Once the patient begins to recover, he is more able to accept limitations imposed by life situations, for he realizes that there are alternate plans available for living successfully and comfortably.

Health workers should admit the patient as calmly, quickly, and with as much interest as is humanly possible. They should extend every effort to make the patient feel at ease, and to convey the impression that they know what they are doing and are in full command of the situation. If the patient is up to it, a brief history of problems and precipitating circumstances should be obtained. The patient is given every opportunity to talk about what is on his mind and to discuss his feelings and problems. It is also desirable to take him on a brief tour of the unit and explain hospital policies. Reassurance and information regarding the kind of help the patient will be receiving does much to alleviate his fears and unfounded expectations. Some patients expect to be locked up, tied down, physically abused, and denied visitors, mail, and their own clothing. Knowing about the frequency of visiting hours, the necessity for adequate everyday clothing, and the advantages of the hospital environment in helping to reduce tension does much to calm the patient, to establish rapport, and to gain his trust.

Often health workers will have to anticipate the needs of the disorganized patient. In the emergency situation, the workers assume an active, assertive, and directive approach. If the patient physically lashes out or becomes violent, additional help may be needed to restrain him until he becomes manageable. The admission procedure should then be continued and the patient queried about the incident. By showing a willingness to understand, the workers often enable the patient to reveal more of what bothers him. The patient may be able to describe the way in which he sometimes upsets others, as well as difficulties he has in controlling himself.

Sometimes a patient balks at accepting hospitalization. There is a moment of, "I don't want to. Oh, no, I'll manage alone"; "What will everyone say?"; "What does it matter; I'm sure I'll never get well"; "This is the end of the line." The workers' attitudes and efforts should be directed to persuading and encouraging the person to accept admission, since it may have been decided on as a last resort. If not admitted at this time, the patient's only hope for care may be destroyed. It may confirm for him that no help is available—that he is totally abandoned.

Psychiatric emergencies are crisis situations. This means the patient is unable to solve his problem by his usual means of coping. Therefore, he feels that the problem is insurmountable. The patient requires immediate intervention in terms of decreasing the environmental stimulation. He needs help in pinpointing what is happening currently in his life. It is important to establish which people are closest to him, and to engage them in the formulation of an immediate plan to provide support and guidance until the acute emotional state subsides.

Health workers may, on occasion, receive telephone calls from patients who present an urgent situation. They may state that they are going to kill themselves or someone else, or that they have taken an overdose of pills. The workers must give immediate attention to these calls since they, too, may be a person's last resort before either killing himself or completely losing control over his impulse to destroy others. When such a call comes to the hospital unit, the health workers must have a quiet place in which to handle emergency calls without distraction. They must keep calm and obtain the caller's name as well as the address and phone number from which he is calling. It is also advantageous to obtain the name and telephone number of nearby relatives or neighbors.

If the patient states that he has taken an overdose of some drug, obtain information regarding the drug taken, the amount, and the time it was taken. The workers should tell the caller that help will be sent directly to the place of the call and that a staff member will call back immediately after arranging for help. If the person objects to giving information or to having help sent, the workers should tell him that he must want help or he wouldn't have called, and in order to receive help, the person must supply the needed information. Workers should inform the caller that he may have swallowed a lethal dose of pills and that action must be taken immediately to save his life. Workers should stress that they will continue to help. If the caller still refuses to say where he is, a worker should continue to talk to him while someone else makes arrangements to have the call traced in order to discover the location.

A final word about patients who present themselves at the clinic but who are not admitted to the hospital unit. Make sure that a plan is formulated before the patient leaves, initiating help for him. Relatives and friends who accompanied the patient to the hospital should be involved. The plan might entail arranging transportation to and from the clinic so that the patient can keep future appointments, or providing child care during scheduled visits, or for someone to be at home with the patient on a temporary basis. Arrangements for a leave of absence from a job or school may also have to be made. Realizing that help is really available encourages the patient to keep his next appointment. However, despite such efforts, there are some emergency patients who subsequently change their minds and refuse any help which is offered. These patients should be advised of all resources available to them should they desire help in the future.

THE APPROACH TO THE PATIENT WITH A PSYCHIATRIC EMERGENCY

Immediate Intervention by the Patient

SELF-MANAGEMENT TECHNIQUES

If the patient has had similar episodes before, use them to teach the patient to recognize feelings or situations that may initiate an emergency situation. If there have been no prior episodes, help the patient become aware of those trigger situations and the feelings that result in an emergency situation.

Alert the patient to the need for an immediate contact with a person who can be helpful. Because the patient may be at home, school, work, or a public place, he should make anyone with him aware of his feelings. If he is alone, he should call the police or other individual and ask them to get him to an emergency room immediately. If he has any lethal weapon with him, it should be surrendered immediately to the person who is providing aid.

Professional Intervention

Immediate Action

Make certain the individual relinquishes any dangerous or lethal equipment, including weapons, sharp instruments (even a restaurant butter knife), pills, rope, etc.

Speak softly, move slowly, touch gently, and do not make any threatening gestures. Remember the patient wants help, or he would not have asked for it.

Protect yourself from any dangerous actions by the patient. If you want to hold him, place your hand on top of his arm so that he cannot grab you. Get help from others if necessary.

Maintain a calm, collected, and assured demeanor. Show sincere interest in the patient and his problem. Do not allow yourself to be immobilized by the emergency. Encourage the patient to accept hospitalization and offer reassurances by telling the patient, "You will feel better in the hospital, and will be able to resist your impulses, eliminate the voices you are hearing and the unpleasant thoughts you have." Also tell him, "You *can* be treated, and will recover as many other people have."

Sustain the patient in his need to be dependent. Offer him any necessary assistance. If he is crying, offer him a tissue. If he is hungry or thirsty, offer him food or drink. If he is unable to stand securely, offer him an arm to lean on. If necessary, help him remove his outer clothing. If he is unable to reach a decision, or make a selection, take over for him.

Talk with those who accompany the patient, and include them as resource persons. They are often invaluable in helping to formulate a follow-up plan.

Allow privacy so that the patient can speak to you alone. But do not add to patient's fears by blocking or closing the door to the room in which you are talking. This can make the patient feel trapped, and can provoke violence.

Be direct in your approach and assess the potential for suicide. Ask the patient, "Have you ever attempted suicide before?" "Do you have thoughts of suicide now?" Be alert to a family history of suicide or actions of the patient which indicate that he expects not to live—for example, planning to sell his house, giving away jewelry, writing letters to deceased persons, and taking out an insurance policy.

INTERMEDIATE ACTION

Take the individual to an emergency room for evaluation and treatment. Do so calmly, reiterating that whatever you are doing will help the patient return to a positive state. Contact his relatives or significant others if possible, and ask them to meet you at the receiving facility.

Hospital professionals should be aware that emergency arrivals are usually very frightened, and may exhibit abusive behavior. Do not react to abusive words or actions by becoming irate or abusive. Remember the patient is out of control, and needs to be assured that those offering help will understand and show compassion. Make certain that the person is not harboring any dangerous materials.

Reduce the patient's anxiety by discussing some of his symptoms. Telling the patient to "try and take it easy" is totally ineffectual. But telling him, "Sometimes if a person is upset he may have a rapid heartbeat, breathe more quickly, or feel faint," helps him to understand what is happening. If he is very confused, introduce yourself by name and role each time you approach him. Attempt to eliminate distractions and get the patient to look directly at you as you talk to him about what is happening.

Reduce the patient's fears by pointing out the reality of what is happening. Or elicit from him what he thinks will happen and what he anticipates it will be like. For instance, if the patient fears that he will lose his mind, the worker can point out that his fear is due to his discomfort, and that preventing and arresting further discomfort will lessen and perhaps eliminate the fear. The patient may also feel that he can never leave the hospital if he accepts admission. Reassure him that he can leave a voluntary unit under his own signature, if accompanied by a relative or friend.

If it becomes necessary, obtain an order for medication with which to calm the patient.

LONG-TERM ACTION

Explain all treatment and medications to help the patient understand what is happening. The patient may believe that he is being held prisoner, particularly if the police have brought him to the facility. If family or friends come to the emergency room, explain whatever is being done so that they can reenforce the information concerning the help that is offered by the professional staff. If the patient is discharged, be certain that he and those who will be with him understand the symptoms that may indicate the need for an immediate return to the emergency room.

Evaluate the patient well before discharging. If the patient is likely to harm himself or others, he should not be sent home, regardless of his wishes. He should be evaluated for hospitalizations, with adequate explanation for that decision given to him and his significant others.

PART THREE

Approaches to the Psychological Effects of Special Circumstances

22

The Person Who Is a Victim of Abuse

Abused patients may appear in any setting and be of any age and either sex. The abuse may be due to physical or emotional actions of strangers, teachers, friends, enemies, health providers, relatives, or spouses. In some states, health workers must report evidence of abuse to a specific authority.

In New York State, the law requires that incidents of abuse, neglect, or mistreatment of patients in residential health care facilities be reported by the agency administrator or any licensed professional. This is so regardless of whether or not the professional is employed by that facility. Nonreporting is punishable by a fine of up to $1,000 and possible disciplinary action by the licensing boards under New York State Public Health Law. The only abuse that is *not* reportable is that committed by one patient upon another. Obviously, every effort should be made to protect patients from others who are abusive, even though the abusers may not be legally responsible.

Mistreatment in residential facilities that is reportable includes the inappropriate use of restraints (physical or chemical), isolation instituted as punishment, or medication used not for treatment but to calm disruptive patients for the convenience of the staff. Neglect that is reportable embraces inadequate treatment services or care, including cleanliness, nutrition, therapy, medication, and usual activities of daily living. Reportable abuse may be any inappropriate physical action, including hitting, kicking, punching, pinching, bumping, shoving, or sexual molestation.

Physical abuse should be suspected when patients have bruises, hematomas, broken bones, burns, bleeding, or symptoms of sexual molestation. Some patients may be reluctant to blame others for their injuries, fearing retaliation that will be more severe than the original abuse. They may, therefore, blame the injuries on a fall or other self-induced action.

Patients who have been sexually molested or raped by a spouse, relative, or friend may refuse to name the abuser, or may be prevented from doing so by other family members who fear publicity. Other deterrents to reporting sexual abuse (especially incest) are fears that the family will be broken up during and after the legal proceedings, or that there will be a loss of income to the family if the breadwinner is accused of the crime.

Until recently, accusations of sexual abuse were not taken seriously. The victim was often viewed as having provoked or seduced the accused, or of making up a story. This resulted in a double insult to the victim—first undergoing the pain and indignity of the attack, and later the pain and indignity of not being believed.

Children are especially vulnerable to any kind of abuse since they often are unable to protect themselves. They may keep the attacks secret because of threats of harm to themselves or their loved ones. Incidents may go on for years before being discovered by people in a position to offer help. One way of encouraging early recognition of child abuse would be the establishment of a central reporting agency in each community, to which reports of all incidents of possible abuse (broken bones, bruises, lacerations, or other complaints) would be mandated. Repetitive reports concerning a particular child would then alert the proper authorities to the possibility of a problem.

There are at least a million children abused each year in the United States, of whom about 10% will die. About 75% of abusive parents are mentally ill, retarded, or addicted to drugs (including alcohol). About 25% of abused children grow up to become abusive parents, which indicates the imperative need for early and proper intervention.

Child abusers may lack understanding of normal childhood developments, and may become angry or frustrated when a child cries, wets himself, spills things, or does something which may be dangerous, such as lighting matches or pulling dishes or sharp knives from a countertop. The abuse may actually be an inappropriate way of trying to educate the child about danger. In addition, there may be an inability to recognize or meet the child's needs, with little, if any, understanding of normal mental, physical or emotional patterns. The caregiver may also be emotionally unresponsive to the child, unable to differentiate between the many levels of a child's happiness or distress.

A major reason for unresponsiveness to the child is parental depression. Afflicted parents are more likely to withdraw from their children, resulting in emotional deprivation for the child. The lack of secure attachment to the mother by one year of age often leads to a major decline in a youngster's functioning between 12 months and 4 years. The older the child, the more affected he is by rejecting or unresponsive parents.

Health care professionals should observe mother-child interactions whenever possible. The nonabusive mother interprets a youngster's cry as an indication that something is making him unhappy, and will then try to rectify the situation. The abusive mother interprets the cry as a sign that the child is no good, or that she is an inadequate mother. She looks to the child for nurturance, a task that the child cannot handle. This results in the youngster developing low self-esteem, seeing himself as "bad," and therefore deserving any abuse that he receives.

Once in a foster home or school situation, a previously abused child may unwittingly attempt to recreate the pattern with which he is familiar. He is used to abuse, and may not know how to react to kindness or respect. He may, therefore, do the very things that will anger teachers or caretakers, leading to punishment that reinforces his low self-esteem. In later years, the child may become involved in situations or with friends that lead to an even greater sense of low self-esteem. As they grow up, these children become prime targets for drug and sexual abuse, often becoming involved in relationships that carry through their sense of not deserving anything or anyone better.

The battered spouse is often a person from a background that led to low self-esteem and may be unable to see any options for escape from the marital situation. Whether or not the victims, usually women, are educated, they see themselves as unable to succeed on their own, dependent upon their mates for care, and deserving the abuse to which they are subjected. It becomes a trade-off—the security of having a mate is worth the abuse, regardless of the frequency or severity.

This problem has become so rampant that a National Task Force on Battered Women/Household Violence was formed in the United States in 1976. During the same year, an International Tribunal on Crimes against Women convened in Brussels, attended by 2,000 women from 33 countries.

In many places, police are no longer permitted to regard battering as a private family matter, but have been instructed to arrest the abuser. Shelters are increasingly available for battered women and their children, providing them with an escape from the immediate situation and time to think about their alternatives for the future.

Abuse of the elderly is a growing concern as more of the population lives to an older age. The abuser may be a spouse, child, care provider, or other person. Since the elderly tend to have memory deficits or episodes of paranoid ideation, their stories of being abused may not be believed. As in childhood, emotional abuse may be far more harmful than physical abuse. Those who have been loved and trusted in the past may suddenly carry out actions that leave the victim in a state of shock, vulnerable to future episodes of abuse. Often too fragile to fight back, or dependent on the abuser for financial aid, the victim may not complain or resist.

   Those who abuse the elderly may do so out of anger or frustration at having to accept responsibility for the victim's care. There may be resentment at being forced to be available to someone who is physically weak, intellectually impaired, or overly demanding and unable to express gratitude. There may be an inability to accept the victim's deterioration, with a buildup of frustration resulting in physical or emotional actions that are abusive.

THE APPROACH TO THE PERSON WHO IS A VICTIM OF ABUSE

Immediate Intervention by the Patient

SELF-MANAGEMENT TECHNIQUES

Help the patient recognize the usual first actions of the abuser. Help plan an evasive action to protect the patient from further abuse. (When the patient is able, the first action should be to report the abuse to the proper authorities.)

Professional Intervention

IMMEDIATE ACTION

Evaluate the physical and emotional status of the patient. Document any physical injuries that are evident, noting the size, shape, color, and location of the area(s), as well as the time the abuse is reported to have taken place. Document the patient's explanation of the occurrence, noting his affect (mood), as well as the content. Remain nonjudgmental, but keep in mind the possibility that there may be omissions or distortions in his story, to protect the abuser.

Encourage the patient to talk about his relationships with significant others. It is better to interview the victim alone because the person who brings him for care may be the abuser. As victims talk, they may gain enough strength to share the incident fully with the health care professional. Again, documentation is important.

Remember that children, and even some adults, may be reluctant to use anatomical terminology. Using the same terms as the victim increases rapport, and focuses on the issue of the event, rather than how it is verbalized. The use of anatomically correct dolls may help children describe the incident more accurately. Be certain not to coach victims (particularly children) into making false accusations.

INTERMEDIATE ACTION

Stress the fact that the victim is not to blame for what happened. Emphasize the idea that the abuser is an individual who needs professional help. As painful as it may be, making the accusation is often the first necessary step in getting that help.

LONG-TERM ACTION

Reinforce the ego strengths of the victim, encouraging him to verbalize his anger. Once victims feel safe enough to express anger, they can begin to mobilize themselves for action. They can then be helped to examine their options rather than allow the abusive situation to continue. Children are at particular risk, since they may have to be removed from the home to prevent future parental or sibling abuse. They need tremendous emotional support to offset the sense of disloyalty involved when accusing a family member of abuse.

23

The Person With a Sexual or Reproductive Disorder

Knowledge of sexual development and sexual behavior has become increasingly important to health care providers as public standards have changed. Behavior that was once considered perverted is perhaps now regarded only as deviant and may in the future be looked upon as an acceptable alternative to "normal" sexual activity. No longer is sexual behavior an important factor in determining an individual's value, although there is a continuing interest in the acts of private and public figures. In general, people are more willing to accept their own sexuality, recognizing that this is but one facet of their personalities.

Before 1972 scientists believed that an individual's sex was solely determined by the X and Y chromosomes that were linked as the sperm fertilized the ovum. This meant that if an X chromosome from the ovum joined the X from the sperm, a female would result. But if the ovum's X met with the sperm's Y chromosome, a male would result. Although these facts are basically correct, newer information includes factors that affect the intrauterine development of the embryo and fetus. It is now believed that the fetal gonads begin their development as ovaries and that fetal and paranatal androgens must be present as inductor substances to change the fetus to a male. These same fetal androgens appear to help the brain organize for future specific sexual behavior. This provides some clues as to why women receiving certain hormones during pregnancy may deliver children with anomalies of their external genitals. This area is also being explored as a possible physiological basis for homosexual behavior.

Sexual development continues after birth. Infant boys have erections, while infant girls have been observed rubbing their thighs and moving their pelvic areas in multiple thrusts. In both, the activity ends with a relaxed period of sleep. There also seems to be an imprinting of sexual expectations on children from birth by the behavioral patterns of their care providers. Little girls are handled more tenderly, are expected to be more gentle and cleaner, and may be dressed in frillier clothing.

From eighteen months to five years, children can be expected to be involved in self-exploration, including their genitals. Parents usually do not voice displeasure when a child feels his nose, ears, or lips, but may pull a child's hands away as he explores his "private parts." This definitely gets a message across—the genitals are dirty, naughty, and should not be touched. The child then meets his first big conflict. Does he provide himself with the pleasure he enjoys through autoeroticism, or should he live according to parental standards? If he chooses pleasure, will he be overwhelmed with guilt?

In today's permissive society, youngsters may become involved in sexual activity as early as eight or ten years of age. Males are capable of experiencing orgasm within two years of puberty, and may engage in masturbation on a frequent basis to achieve sexual release. Girls may become involved in unprotected sex to become part of the "gang," or as a way of attaining closeness. The health professional can help youngsters realize that delaying sexual activity until emotionally ready is acceptable, even preferable.

At present, there are almost a half million pregnancies per year in unwed females, and about half of these are in teen-agers. Although some elect to terminate the pregnancy or give the baby up for adoption, most decide, although single, to keep and raise the baby. Often this means the end of the mother's education, sealing her fate in terms of low-level jobs. These mothers have a high potential for child-battering (they, too, may have been battered as children), and are likely to become pregnant again. They may be knowledgeable about the anatomy and physiology of pregnancy, but tend not to integrate the facts that they have learned in sex education classes with the ways in which their own bodies function. Therefore, although they may have learned about contraceptive measures, they may not apply them properly in practice. Many refuse to use contraceptives because they don't wish to acknowledge any thoughts about intercourse. For them, lack of protection is equated with spontaneity of action, for which they do not feel guilty.

Some pregnancies are quite deliberate and are used to prove that the "girl" is truly a woman. For others, having a baby represents an important goal: at long last, the individual has someone of her own to love. Unfortunately, the area of responsibility is not recognized, and little thought is given to aspects of day-to-day care that will be needed by the child. Still others see pregnancy as a hold on a man that will lead to marriage, without realizing that about 50% of such marriages end in divorce. Some choose pregnancy as a way to punish overly strict parents, while others may choose pregnancy as a way to meet their own parents' need to have a baby in the family. (This is particularly true in families where the mother works to provide support and her child is raised by the grandmother or other caregiver. This skipped-generation upbringing deprives the mother of closeness with her own child. In effect, if the grandmother takes over, the mother becomes a sibling to her own child, rather than acting as the parent.)

Coitus used to be delayed until later in adolescence (sixteen to eighteen years), but has steadily been increasing as an activity among younger adolescents. Often the naive youth who is over eighteen finds that he is unprepared to handle the sexual pressures to be found in college life. He may not be ready to become involved sexually, yet may be fearful that classmates will jeer at him for remaining a virgin. As a result, he may develop symptoms that relieve him of the necessity for sexual involvement. He may complain of headaches, gastrointestinal symptoms or anxiety attacks that allow him to withdraw from social activities. His problems may be severe enough to result in hospitalization, yet so covert that the underlying cause is not suspected.

During the period of more or less permanent relationships, the young adult (23 to 30 years) may enjoy lovemaking or may be so concerned about his level of sexual performance that he is immobilized and cannot perform at all. Both sexes are very aware of their right to orgasms and may complain of feeling inadequate if both partners are unable to reach the common American myth of equal orgasms at the same time. One partner may have a more extensive sexual appetite than the other and may desire more experimentation with different aspects of sexual behavior. This may or may not be acceptable to the other.

Venereal diseases have risen sharply as more individuals are involved with a variety of partners. Gonorrhea is the most common, with an average of ten to fifteen million cases a year being suspected. Of these, 25% involve teen-agers. Chlamydia is another venereal disease that is very common, causing many of the same complaints as gonorrhea (discharge, pain, pelvic inflammatory disease, sterility). Some organisms that were limited to mouth, anus, or genitals may now be found in other areas, as oral-genital, anal-genital, or genital-genital sex are practiced. Anyone with a venereal disease must be treated as soon as possible, along with any sexual contacts who may have contracted the disease, to lessen the chance of future transmission of the disease. (AIDS is discussed on pp. 00.)

During middlescence (thirties to seventies), sexual performance is often related to work performance. If the individual sees himself as potent in life, he will probably continue to be effective sexually. Conversely, if he sees himself as having failed, as unable to attain his goals, he is likely to be less able to perform sexually. The longer the period of abstinence, the more difficult it will be to perform well. During these years, male interest may decrease, while female interest increases. The menopause, with its freedom from possible pregnancy, may allow some women to enjoy lovemaking more than ever before. But for others, the end of childbearing, as well as some unpleasant physical symptoms of menopause (vaginal dryness, hot flashes with perspiration, breast and bone pain) may lessen the desire for intercourse.

Sexual activity continues for healthy adults through their 60s, 70s, and even later years. Some are made to feel guilty or ashamed by their children, almost as though they had reentered adolescence. They may lose mates through death or divorce, and enter into repeated instances of sexual involvement with numerous partners, as they seek closeness and intimacy. Too often, feelings of emptiness, distrust, disgust, and guilt follow these meaningless sexual encounters. For some, the loss and grief reactions may be so severe and prolonged that restructuring of their lives is delayed for a period of years, or perhaps forever. Again, physical symptoms may be a sign of emotional problems. For those who are fortunate, a new significant other may be found, and once again life becomes fully satisfying. Some of these couples decide to marry, whereas others choose to remain monogamous without marriage.

In today's society, many sexual variations exist. Sexual identity is determined by the external genitalia—male or female—while gender identity depends on the individual's orientation to the masculine or feminine role. Disturbances in sexual orientation may cause social problems, as the person determines whether he wants to be heterosexual, homosexual, or bisexual. Regardless of his decision, he may be hypoactive or hyperactive, or may have problems with impotency. Men may suffer from premature or retarded ejaculation, while females may complain of dyspareunia (pain upon inter-course), vaginismus (contractions of the vagina that may prevent admission of the penis), or orgasmic dysfunction. Some may decide on transsexual changes to reverse what they see as a "mistake" by nature in their sexual iden-tity. This may involve surgery, hormone supplements, electrolysis, and learn-ing the gestures and voice modulation of the chosen identity.

Sex crimes result in severe problems for some patients. Rape is one crime which can involve a victim of either sex and any age. In past years rape victims were often considered as guilty as the offender, particularly if the individual was a young, attractive, unescorted woman in a locality of questionable safety at a late hour. Today the victim is no longer equated with the rapist in terms of being a partner in the crime. Health professionals often work closely with law enforcement officials as they question and physically examine the victim, usually a female. Evidence that can be used against the offender must be saved and handled in a nondestructive manner. Fragments of the offender's clothing, skin, or hair may be present under the victim's fingernails, in her mouth, or vagina. There may or may not be an ejaculate specimen, since offenders are often impotent.

Rape, contrary to common thought, is not a crime of love, but is an act of hostility, meant to hurt and demean the victim. She may be bruised in any area of her body, and may be bleeding from her mouth, vagina, and rectum. Beyond the physical damage, and perhaps more important, is the psycholog-ical damage that results from twisting what should be an act of love into an act of hate and pain. The approach of the health care provider should be gen-tle, understanding, and supportive. The patient should be encouraged to talk about the incident as fully as possible, in order to lessen the possibility of long-term emotional damage. If there has been more than one rapist, each incident should be discussed separately, since the victim's reaction may have differed with each. In one case, the teen-aged victim reacted most hysterically to the offender who initially made her feel that he would help her escape and protect her from further attacks by the others. He then took her to another room and proceeded to rape her. She saw this as more deceitful than the acts of his four companions, who had threatened to kill her as they raped and sodomized her.

Young children present the most difficult problem when they are rape vic-tims, since they may not understand what the brutality meant. They may be the victims of that most specialized form of rape—incest. Again, the victim is usually a girl, and often preadolescent, so that pregnancy is not possible. The emotional load of having a loved and trusted relative take advantage of a child is extremely traumatic. The child has usually been sworn to secrecy, so that telling a parent (or another person) becomes an act of disloyalty. In addition, the child may enjoy the closeness, and be afraid that it will stop once discovered. Another fear is that the offending relative (usually a parent or sibling) may be removed from the home and punished by the authorities. Even if the child does complain, the accusation may not be believed and the child punished for telling a falsehood.

Sexual problems may also result from medical disorders or surgical procedures. Most patients are disinterested in sexual activity when acutely ill, but may be concerned about what the future holds. Many are afraid that health personnel will reject them if they voice worries about sexual limitations. It is therefore important to anticipate such concerns and bring them into the open. Patients with heart disease may mistakenly believe that their sexual activity is ended forever, and may become deeply depressed. Health workers should clarify any prohibitions and make suggestions that will help the patient function in a way that he finds acceptable. Most patients can resume sexual intercourse when they have recovered to the point where they can climb two flights of stairs and walk rapidly. Some may require nitroglycerine before sexual relations to prevent angina. Comfort may be increased if the partner is on top and assumes most of the physical exertion.

Decreased blood flow to the genital area (as in diabetes) or neurological problems that prevent an erection, as well as the use of certain medications, or performance anxiety are other factors that may affect sexual enjoyment. All should be discussed, perhaps with a sex therapist, and various solutions leading to mutual satisfaction explored. For example, radical surgery for cancer may result in castration. The patient and his mate should then be encouraged to explore various ways of finding (and providing) sexual satisfaction. Kissing, touching, and physical closeness may become as meaningful as intercourse. The absence of a penis, testicles, uterus, vagina, or breast will undoubtedly affect the individual's vision of himself. Plastic surgery or prostheses have been used successfully to refashion missing parts, but the resulting emotional state is even more important for most patients. Much help may be needed to help the patient recognize his own continuing worth in light of his changed body. He may need tremendous support to believe that life is still worth living.

Sexual incompatibility may be the result of incorrect sexual education. One woman had been told that masturbation was sinful and that having an orgasm would cause her to die. She entered into therapy, and was able to gain insight into her fears and misconceptions. She was eventually able to masturbate and use a vibrator. She also learned to enjoy clitoral stimulation. Exercises to strengthen the vaginal muscles as well as the use of the sensate focusing also helped enable her to enter into an enjoyable sexual relationship.

Reproduction is another area in which sexual concerns abound. The very state of pregnancy may cause emotional problems for the mother- or father-to-be. Even when a pregnancy is desired and planned, it may cause a high level of anxiety as an acceptable life style is changed. This is particularly true when a woman is involved in a successful and satisfying career. It also occurs when there is a history of previous miscarriages, loss of a fetus or child, previous birth of a child with anomalies, or a period of infertility. The couple may be supportive of each other as they endure limitations of sexual activity or are concerned about what the future holds. Perhaps the greatest difficulty occurs when a fetal death has occurred in utero and the mother is told that she must wait until labor starts in order to deliver a dead baby. She may be asked to wait at home, possibly for several weeks, before delivering. This is considered the safest procedure in terms of the mother's physical state, but is devastating emotionally. Those who are unaware of what is happening will continue to inquire about the pregnancy. Others who do know may avoid her, fearful that any questions will distress her. In either case, her reaction will be an indication of her deep emotional turmoil. The fact that she has a dead body within her uterus is understandably unacceptable. Most women in such a situation are deeply sedated for the delivery, since the fetus will probably be macerated and odorous. They need to talk about the event and their feelings, and should be warned that they may have nightmares about the event, difficulty in sleeping (perhaps to avoid the bad dreams), and marked depression as they work through their feelings of grief. Almost all search for reasons and may not be satisfied when none are available.

In order to help patients with sexual problems, health professionals need to have a positive sense of their own sexuality. It takes practice to be comfortable when discussing such matters, particularly if one has many inhibitions in this area. This does not mean that the professional has to be sexually active in order to help others, any more than one has to have an infarct, a stroke, or cancer before counseling patients with those disorders. The health worker can learn a great deal from reading on the subject, as well as from watching films geared to providing helpful information. The more knowledgeable the worker, the more valuable his input will be.

THE APPROACH TO THE PERSON WHO IS A VICTIM OF ABUSE

Immediate Intervention by the Patient

SELF-MANAGEMENT TECHNIQUES

Help the person recognize the target symptoms that interfere with sexual functioning. Approaching, or being approached by, someone socially may arouse marked anxiety. Concentrating on what that individual says and realizing that it is innocuous may enable the patient to relax rather than fearing that there may be sexual overtures before he or she is ready.

Professional Intervention

IMMEDIATE ACTION

Recognize the possibility of sexual problems resulting from medical disorders or surgical procedures. Help the person verbalize his feelings.

If the person is a victim of rape or incest, collect and label physical evidence carefully and keep it available for law enforcement officials. Be supportive, encouraging the person to discuss the situation as fully as possible. Keep a written record of the person's description of the individuals involved or of the event because the victim may be unable to recall details later. Help arrange for follow-up care to lessen the emotional turmoil that the individual is experiencing.

INTERMEDIATE ACTION

Recognize the sexual problems associated with the reproductive process. Infertility, miscarriages, fetal anomalies, or death each present special problems. The patient and her mate need support as they work through their feelings.

Come to grips with your own beliefs and feelings about sexuality and sexual behavior. Reading and film attendance may be helpful. Separate your personal standards from those of the patient without being judgmental.

LONG-TERM ACTION

Be available to persons who want to discuss sexual problems. There are several national organizations with local branches which can provide additional information and specific help.

24

The Person With an Eating and Weight Disorder

Weight concerns are big business in the United States, as evidenced by the involvement of many large companies in sales of diet aids and foods, low-calorie beverages, various nutritional supplements, exercise equipment, and video tapes for home exercise programs for those who overeat or are overweight. It is virtually impossible to pick up a newspaper or magazine that does not provide information or advertisements about weight reduction classes or groups, or articles about food preparation for dieters. Concerns for the underweight tend to focus on the harmful effects of anorexia nervosa or bulimia, with emphasis on those who are very ill or who have died as a result of those syndromes.

The news media have focused on anorectic patients during the past few years, leading many to believe that this disorder is peculiar to our times. In fact, it is an entity that was described as long ago as 1689, when the relationship between anorexia, constipation, amenorrhea, and overactivity was recognized. Although the condition is usually considered benign by lay people, fatalities were recorded as far back as 1789.

There are a variety of approaches that have been used in treating the anorectic individual. A purely somatic approach has been taken by some health professionals, increasing the caloric intake from 1,500 to 5,000 calories per day over a 2-week period. If the patient refuses to eat willingly, the decision may be made to force-feed her by means of tube feedings. In other instances, electrostimulative therapy has been used in an effort to produce an anabolic effect on the diencephalic centers of the brain. For some, hospitalization is ordered to separate the person from her family. For others, family therapy on an outpatient basis is regarded as the treatment of choice. Behavior modification is another modality that may be utilized, giving permission for increased physical activity as a reward for weight gain. The fact that the approaches are so divergent is an indication that this is a very difficult disorder to treat.

Why should a person (almost always an adolescent female) choose to starve herself when food is readily available? What kind of person would torture herself in this way? What kind of family would allow this to happen? Health professionals are often at a loss to understand the emaciated patient who forcefully states that nothing is wrong and who is uncomfortable if she gains a few ounces. Nor are they likely to recognize the distorted relationships between the patient and other family members. The patient may exhibit extremely antagonistic behavior to her relatives, yet will fight any attempt to remove her from the home, whether to a hospital, residential school, or other place. She clearly has difficulty in separating, particularly from her mother.

Anorectic patients arouse many negative feelings in care providers. Although the patient sees herself as being appealingly slim, she is more likely to be painfully emaciated. She looks like a skeleton covered with skin, with some ptosis of the abdomen. She often has rampant tooth decay, bluish mottling of her hands and feet, abnormally brittle nails, and very slight breast formation. One eighteen-year-old, who was five feet three inches tall and weighed 76 pounds, denied that she was underweight. The fact that she resembled a concentration camp victim, with her skeletal structure clearly visible under her skin, was not apparent to herself. However, regardless of her physical appearance, it is usually her behavior which alienates those who are trying to help. She is absolutely determined to maintain an emaciated state, denying that she is ill, even appearing somewhat euphoric about her ability to refuse food. She tends to have a very cold manner, an unchanging facial expression, and resists any attempts of the professionals to be friendly. She avoids sharing pertinent information about herself, rarely telling the whole truth about anything. She buys, collects, and stores an oversupply of items that she uses, such as shoes, underwear, linens, or household articles, yet does not use more than two or three of each. She needs the reassurance that things are available should they ever be needed.

Recently it has been noted that anorectic patients who have started to maintain weight that is more appropriate for their height will revert to their previous behavior unless additional help is provided. The use of the antidepressant drug fluoxetine (Prozac) has helped some maintain their new weight level. Because many patients also have symptoms of a major depressive disorder, including irritability, insomnia, a depressed mood and a lack of desire to maintain social or sexual relationships, it is understandable that this drug will help. However, it is not helpful before patients begin to change their eating patterns.

Patients with anorexia nervosa often demonstrate an interest in food and its preparation. They collect recipes, cook, help with the serving, and clean up. In these activities, they appear to emulate the mother/woman role. They will often appear panic stricken if the refrigerator or cupboards are not well stocked with food. Yet when food is served, they eat little, if anything. They manage to push the food around on their plates to give the appearance of having eaten. They also resort to hiding food in their napkins, discarding it in receptacles when unobserved, or eating well and then disappearing into the bathroom to stick their fingers down their throats and forcibly vomit whatever they have swallowed. They use laxatives and enemas as other ways of purging their bodies of food, and exercise vigorously to lose weight.

It is important for health workers to realize that anorexia is only a *symptom* of a pathological state. The use of this particular symptom may be the patient's defense against more overt pathology, such as deep depression or suicidal thoughts. She may use starvation as a way to exert control over herself, her family, and her friends. To cure the symptom without treating the basic problem may well lead to an even more destructive behavior pattern.

Most patients with anorexia nervosa are described as having been very cooperative, pleasant, and highly disciplined during the premorbid phase. They tended to be involved only superficially with others, often fearful of new situations, but deeply entwined with family members. They did as they were told, dressed according to parental wishes, ate as much and as often as they were directed to, and went to bed or arose in accordance with the family rules. They never developed a sense of their own selves or had the opportunity to determine, among other things, whether or not they were hungry or satiated, hot or cold, sleepy or wide awake. If they did attempt to express some feeling, such as, "I'm very cold," it was likely to be invalidated by a comment noting, "You *can't* be cold. It's much too warm in here."

Often the anorectic behavior began the first time the child lived away from home, perhaps at a school or camp. Unable to recognize her satiation point, she continued eating as long as any food was available. In time, it became apparent that the only way to prevent overeating was not to eat at all. If she could not trust her own body to tell her when to stop, it was safer not to start.

In a society which emphasizes youth, beauty, and slender bodies, it is often mothers who coax their daughters to diet. The message, which is also stressed by the media, is that thin is preferable. Still compliant, the young, overweight adolescent begins to diet, and enjoys the praise that she receives from those around her. As time goes on, it becomes apparent to others that the degree of slenderness for which she strives is pathological, that her pursuit of thinness is an obsession as well as a compulsion. The individual's behavior about food changes radically. She refuses any plea to eat, appearing negative and obstinate. The stronger the command to eat, the more resistant the patient becomes, resorting to deceit and trickery if necessary so that she will appear to be eating even though she is not. The household begins to revolve around her.

The patient who is anorectic often recalls the teasing received as a youngster for her obesity, and blames her weight for rejection by friends. The more she was rejected or teased, the more she ate to ease the emotional pain. Although her mother may have appeared to be a caring person on the surface, doing whatever society deemed necessary in terms of household tasks, the history may reveal a lack of closeness between them. Food became a replacement for the missing emotional relationship; if the daughter ate, she accepted the "good" mother who prepared the food. The mother may have been ambivalent about her own role, absenting herself from the home because of work, recreation, or illness. On the other hand, she may have been a compulsive, rigid woman who forced her opinions on the family, demanding that the daughter do as she was told in every area of life.

Control is a very large issue in the life of an anorectic patient. She chooses self-starvation as her ultimate weapon, viewing it not as a self-destructive act, but rather as a way of controlling her own impulses. By not eating, she is making a statement. Even though she may crave food, she will not take it into her body. She alone is in total control of what will enter her body. She, rather than those around her (including her mother or the health care providers), is making the decision.

There are several other components at stake for the patient. Rejecting food, particularly that which has been prepared by her mother, is a covert way of rejecting her mother. The person who finds it difficult to develop an identity of her own within the family may not have the courage to separate from the other members. By rejecting the food provider's offering, she creates hostility in only one area of life. The family rallies around to get her to eat, yet their anger at her continuing use of starvation creates space between them and the patient. It is easier for the anorectic individual to deal with the family's hostility than to lose her hard-earned control over her own impulses.

Sexuality may be another issue for the patient. Most anorectic patients are adolescents who are uncomfortable with their new sexual awareness. They have never become sensitive to their other feelings, such as hunger or exhaustion, because their needs were met before they could be acknowledged. This new sexual sensation, for which they have not been programmed by mother, alarms them. If eating food may lead to a binge, then might a little sexual activity lead to promiscuity? Abstention is clearly the best course. Some adolescents fear pregnancy, equating it with an enlarged abdomen, and thus with eating. For them, self-starvation may be used as a contraceptive action to prevent oral impregnation. Once again, the patient sees herself to be in control of her sexual impulses, which she rejects as unacceptable. In addition, her anorectic state causes amenorrhea, and prevents breast development indicative of womanhood.

One patient recalled viewing her parents in the act of love-making when she was a young child. She heard her mother make sounds which she interpreted as groans of pain, and thought that her parents were doing "terrible and dirty things." She never talked about what she had seen. When her mother's subsequent pregnancy became noticeable, the patient associated it with the primal scene. She unconsciously feared that some man would do "dirty" things to her when she grew up. At the same time, she remembered her mother urging her to eat "so that you can be a mommy like me." Consequently, the patient stopped eating.

The parents of the anorectic patient frequently have a dysfunctional marriage. The patient may view each as having deficiencies and may feel responsible for providing sufficient attention to both to make up for their mutual deprivation. If the mother is away for a length of time, the daughter may be placed in the position of taking care of siblings and father. In one respect she delights in her pseudowifely role, for she can now give her father the understanding that he deserves. On the other hand, she resents being placed in the difficult position of acting as a parent to her siblings. She may have anticipated plaudits from her father for her efforts, but he may be too engrossed with responsibilities or concerns about his wife to offer recognition to the patient. He may repeatedly mention how much he misses his wife and how eager he is for her return. Moreover, the mother may not acknowledge her daughter's efforts either. The patient will see this as further proof that no one, not even a parent, is able to give her the affection and approval that she wants, even if she assumes a womanly role. Again, her anorexia will prevent her from developing or maintaining physical signs of womanhood, menstrual periods and breasts, which are present in her mother.

One hospitalized anorectic patient clearly demonstrated the cause and effect of family problems on the patient. She told of the 2 years her mother spent in a psychiatric hospital when the patient was 5- to 7-years-old. During visiting hours, the mother was too ill to talk to the daughter, which the child then assumed meant that her mother hated her. The father was involved with the five other youngsters in the family and was unable to fill the patient's needs for affection and reassurance. The patient recalled that her father teased her and called her chubby at one point. Even though she was young, the patient was expected to assume some household duties and responsibilities for her younger siblings. She deeply resented this, but said nothing.

At the age of 14, the patient embarked on a self-imposed starvation diet and exercise program, which she was unable to recognize as a self-destructive weapon. She later said, "I felt this was the only way I could exercise some control over my life." The patient began therapy after medical advice had been sought for amenorrhea, hair loss, and her refusal to stop a fanatical exercise routine. Over several years of treatment, she recognized the relationship between her compulsion to be thin and her unconscious anger at her mother, her anger regarding home responsibilities, her need for affection and approval from her father, and her fear of growing up to be a woman like her mother.

Because many health workers are engaged in a personal battle against obesity, they may secretly admire the patient's adherence to a starvation regime. One overweight professional, on seeing the emaciated patient, said, "I'd like to have your illness for a few days." Attitudes such as these reinforce the patient's pathology and render the health worker ineffective in any treatment approach. In addition, the worker may not recognize the manipulative aspects of the patient's behavior, because he identifies with her. For example, the patient may complain relentlessly that she has not been able to defecate, and demand a laxative. The professional may accede to this request, not realizing that the laxative is being used to prevent any weight gain, rather than to treat constipation.

The anorectic patient reacts negatively to authority figures, since they represent the negative parent figure and threaten the control that the patient is exercising over herself. At times, the patient appears to cooperate, perhaps overeating ravenously, in order to make the health workers believe that she is cured. She will then return home and resume her chronic behavior very quickly. She has outsmarted the professionals, which lowers her regard for them and makes her feel that no one can really help her. She again has control of her body through her behavior.

Starvation is an effective fortification of the patient's precarious psychological balance and cannot be stopped for too long. When this symptom is taken away, she finds herself unable to control her other impulses. Having lost her control, she may demonstrate increased pathology, including suicidal behavior. In essence, the control, which she sees as absolute, is really quite tentative. It is an all-or-nothing situation—starvation or binge, with little hope for maintaining a middle road.

Often health workers assigned to anorectic patients resent the fact that they are cast into the role of law enforcement agents, having to check the patient's room and wastebasket for discarded food. They often voice anger that despite their own attempts to be helpful, the patient is unappreciative. The more effective they are, the more deceitful the patient becomes. Yet the involvement of a warm, supporting, and consistent health worker is essential in helping the patient establish her own identity.

Patients with anorexia nervosa object to hospitalization for good reason. An institutional setting encourages regression to a state of greater dependency, the very situation which they are fighting. However, there are times when the patient's physical state has deteriorated to such an extent that immediate medical intervention is required to maintain her life. She may require intravenous as well as tube feedings to supply sufficient fluid and nutrients. She will also need intensive psychotherapy to provide support as she is deprived of her most precious possession, her ability to control what goes into her body. One 16-year-old, enraged by her weight gain and the continuous supervision, proceeded to throw herself down a flight of stairs. Immediate intervention prevented any injury, but the patient announced that she intended to kill herself if necessary in order to escape from the restrictive hospital environment.

Family therapy is often used to change the emotional climate of the home environment. Improvement of the relationship between the parents, as well as between each parent and the patient, is necessary. The family may appear very resistant to this, offering a variety of excuses as to why they cannot institute any changes. If this occurs, it may be helpful to use a therapeutic paradox. To do this, the professional should insist that each family member, including the patient, continue using the same behavior patterns as before.

The patient is once again placed in the position of being told what to do by an authority figure. Because control is the basic issue, she is likely to rebel by refusing to obey to continue her starvation pattern. To do this, she must give up her symptom and eat. The coalition of family against the professional's order is a healthy first step. Therapy with the family has to continue until the relationships are healthier, and the patient is recognized as an autonomous individual, capable of making decisions for herself.

Overeating is another self-destructive behavior that incorporates many of the same patterns as anorexia or bulimia. Patients who are very obese may use overeating to meet psychological needs. Food intake may bring back happy memories of family life, or of childhood rewards for good behavior (lollypops for not crying during a medical examination, cookies for having helped with household tasks). In these cases, food is not associated with hunger, but rather with an attempt to provide feelings of inner warmth and emotional satiation. The compulsive eater is unable to restrain himself, and will continue to eat even though uncomfortable, in an effort to meet his emotional needs.

Patients with bulimia, who binge by overeating and then purge (vomit or use laxatives and/or enemas) to prevent weight gain, tend to have the same manipulative characteristics as anorectics. Their need to control is the same, but they use weight maintenance rather than starvation as their measurement of success. Therefore, although they are *out* of control when they binge, they are *in* control when they purge to maintain the same or lower weight.

Obese patients on diets often suffer bouts of anxiety and depression, and may end their efforts to lose weight because of the ensuing emotional problems. Some become so depressed that they may entertain thoughts of suicide. Some develop a defeatist attitude about dieting because about 50% of dieters return to their initial weights within 3 years, and fewer than 10 percent can be expected to remain below the initial weight for 9 years. Some dieters not only regain the weight, but reach an even higher level once off the diet.

One theory of weight maintenance is that each person has a physiological set point for weight which can be maintained with relative ease. Attempts to lower that set point (dieting, starvation, purging) or to raise it (overeating, bingeing) may be successful, but only for a short period of time. When the individual returns to a free selection of food, he is likely to find himself back at his original weight within a relatively short time. Permanent maintenance of a change in weight requires retraining of the body to a new set point, a difficult and often discouraging task.

Gaining weight, for most people, is far easier than losing, since gaining can incorporate junk foods associated with pleasurable experiences (ice cream, cake, candy), while losing may be equated with self-deprivation and physical discomfort (headaches, hunger pangs, weakness, and ever present thoughts of food).

Many approaches to weight control have been used. Keeping an accurate diary of food and beverage intake usually makes the individual aware of when, where, why, and how much he has eaten. Once the pattern is examined, foods of lower caloric content can be substituted, gradually bringing down the total daily intake. However, unless the patient really *wants* to lose weight, it is unlikely that this or any other method will work. The health worker should remember that overeating may be one way in which the individual can prove that he can do as he pleases with his body, and that taking that control away may cause him to feel helpless, hopeless, and even suicidal.

Some dieters become extremely anxious as they lose weight and receive compliments from others. They may be afraid of being more attractive, with the possibility of becoming actively involved in a love relationship for which they are emotionally unprepared. Others are unhappy at being evaluated for their weight level, feeling that it emphasizes their physical state and ignores their unseen but important inner core. There may be a high level of self-hatred for being obese, but an even greater fear of the consequences of becoming thin.

THE APPROACH TO THE PERSON WITH AN EATING AND WEIGHT DISORDER

Immediate Intervention by the Patient

SELF-MANAGEMENT TECHNIQUES

Recognize the symptoms that activate thoughts about food and refusal to eat, or overindulgence in exercise by the anorectic, and overeating by the obese person.

Professional Intervention

IMMEDIATE ACTION

Be clear about your expectations of the person. Make sure she knows that her participation in treatment is essential. Clear, consistent guidelines reinforce the patient's sense of self-control and increase her confidence in the health workers.

Explain to the patient that room checks may be necessary to validate whether food was eaten or hidden.

Do not become angry at the person's deviant behavior, which may include spilling food on the floor, hiding food in her room, eating in binges, or forcing herself to vomit.

Approach the individual several times daily to assure her of your personal interest. Be consistent when responding to her. Patients with eating disorders tend to be manipulative, playing those involved in their care who are inconsistent against one another.

Give positive reinforcement when the person cooperates.

INTERMEDIATE ACTION

The person should be confronted with her role in any negative behavior while she is being treated. The anorectic may have been riding an exercise bike for several hours, doing vigorous calisthenics, or taking laxatives to lose weight, or, if obese, may have been eating high calorie foods while supposedly on a diet. *Encourage participation of the individual in her treatment by including foods she requests.* Include other items that contribute to a well-balanced diet.

Be aware of your feelings and responses to the patient. If the person uses flattery in an effort to get a special privilege, calmly inform her that you recognize what she is doing. Do not react in an angry manner because that would not be therapeutic.

Engage the patient in a relationship that emphasizes her value as a human being. If the patient can accept you as trustworthy and reliable, she will be more amenable to giving up her symptom on a permanent basis.

Substitute positive activities for concerns about food and exercise. Whenever possible, patients should be encouraged to become involved in volunteer activities that help them concentrate on others, rather than on themselves, and put them in a position of control. If they have the background to do so, they could help tutor students who are falling behind in their school work, or assist the elderly, who need help in daily activities of living.

LONG-TERM ACTION

Encourage the individual to recognize her feelings about her body including hunger, sleepiness, anxiety, and so on.

Keep discussion of food and its intake to a minimum.

Make clear to the person that responsibility and determination for her care is mainly under her control rather than yours. Give the patient choices in as many areas of her care as possible.

Follow up on the techniques utilized by keeping in touch and giving support.

FREQUENTLY PRESCRIBED PSYCHIATRIC DRUGS

Psychiatric drugs frequently prescribed for eating disorders include the following:

Bulimia: amitriptyline (Elavil, Etrafon, Triavil), desipramine (Norpramin)
Anorexia: fluoxetine (Prozac)

25

The Person With a Substance-Related Disorder

An individual with a substance-related disorder can become dependent on anything that strikes his fancy. He spends as much of his waking time as he can pursuing that substance, often causing changes in his "normal" life patterns. Often there is a large component of denial, with the person unable to accept the fact that he is in the grips of an addiction.

Some actions are seen as having positive components. For example, a liquor salesman is expected to treat his buyers to a drink as he extols the virtues of his product. If, however, the salesman drinks too much, so that his speech is slurred, his actions become unacceptable, and he is noticeably out of control, what was positive becomes negative. If he refuses to accept his actions as indicating a problem, he may enter a state of denial, stating that "everyone does it," and that all liquor salesmen drink as much as, if not more than, he does.

Another part of denial is evident as the individual refutes the problem by stating that the substance use is limited to certain days or hours, and that he can stop whenever he chooses. The good feelings associated with the substance use reinforce the belief that it is all right to continue the pattern. The use of illicit drugs may help blunt feelings of loneliness or alienation, or the sense of having been abandoned or abused by an uncaring family. The drugs may also lessen his belief that he is a failure at work or in school, dulling his feelings to the extent that he does not have the energy to solve the causative problem.

Difficulty in abstaining often occurs when the person suffers a loss of energy, a lack of feeling, and/or irritability. He may place the blame for his continuing substance dependence on his spouse, friends, or coworkers, stating that they are provoking him. He then depends on the preferred substance to return himself to his normal demeanor and activities. As long as he continues this self-destructive pattern, he will not be amenable to treatment. Once he understands the relationship between his actions and the underlying problem, he may decide to seek help.

Some people have great difficulty in understanding how others can become addicted to drugs including alcohol. For them, "just say no" makes sense. By the same token, they may not recognize the addictive properties of tobacco, nor the multiple dangers attached to its use. They connect tobacco use to lung cancer, but are unaware that it may also cause cancer of the bladder, cervix, esophagus, cheeks, mouth (lips and tongue), and throat. It is also associated with emphysema, chronic bronchitis, heart disease, cerebrovascular accidents, and the signs of aging skin. It is a dangerous substance, capable of raising blood pressure, increasing blood clotting, reducing the supply of oxygen to the heart and other organs, damaging arterial walls, and causing peripheral vascular disease.

Nor does the damage stop with the smoker. If the patient is a pregnant woman, she is at risk for a miscarriage or difficult delivery. Her child will probably be smaller than average, and be at greater risk for upper respiratory problems, and even for the possibility of dying. In addition, those nonsmokers who are in close physical contact with smokers may absorb some of the contaminants found in second-hand smoke, products that are responsible for thousands of lung cancer deaths in those innocent bystanders.

Presentation of the facts does not result in an end to smoking. The ease with which cigarettes can be obtained, the fact that they are legal, and their relative inexpensiveness all lessen the sense of importance concerning giving up the habit. For some, the benefits of smoking make them reluctant to give up the use of tobacco. Those with weight problems may rely on it to curb their appetites. Some schizophrenic patients may have a temporary improvement in sensory gating with less confusion caused by their inability to block out the overstimulation they sense from extraneous environmental stimuli. They may also find their ability to concentrate improves, and that they have increased relief from their antipsychotic medications when smoking.

Those who try to stop smoking have described the habit as more difficult to give up than heroin or cocaine. Years after trying to give it up, they may still relapse, with cravings suffered even 10 years later. It is estimated that there are about 45 million smokers in the United States, and that another 50 million have stopped but with difficulty. The aim of the federal government is to prevent today's adolescents from starting because those who smoke two or more cigarettes a day are likely to become addicted.

Whenever one uses a prescribed or unprescribed drug (including alcohol) on an excessive and continuous basis, one flirts with the possibility of becoming dependent on that substance, unable to function properly or get through the day without it. The need for the drug interferes with many aspects of life. For instance, the individual may be so physically ill without the drug that he is unable to work. Or, if he is working, he may crave more of the drug to keep up his mood. He may become irritable, nasty, short-tempered, and rude to his friends and coworkers when unable to have it. At home, his family may feel that he is a bit secretive about himself. They don't appreciate his not coming to family gatherings, hardly ever showing up for dinner, and not pitching in with the household duties. But they excuse him because, "Well, that's his nature," and besides he probably is just "going through a stage." It certainly seems that way when one minute he seems happy and content and only a few hours later is miserable and desperate. Other changes may be noticed: his appearance is unkempt, schoolwork suffers, interests and hobbies aren't sustained.

All too often the health worker views the person as resistant, hostile, and ungrateful. This has validity because when a person is under the influence of an addicting substance, he can indeed be difficult, and can be expected to deny his problem totally. This is part of the illness, and demands frequent exploration by health professionals.

If health professionals are very sympathetic, viewing the dependent person as one who "drinks only as much as I do," or as someone who is "only enjoying himself like my old grandfather did," they are unlikely to convince the patient that he needs treatment and rehabilitation. If, conversely, health professionals are judgmental, viewing the person as weak, sinful, degraded, and worthless, they are also likely to be unsuccessful in approaching the patient therapeutically.

Each health professional should develop an awareness of his own attitudes toward drug use. These usually stem from his association with members of his family or significant others whom he may have met through social, educational, religious, political, or professional affiliations. For example, if the health professional had an assaultive parent who abused alcohol, the worker is apt to view the alcoholic as a disgusting, and hateful person to be feared.

Our society imparts conflicting messages. Some drugs and alcohol are all right but only if you don't get "hooked." Once dependence develops, the individual is often regarded with disdain. It is vital that the health worker accept substance-related disorders both on emotional and intellectual levels, as a treatable disease.

The addicted person loses his willpower as a result of the substance on which he is dependent. Most want to get well but don't know how. The help and guidance of the health worker who has already worked through personal conflicts and received proper education regarding addiction is important. No group, race, religion, or profession is immune to the disease. Everyone is vulnerable. If drug or alcohol use leads to misuse and then abuse, it becomes an illness that can shorten the patient's life.

Some drugs have a calming effect (downs), and others have a stimulating effect (ups). Taking drugs seems to be more common with the adolescent and young adult, while excessive alcohol consumption seems to be more common as one approaches middle age. However, no age group is immune from the possibility of becoming addicted to either drugs or alcohol. It is rare to find a family that has not been personally touched by some aspect of the addiction problem.

Most substance-dependent individuals have had some psychological problems before starting to use drugs. Many first tried drugs or alcohol to help cope with their troubles, or to be accepted by their peers. Still others felt that certain substances helped ease some of their daily tensions or handling of responsibilities, providing a way of coping with stress.

Sometimes the effect of a drug on an addicted individual is visible to others who note a definite change in the person's behavior. The drinker may become very jolly, sociable, outgoing, and assertive. Or he may become nostalgic, sad, weepy, and retreat from others. Users of the so-called psychedelic drugs (amphetamines, LSD, marijuana) hope to feel a stimulating, exhilarating (high) effect. At times, they may have an unexpected effect (a "bad trip"), with terrifying feelings and depression that may lead to a psychosis.

The benefits of using the substance, according to the user, are the gaining of an ecstatic feeling, a sense of being in touch with one's unconscious, and an ability to think more clearly and relax completely. Whatever a person's reasons, there seems to be a relationship between dependency and the personality of the user. The more immature and unstable the person, the greater is the risk of substance dependence or abuse.

Generally, the person who is addicted is one who usually feels "low," centers his thoughts on himself and his needs, is bored easily, has difficulty tolerating any anxiety or coping with any frustrating situations or drives, finds few satisfactions in life, and seeks a continual state of bliss. It is not unusual for the patient to tell the health worker that he was first introduced to drugs by friends and that he really isn't addicted. He will defend the viewpoint that drugs are helpful to him, not harmful. He will steadfastly maintain that he really doesn't need them, despite the fact that he seeks drugs at every opportunity.

In the general hospital, it is not uncommon to meet an addict who was admitted to the hospital for some condition other than his addiction—backache, abdominal cramps, possible gallbladder disease, intestinal obstruction, or a severe headache. Only after nothing is found to be wrong organically does it become apparent that the patient is requesting pain medication every three to four hours.

On the psychiatric unit, the health worker may come into contact with individuals who have developed serious psychiatric complications because of the excessive use of drugs or alcohol. Many of these patients have had longstanding problems because of an unstable personality. The effect of the drug may increase the difficulties, bring out problems that were not obvious previously, or result in a psychosis. One patient who was experiencing a severe depressive reaction took some drugs, thinking that perhaps they would help her. Instead she had auditory hallucinations that coaxed her to run into the path of an oncoming bus.

Whether the patient with a substance-related disorder is on the psychiatric, medical, surgical unit, or in the community, the health worker will usually find him very demanding, wanting what he wants when he wants it, particularly his pain medication. He is easily upset at having to wait, and threatens to sign himself out of the hospital, or calls his doctor, or reports the staff members to the supervisor. His need for attention is always urgent, as are all his requests. He finds the change of shift a particularly desirable time to renew requests and complaints because the fresh staff is less likely to check thoroughly on how many previous doses of pain medication he has received. The staff may even feel that unless they comply with his demands, there will be a scene that will prolong their time on duty. The patient will tell the staff coming on duty how terrible those on the other shift were. Lying convincingly, he will swear that he has been promised medication anytime he wants it. His idea is to manipulate the staff into meeting his needs through flattery, inducing guilt, or questioning their competence. Incidentally, these patients have a glib tongue and are rather persuasive. Everything they say or swear to should be taken with a large grain of salt.

At the same time, the patient is easily provoked. He will walk away, become angry, yell, become highly indignant and even abusive when he is confronted or thwarted. His tolerance for frustration is practically nonexistent.

Because most of those who are substance dependent or abusers deny that they need drugs or alcohol, it is not uncommon for them to resent any help. They often view the health worker as a threatening person, an authority who is out to catch them. Thus the individual may be very careful and guarded with the worker. He does not want to be judged or rejected, as he may have been by others.

The health worker should bear in mind that the person has developed a physical dependence on the drug. Whether his continued need results from his psychological difficulties and/or is due to a neurochemical imbalance, which continues even after detoxification, is currently being investigated. If it is due to an imbalance, then the addict will need continuous treatment, much as a diabetic requires insulin. An example of this is the use of methadone to curb the desire for heroin. However, regardless of the cause, the health worker's feelings, attitudes, and interest in this illness are crucial to maintaining a sustained and helpful approach to the patient who are addicted or dependent.

THE APPROACH TO THE PERSON WITH A SUBSTANCE-RELATED DISORDER

Immediate Intervention by the Patient

SELF-MANAGEMENT TECHNIQUES

Recognize the discomfort associated with not having used the substance recently, and of situations or places that trigger his desire for the substance. Teach him to substitute more helpful activities when feeling stress, such as walking, running, reading, listening to music, playing an instrument, or using a computer.

Learn to avoid areas or friends that will make the substances readily available or acceptable. Recognize those behaviors likely to promote the use of a substance. For example, if the individual has gotten into the habit of lighting a cigarette when speaking on the telephone, watching television, reading, or relaxing, sucking on a straw or a noncaloric candy may be helpful.

Professional Intervention

IMMEDIATE ACTION

Remove any substances that may be involved with the patient's dependency problem.

Support the friendships and activities that are not associated with the substance.

Help the patient become aware of any depression that precedes or follows his substance use. Life stresses may result in an overdose that will lead to death that may or may not be accidental.

Distract the patient as soon as he appears to want to revert to the undesirable behavior. Make him aware of the target symptom.

Support the patient in his effort to abstain. Discourage him from substituting another unacceptable behavior, such as overeating.

Help the patient find alternative behaviors that are acceptable to him.

If you are a substance user (e.g., a smoker), try to stop. Above all, do not let the patient see you smoking or using any other substance.

Remember that treatment is usually long term and slow. Those who care for substance abusers or addicts must have a great deal of patience. Be aware of your own feelings. If you dislike, feel angry toward, or look down on those with substance-related disorders, do not work with them if you can avoid the assignment. Do not argue with the patient when he defends his right to do as he pleases.

Set up a flexible but consistent therapeutic schedule. This will provide opportunities for the patient to find ways to fulfill himself without resorting to his usual addictive pattern. Promote activities and interests that provide a feeling of satisfaction. Use films and documentaries that do not make substance use appealing and that stress moderation in all activities.

INTERMEDIATE ACTION

Talk to the patient about previous substance use. Help the patient recognize his substance use as an unacceptable aid to socialization or increasing his self-esteem.

Help the patient realize the extent of his reliance on whatever the substance is. Help him discover other ways of meeting his emotional needs.

Help the patient focus on the underlying causes of the involvement with substances. Teach him how to cope with or avoid situations that threaten his abstinence. Stress the importance of ongoing involvement in individual or group therapy, or, if appropriate, the use of agonist medications.

Give attention to the patient's physical condition, appearance, and safety. Involvement in drug use or alcohol tends to diminish interest in many aspects of self-care. Be aware of other actions that are also associated with abuse: cigarette smokers may have burns on clothing as well as on furniture. (Smoking in bed may result in fires leading to severe body burns, even death.) Gamblers may forgo eating for days when deeply involved in games involving high stakes. Those addicted to food may eat nonstop, even though not hungry, ignoring the possibility of physical illness from their excessive intake. Joggers may continue to run even in the throes of exhaustion or physical pain.

Firmly but kindly describe any episodes that occurred while the patient was under the influence of drugs or alcohol. Video tapes of patients during such episodes offer irrefutable evidence to those who deny their behavior. If the patient refuses help, saying he can do it himself, encourage him to evaluate his progress at intervals. In time, he may agree to enter treatment.

Be aware of your own drinking and drug habits. Do not use them as a guideline in determining whether or not the patient has an addiction or dependency.

Educate the patient regarding the disease. Don't advise a patient to "cut down." If he could, he would have done so long ago. This is the crux of the patient's difficulty. Once he starts drinking, taking drugs, or engaging in the activity to which he is addicted, he loses all control and is unable to stop.

Remember that most addicts have unresolved emotional problems. Initially, the addict may have used drugs as a way of asserting his independence or to express anger toward his parents or other authority figures. He may also have deep-rooted feelings of inadequacy, and is using drugs to make himself feel more able to cope. Since drinking or drug use most often begins in the home, family members also need education. Let the family know that covering up the addiction problem out of guilt and shame only adds to the problem.

LONG-TERM ACTION

Remember that the patient has a deep problem that he is trying to solve through drink, drugs, or destructive actions. Do not moralize or scold him for his behavior. Others undoubtedly have done this, and it is not effective. Help him realize that his behavior is a symptom of his illness. If addicted to drugs, he is also likely to be depressed and anxious and to suffer from insomnia, gastritis, and unexplained bruises that are often due to unremembered falls.

Do not directly confront the patient because he has a low tolerance for frustration. He probably will balk and reject any confrontation. Do not involve him in anxiety-producing situations. Instead, begin with an individual interaction to let him know that you are concerned and interested in him. Discuss his acting-out behavior as it occurs. Help him develop some awareness of his strengths and abilities. This builds ego strength and improves his self-concept.

Realize that relapses can occur, as with any illness. Do not expect the addicted patient to always be in control. Remember that loss of control and an irrational need to use drugs, tobacco, or alcohol or to continue his addictive behavior is a prime manifestation of his illness.

Help the patient set up a reward system for himself if it appeals to him. Women may find it helpful to reward themselves with a cosmetic treat; men may want to buy something in relation to a hobby with the money they have saved by not purchasing substances related to their problem.

Encourage the patient's participation in community groups, such as Smoke Enders, Overeaters Anonymous, Gamblers Anonymous, or Alcoholics Anonymous. His family should be encouraged to join the companion groups, such as Alanon or Alateen.

Encourage patients who are addicted to excessive work, sports, or other activities to develop additional interests while practicing moderation in all.

FREQUENTLY PRESCRIBED PSYCHIATRIC DRUGS

Psychiatric drugs frequently prescribed for substance-related disorders include the following:

Alcoholism: disulfiram (Antabuse), acamprosate

Cocaine withdrawal: Desipramine (Norpramin)

Anti-Tobacco aide: The nicotine patch, special chewing gum, cigarettes used in series with decreasing amounts of nicotine (Nicorette), or bupropion HCI (zyban)

26

The Person With Post-Traumatic Stress Disorder (PTSD)

Stress following traumatic incidents can cause acute or chronic symptoms that leave the individual psychologically impaired for many years, possibly for life. The symptoms of this disorder may not become apparent until years after the causative event and, therefore, may not be recognized by the health professional. In addition, this disorder usually has an effect on all those who are involved with the patient, and may be a major factor in emotional illness found in the patient's offspring.

Victims of PTSD have been exposed to a situation capable of producing an intense reaction of distress in anyone facing a similar circumstance. Examples are (a) victims who have been tortured or beaten savagely, without provocation; (b) survivors of the Holocaust in Germany, or of the atomic bomb explosions in Japan at the end of World War II; (c) the survivors of starvation and disease, such as occurred in Ethiopia in the mid-1980s; (d) the surviving victims of political outrages in various parts of the world, including those who have been kidnapped or held incommunicado for periods of time; (e) survivors of freak car, train, or aircraft accidents, fires, or collapse of buildings or other structures; and (f) victims of environmental catastrophes. The most recent publicized evidence of PTSD has been associated with the Oklahoma City bombing.

In 1995, a U.S. terrorist bombed a federal building in Oklahoma City, leaving 168 dead victims and an additional 500 wounded. The most difficult emotional involvement of all who were there was due to the injuries and deaths of the many children at the day care center in the building where the bomb exploded. Many of the survivors or relatives found themselves unable to concentrate on anything but the disaster over a long time. Any loud noise or explosive sound brought back the memories and terror connected to the bombing. Even citizens who were not directly affected, but who had seen the event on television, became concerned for their own and loved one's safety. Radio and newspaper reports added to the immediacy of the reaction.

The definition of PTSD has undergone revision since it was first described in the 1980 Diagnostic Manual published by the American Psychiatric Association. In the earlier version, it was thought to be a somewhat normal, predictable reaction to an overwhelming, terrifying experience. Presently, it is recognized as trauma not only as experienced by the individual, but as it may potentially affect others who hear of it, or are spectators, depending on their vulnerability. Those who have suffered previous trauma are more likely to be affected by this additional stress, again feeling helpless in the face of the event. For example, women who have been raped are three times more likely to develop PTSD if raped again. About a quarter of Vietnam veterans with PTSD reported they had suffered physical or sexual abuse as children.

Nurses who reported to the emergency areas after Hurricane Andrew or the Oklahoma City bombing did whatever was necessary to help the other emergency workers. The specialists in trauma care found their skills were invaluable at the onset, setting up and working in makeshift operating room areas. Psychiatric nurses initiated and staffed critical incident stress management units, going from area to area as they were needed. Their treatment was available for the wounded, the survivors, the families and the rescue workers, around the clock. In Oklahoma City, parents searching for their children were particularly traumatized as they realized that many of the youngsters would not be able to supply their names or other identifying information, forcing the parents to rely on descriptions of children that might lead them to the right hospital or morgue area. Those whose children died, or were severely wounded, found themselves unable to function, eat, or sleep as they tried to comprehend their loss.

Other nurses, with or without specialty training, joined in by calling on skills long unused, but now needed. Regardless of how demeaning the tasks might be, the volunteers carried them out as well as they could. Dr. Patricia

Ann Clunn of the University of Miami School of Nursing, observing the after-effects of Hurricane Andrew, found that those survivors who did something active, who touched or were touched physically, who accepted themselves and their own reactions fared better than those who tried to participate as uninvolved and detached workers. In many instances, symptoms of PTSD did not appear until 2 years after the hurricane.

During the actual event, some victims dissociate from the experience by imagining that they are watching someone else as victim. In this way, they do not bear the full brunt of the experience. If this becomes chronic, it prevents the resolution of the sense of helplessness and may even result in amnesia for the event. For some who have been abused over a long period, the use of dissociation may result in the development of alter egos unaware of each other's existence. This dissociative identity disorder (formerly called multiple personality disorder) prevents the resolution of the underlying problem.

There are rarely sufficient professional workers to care for all the victims in a catastrophe. Untrained volunteers must be integrated into the numbers of health care professionals, helping under supervision. Some professionals later feel a great sense of guilt that they had to rely on those volunteers rather than recognizing the importance of including nonprofessionals. In some geographical areas, the victims may be primarily from another culture, with little understanding or trust in what professionals are doing. It is important to include any volunteers from that population, using any safe suggestions that they may offer, to help victims accept the professionals' treatments. The sense of helplessness and inadequacy experienced by some of the professionals may result in even their showing the recognizable symptoms of PTSD.

Three levels of symptoms become apparent among those with PTSD. At first, the victims show signs of hyperalertness or hyperarousal, are easily startled, irritable, unable to sleep well, possibly agitated and unable to concentrate on the tasks at hand. During the next level, there are episodes of involuntarily reexperiencing the episode in flashbacks, nightmares, and memories, particularly when confronted with sounds, sights, or odors reminiscent of the event. On the third level, the victim may endure emotional numbing or constriction as the effort to block all thoughts and feelings becomes paramount. Some try to do this by turning to alcohol or other drugs. Some can no longer trust others, and find themselves feeling shame and guilt about what they have gone through.

One Vietnam veteran remembered shooting children who would invade the combat area at night, as they threw grenades at the sleeping soldiers. He remembered the screams of the wounded children as they were dying. After returning home, he would react to his own screaming children, reliving the nights in Vietnam. Even years later, the sounds of screaming children would fill him with terror and fear that he would harm them. At the urging of the therapist, he visited the Vietnam War Memorial in Washington, D.C. There, he was able to cry as he recognized names of comrades who had died. This was the first step in getting in touch with the emotions bottled up for so long.

Vietnam veterans, like other PTSD victims, are frequently beset by memories of past events. Their reexperiencing of events that occurred while in Vietnam intrudes into their dreams, resulting in flashbacks so real that they may physically abuse others in a reenactment of an incident. Some veterans, fearful of the possibility of violence while dreaming, develop sleep disorders, including difficulty in falling asleep or frequent episodes of wakefulness during the night. There may be times during the day in which an occurrence, sound, or thought stimulates memories all too vividly, distracting the individual from working on the tasks at hand. This contributes to difficulty in holding on to jobs.

Some PTSD victims resort to drugs (including alcohol) to deaden their thoughts, pain, and memories, with the hope of a night of dreamless sleep. They may also be deeply depressed, primarily as a result of unresolved anger at having been in a situation over which they had no control. A sense of hopelessness is another frequent symptom, as is a psychic numbing that prevents trusting or caring for others.

Most PTSD victims detach themselves from others, fearing closeness. One of the contributing factors may be a sense of guilt for having survived, while others (friends, relatives, associates) did not. Even though it might have been impossible to prevent the deaths of others, as in the gassing of Holocaust victims or the slaying of a comrade by the enemy in Vietnam, the survivors may believe that they, too, should have died.

The sense of loss is often so great, the pain so unbearable, that it becomes safer for those with PTSD to remain isolated and never again have feelings or concerns about others. This detachment even prevents closeness with spouse and children, and often results in marital and familial discord. Their children often grow up with a sense of never having loved or been loved by that parent, and are likely to perpetuate the same sense of detachment in their future personal relationships.

Some survivors are guilt-ridden about the actions that they took to remain alive. Disasters and wars are never "nice" events, and often require antisocial actions (brutality, killing, ignoring the injured) that are acceptable only in the context of the moment. PTSD victims are often horrified and sickened by the actions they either undertook on their own or carried out under orders from those higher in command. Thoughts about these actions may have been repressed or suppressed to survive at the moment. It is only later, when the pressure of the situation is gone, that moral judgments come into play and the full horror of what they have done comes into consciousness. Some, perhaps most, are unable to discuss their experiences fully, fearing the disgust and disapproval of the listener. Health care professionals must be capable of listening without placing value judgments on any material that the victim is able to share. Unless this is so, the patient will remain isolated and unreachable.

PTSD victims must be treated individually, with consideration given to their pretrauma personalities. Those with stable backgrounds have a greater chance of overcoming (or never developing) disabling symptoms. Those with unstable backgrounds may not have developed coping mechanisms to deal with every-day stresses, let alone catastrophic occurrences. The health worker should be aware of any contributory life experiences in order to help the victim understand his reactions.

THE APPROACH TO THE PERSON WITH PTSD

Immediate Intervention by the Patient

SELF-MANAGEMENT TECHNIQUES

Help the patient to recognize the target symptoms that cause him to remember the original trauma. Teach him to use abdominal breathing and relaxation exercises to help him relax whenever the thoughts recur (see p. 00). Encourage him to talk about the experience. Whenever feasible, he should try to help others going through the same type of trauma.

Professional Intervention

IMMEDIATE ACTION

Evaluate the symptoms demonstrated by the patient. Depression, guilt, hopelessness, and grief, as well as unrelenting and free-flowing rage, are all symptoms that may be present in varying degrees. Some feelings may be repressed and will require an atmosphere of acceptance by the health professional before they are likely to be expressed.

Establish trust by accepting the victim's story nonjudgmentally. Remember that whatever occurred was beyond the patient's control, and something for which his normal coping mechanisms were inadequate. Do not express shock or revulsion at his description of events or his own responses or actions.

INTERMEDIATE ACTION

Encourage the patient to regain control of his life. The patient should be helped to discuss situations that have resulted in loss of control, recognizing the precipitating factors as well as any contributory experiences from his pre-trauma life. He may need help in devising strategies to cope with future events that might cause him to lose control.

Encourage the patient to express anger in an acceptable way. Expressions of anger should be converted from possible abuse of individuals to physical activity vigorous enough to displace it, such as chopping wood, hitting a punching bag, or pounding dough for bread. Once beyond the need to strike out physically, the patient should be helped to substitute verbal expression of his feelings for physical actions.

LONG-TERM ACTION

Help the patient to accept and forgive himself for actions taken in relation to the traumatic event. Encourage him to take part in any public events related to the traumatic event as a way of identifying with other victims. Many Vietnam veterans found emotional relief in attending the parade honoring them on the 10th anniversary of the end of that war. Victims of the Nazi Holocaust also find that involvement in yearly observances allows them to examine and express their feelings and come to terms with their experiences.

Remember that caretakers have also undergone severe stress, with exposure to sights and incidents for which they may never have been prepared. It is important to help them through any feelings of guilt as well as an acceptance of their own limitations while involved in the catastrophic events.

27

The Person Who Is Bereaved

Bereaved individuals display a steady, continuous affect of sadness. They cry, have difficulty falling or staying asleep, and eat little or overeat without being aware that they are doing so. Usually they complain of weariness, although they have the strength to manage themselves. They are anxious, and their memory may be poor. Their feeling of being dependent and needing people to help them increases. Sometimes such patients become clinging, almost helpless. However, most grieving patients are well oriented and in good contact with reality. Their self-esteem may not be threatened or appreciably compromised.

Grief is usually due to a loss the patient has already sustained or one that is anticipated. People grieve for various kinds of losses—a very dearly loved person or pet; a material thing such as a boat, house, or diamond ring; or even for an opportunity that has passed them by. The feelings of bereavement resulting from loss usually subside gradually. Sometimes, however, the reaction to the loss does not subside, and hospitalization is required. This does not mean that the patient is not grieving, but rather that there may be preexisting conflicts and difficulties that interfere with resolution of the grief. The new situation uncovers other problem areas that had previously been dormant. The health worker should be aware that anyone with unresolved difficulties may have a grief reaction that can result in a potentially serious depression.

People who have a normal response to grief do not require hospitalization. Their extreme distress abates within a reasonable period (rarely before six weeks or beyond two months). They adjust to their loss and do not blame themselves for that which could not be prevented. Friends and family help by allowing them to talk about their feelings without feeling ashamed or humiliated.

Those unable to function because of their inability to accept the loss, who continue to dwell on it while berating and condemning themselves, probably need psychiatric treatment. Such a reaction to a permanent, irretrievable loss is illustrated by the following cases: a young woman whose lesbian partner deserted her for someone else was beset by a constant feeling of sadness and inability to concentrate on her college courses; a mother whose child died from leukemia was unable to have satisfactory sexual relations with her husband; and a woman whose dog was killed by a car cried openly for weeks.

Anticipated losses may also trigger a grief response. Examples of mourning for losses in advance include the college-bound adolescent anticipating the loss of family life; the woman whose husband is drafted to serve in the army anticipating changes in her life pattern; and the man transferred to a new job fearing the loss of old friends and status.

A loss usually involves someone or something that has a special meaning or significance for the loser. Without the loved one, the bereft individual feels he will be less capable, less able to function, and less happy. The loss may be interpreted as a rejection, causing concern about possible rejection by other meaningful people in the future. The individual experiences feelings of guilt. For instance, one woman whose spouse died felt that she had not been warm and loving enough during their life together, and now it was too late; she began to experience deep remorse. Another patient expressed the feeling of not having done enough to help care for his wife during her lingering illness. Still another patient experienced moderate grief but had intense guilt feelings when his wife died from multiple sclerosis in a nursing home; he felt that placing her there contributed to her death.

Some individuals verbalize their anger in their grief. A college student related that his father's death meant that he no longer could continue attending an elite university. His important plans for the future were now interrupted, and he was angry.

In normal bereavement, the individual does not blame himself inappropriately for the loss. Although there may be a feeling of being adrift or empty, the person's self-esteem is not lowered. The grief can usually be worked through with help from supportive friends and family who provide the opportunity to express feelings regarding the loss.

Some individuals show very little overt reaction to the loss at the actual time it occurs, demonstrating an avoidance of emotional discomfort. Instead, they may not react until an apparently minor incident occurs, triggering the grief reaction. One patient accepted her 23-year-old daughter's death from leukemia and returned to work almost immediately, functioning well for more than a year. Then her talkative parakeet died and she became tearful, began ruminating over her loss, and complained of weariness to the point where she could no longer continue in her job. In another case, a man whose son was killed in a car accident continued seemingly well until 6 months later when his car (which had previously belonged to his son) broke down and needed extensive repairs. He became morose, irritable, and wept openly that life would never be the same again. Many individuals are unable to grieve during the funeral for a loved one, but become very emotional during subsequent funerals. This may be so even when those deaths involve people to whom they are not close. In effect, they are grieving for their own loss.

The length of grieving, the intensity of the symptoms, the degree of disturbing thoughts, the relevance of behavior (reality contact), the pressure of delusions, and the extent to which the individual's living is diminished in proportion to the particular loss involved, help the worker to make some conceptual distinction between neurotic depression (a reactive grief) and psychotic depression. For example, an elderly man who lost his wife following a lengthy illness became quite sad and stopped taking part in the many activities they had previously participated in jointly. For a while all he could think about was his wife and the happy times they shared together. He cried a great deal and complained of insomnia and fatigue. This continued for 2 months at which time a close friend insisted that he see a doctor. The doctor advised that he join a bereavement group. In the therapeutic environment, the widower began to accept his loss. He began to interact with others in the group who had had similar experiences and were working on ways of dealing with their difficulties. He found he was able to concentrate when distracted from his loss. Suicidal thoughts related to his sense of hopelessness diminished. His self-esteem increased as the void in his life was replaced with renewed interest in old hobbies and involvement in group activities. Gradually his grief was relieved, and he returned to his normal pattern of life.

If a patient's grief is prolonged, he may begin to idealize the deceased to deny the negative aspects of the relationship. For example, a 45-year-old patient who had lost her husband 5 years earlier claimed that he was the most fantastic, kind, brilliant, caring man in the world. No one could ever be as good a provider, as devoted a husband and father. After many weeks in group therapy, she identified with the angry feelings expressed by another participant who spoke of her husband's authoritarianism and inflexibility. The patient began to recognize her own feelings of having felt stifled during her marriage, as well as her failure to assert herself when it came to making decisions or disciplining her children. Her reliance on her husband, and her passivity, kept peace in the household. As she expressed her previously suppressed anger, her need to deny her feelings and the glorification of her spouse lessened considerably.

When grief is prolonged (as in a reactive depression) the individual continues to dwell on the loss, experiences guilt, and condemns himself for what has happened. His suffering becomes abnormal and, if not treated, may progress to a deep depression. (See "The Person With a Depressive Disorder," pp. 00–00.)

Although a loss may be accepted, the adjustments, disruptions, and changes in other aspects of a person's life may prove to be overwhelming when superimposed on the initial trauma. Such was the case of the patient whose husband was drafted into military service. She dealt with the separation fairly well. However, the subsequent loss of social relationships as married friends no longer extended invitations to "singles," coupled with the financial hardship resulting from her husband's lower income as an army employee, were additional stresses that she responded to with grief. In another case, a very competent woman learned that her husband was going to leave her for a woman older than herself. She blamed herself for not doing enough to hold the marriage together. Besides the loss of her husband, she had to face a disturbing legal procedure. Her previously stable household was destroyed, and the care of her children without their father was overwhelming. She became grief-ridden and dwelt on the loss of her past happiness. Both of the cases cited here involved the effects of harsh and sudden changes in circumstances that caused a reactive depression (grief) which was neither neurotic nor psychotic.

The grief reaction of a person experiencing a loss will vary according to how the loss is interpreted. This is usually dependent on the depth and quality of the relationship involved and past experiences and associations with the lost object or relationship. For example, a patient who had felt deserted by her parents when she was hospitalized for several years as a small child, reacted with uncontrollable grief when they moved to another state, although she was by this time a seemingly well-adjusted adult. She interpreted her parents' move as another desertion and relived the intense trauma of her childhood.

Similarly, a 25-year-old woman was immobilized by grief after her lover ended their 2-year relationship. This rejection rekindled memories of her parents' divorce and her father's remarriage and relocation to another state when she was 16 years old. Her grief was, in fact, based on the earlier incident, which she had never resolved.

One factor which may influence grief reactions is the degree to which the person anticipated or prepared for the loss. Another factor is the extent of trust the person has in his ability to survive alone. Steps taken to assure continuity for the survivor are important. For example, a woman whose spouse was terminally ill with cancer spent the year preceding his death becoming acquainted with all their legal and financial affairs. She enlisted his help in learning how to manage their situation. In addition, she enrolled in a secretarial review course. When her spouse died, she grieved, but the knowledge that she could continue on her own did much to prevent her grief from becoming destructive.

Similarly, all patients who enter the hospital experience a sense of loss. Hospitalization is a stressful period because it entails separation from family and friends, loss of one's normal roles, loss of a familiar and comfortable environment, and possibly loss of income or savings.

Patients who recognize that their reaction to the separation or loss is only temporary are able to find comfort in the knowledge that they will recover. Get-well cards, calls, and visits from friends also help to reassure patients that they have not really been deserted. Thus, their self-esteem is not appreciably decreased, and their reaction is minimal with little real discomfort. For example, one patient may react by complaining of inability to obtain adequate rest at night. Still another may complain of rumbling in his stomach and of not being able to eat as well as usual. Both complaints can be related to the patient's stress during his period of hospitalization.

THE APPROACH TO THE BEREAVED PERSON

Immediate Intervention by the Patient

SELF-MANAGEMENT TECHNIQUES

Teach the patient to recognize the target symptom that increases normal bereavement to the psychotic level (sleep disturbance, appetite changes, disinterest in appearance as well as family and monetary affairs). Immediately institute plans to become actively involved in necessary family matters, nutrition, and appearance.

Professional Intervention

IMMEDIATE ACTION

Accept the person's tears. Halting tears is not necessarily an objective, but if the individual is able to stop his crying, it may be reassuring to him to realize that he has regained a measure of self-control. Ask him to look directly at you, and talk with him.

Express interest in the person as a physical being. Interest is shown by asking when he last showered, how he slept the previous night, and whether or what he ate. This helps the patient feel cared for and enhances his self-esteem.

Supervise the individual's physical care. Gently correct his bathing or mouth care habits; his table manners. Avoid harshness. Remember that maintaining a good physical appearance often influences one's mood. Encourage the patient to use the hospital beautician or barber, if one is available.

Facilitate eye contact by sitting where you can be seen. Although the person may be unable to respond initially, remember that he still needs attention. The worker must initiate the approach. The person feels lost, isolated, and as though he is carrying a burden. He is unable to ask for help. Interrupt his preoccupation by directing him toward former interests. Support his endeavors. Don't rush him or insist that he answer you.

Help the person to confine his thinking to the here and now. Do not talk about the future because he is unable to see that far. Help him identify his present feelings in relation to his loss (i.e., his denial, anger, and bewilderment). Explain that these feelings are common in people who have suffered a loss. He can accept his feelings about his illness better if you allow him to talk about them openly.

INTERMEDIATE ACTION

It is not uncommon for the grief-stricken individual to become angry and blame the health professional for his loss. Do not become defensive. Accept the patient's irritability, while pointing out reality, injecting doubt into the validity of his claims. "Your wife lived for 10 years as a result of medical treatment for her tumor. It sounds as though she received quite a bit of medical help."

Encourage ventilation of the person's feelings regarding the loss and his life with the lost person. Most of the time, others (family and friends) have stifled any expression of feelings.

Try to settle incidents that make the person angry at the time they occur. If the individual seems angry about not speaking to the doctor, not getting a telephone call he expected, or missing snack time, talk with him about it and try to correct the difficulty immediately so that the patient won't brood about it later.

Do not be judgmental or rejecting. Do not view the patient as uncooperative if he is slow to accept his loss. This takes time. The worker should be aware of any degree of acceptance because mobilization of the patient is more likely to occur after that time.

See that the individual avoids stimulating group activities during the evening. The grieving person often has difficulty sleeping and any excitement on the unit should be stopped before bedtime. Keep him on a schedule (e.g., breakfast, rest, activity, lunch, rest, occupational therapy, rest, etc.). Restrict his daytime sleeping by introducing activities that keep him awake. Encourage him to stay up during the early evening so he will be sleepy when bedtime comes. A warm shower or bath as well as sleeping medication a half hour before bedtime are helpful in inducing sleep. Do not offer caffeinated beverages (e.g., coffee, tea, or chocolate) or stimulants.

If the individual wants to overeat, do not dwell on it. Acknowledge his desire, but help him recognize that overeating won't lessen his problem. Offer food, attractively prepared, but in proper amounts.

LONG-TERM ACTION

Provide and encourage an opportunity for the individual to discuss his feelings. When he talks about his loss, accept his remarks. As he talks, the intensity of his feelings will diminish, and it will be possible to distract him by introducing other subjects. Do not tell the patient to "dry your eyes" or say, "Come on now; big boys don't cry"; or "You'll only make yourself sicker by carrying on this way." Such statements reinforce the patient's sense of helplessness (the feeling that he cannot help himself). Encourage the patient to join a community group that helps the bereaved.

Help the person alleviate his guilt or an overzealous conscience. Let him discuss the extent of his suffering in light of what he feels he committed or omitted in the past. The worker might say, "You were not able to drive your friend through the snowstorm because your employer specifically requested you not to leave the office at that time. I can recognize your feelings that resulted from his subsequent fatal accident as he drove to the airport. But isn't it time to call a truce with yourself? You certainly have suffered so much already"; or "If your friend were here, what suggestion do you think he would have for you at this time?"

Remember that children go through feelings of bereavement after losing a family member or friend. Depending on the age of the survivor, the loss may not be accepted as permanent, leaving the child to await the return of the individual. Adults often ignore the needs of children to understand the circumstances and to participate in the rituals surrounding death. In today's society, many violent episodes have exposed children to deaths at home or in the community. Specially trained counselors have helped school children overcome the deaths of classmates resulting from violent incidents. Family members should be aware of the possibility of posttraumatic stress syndrome reactions (see ch. 26) in children as well as adults when violence has occurred.

Remember that the bereaved person faces changes in his life. He may have to assume additional responsibilities and reevaluate his resources, work, residence, social life, leisure time, and status. These are real problems which add to the patient's misfortune.

Be aware that although grief is normal, it can become an illness if prolonged over 4 to 8 weeks.

PART FOUR

Approaches to the Psychological Effects of Physical Illness

28

The Person Receiving Electrostimulative Treatment

Physicians administer electrostimulative treatment (EST) for several psychiatric illnesses. The health worker must be able to respond intelligently and knowledgeably to the patient's questions and concerns about the treatment. He must also be able to reassure and care for the person adequately. In addition, he should be able to convey what he knows to the patient in easily understood language.

Those with severe unipolar depression who cannot take medication because of side effects or for whom medication is ineffective may respond well to EST. It can also be given as a monthly booster to prevent relapses. It is also useful in the treatment of bipolar mood disorders in people who cannot be stabilized and have repeated episodes of mania alternating with depression.

One patient suffered from alternating rapid cycles of depression and mania. During her manic cycles, she became overly active, talking about numerous subjects and projects. During the depressive cycle, she would berate herself for her failed marriage, her dysfunctional family life, her uncontrollable children, and her inability to carry out housekeeping tasks. She attempted suicide on two separate occasions. Each time she was hospitalized and treated with medications. A subsequent relapse was noted at its inception, as the patient spoke of wanting to "end it all" during a group therapy session. The nurse therapist leading the session notified the patient's husband and physician, who agreed that she should be hospitalized immediately. She was then treated with a series of six ESTs, interrupting her suicidal ideation, and ameliorating her depressive symptoms.

EST is now frequently administered in an ambulatory setting. Under those circumstances, a family member, or other responsible individual must follow the same pretreatment routine as for the in-patients. The patient must be accompanied to the facility by a responsible person who can then remain with the patient for the day (or days) after the procedure. It is imperative for that person to be very knowledgeable about the treatment process and have the ability to provide necessary explanations to the patient. The following information should be available to the caretaker:

The health worker can suggest that the family help the patient prepare for the likely episode of transient memory loss by having a list of names, addresses, and telephone numbers of significant others, important appointments, and activities, available for the patient. If the patient has episodes of disorientation and confusion, it is important that he be reoriented frequently as to time, place, the names of his caretakers, and any imminent planned activities. He should be prevented from making any major decisions or purchases during that time, and should not become involved in legal matters.

Patients should be reassured that the memory loss is transient and that memory will return. Assurance should also be given that the treatment, according to current knowledge, should not result in any brain damage. An informed consent must be signed by patients and a pretreatment workup completed. This consists of a physical examination by the doctor who will clear patients for treatment. An electrocardiogram, complete blood count, urinalysis, chest X-ray and serum electrolytes are included. The health worker meets with patients and caretakers before the procedure to explain what patients will experience, answering any questions they may have. Patients have an intravenous line inserted to allow for the administration of any emergency medication that may be needed during the treatment.

Because of the use of anesthesia, patients should have nothing to eat or drink after the midnight before the treatment, which is usually administered in the early morning. The health worker or person responsible for patients should be alert to the possibility of patients hiding snacks in their room, accepting food from others, or swallowing water during mouth care. This is the reason for having someone available to supervise patients the night before and the morning of treatment.

If any medications are absolutely required (antihypertensive, cardiac, etc.), they are usually given with only a sip of water. Remind patients to empty their bladder before the treatment because the muscle relaxants given can cause incontinence. Eye glasses and contact lenses as well as removable dentures must be taken away before the treatment. Patients should not have curlers, hair pins, or ornaments in their hair. Patients who are extremely upset may be given an intramuscular sedative a half-hour before the treatment. A mouth guard will be inserted to protect the patient's teeth, and an airway inserted once anesthesia is begun.

Electrostimulative therapy is the conduction of an electrical current though the head and brain, using electrodes applied by hand to both temporal portions of the scalp. In some instances, only one electrode is applied, usually to the right side, with the hope of minimizing posttreatment confusion and memory loss. An electrolytic jelly or paste is used to facilitate the conduction of the current. The range of electrical charge settings (joules) varies from 5 joules to 103 joules applied for 0.25 seconds. The actual intensity of the electrical charge and the time interval used is determined by the physician. The treatment has been used for acute and chronic endogenous depressions, including those occurring in manic depressive illness, schizophrenic episodes, emaciation, suicidal ideation, and psychiatric illnesses unresponsive to medication or psychotherapy. It is usually used as the treatment of last resort.

Many theories have been proposed to explain the reason for the effects of the treatment. No *one* theory has been accepted as the last word on the subject. The more generally accepted explanation is that the current causes a massive discharge of brain cell activity, thereby interrupting established nerve network connections. It is hoped that this will free the patient of some previously painful and undesirable thought and behavior patterns and allow him to form more helpful and desirable connections and patterns. Medication is given before the treatment to reduce convulsive muscular movements of the body to mere flickers of movement. This virtually eliminates the danger of fractures.

As a result of the treatment, depression should subside, anxiety should be reduced, and disturbing or recurrent thoughts that have bothered the patient should be interrupted. The number of treatments varies with the individual patient, but generally a series of 4 to 10 are ordered to be administered on alternate days, three times a week, until the series has been completed.

The patient who agrees to a course of electrostimulative treatments can be expected to harbor numerous fears and apprehensions before and even during the series. Some of these fears and apprehensions are also partly related to the emotional illness itself. But those related to the treatment can be worked through with the help of the informed health worker, who can instill a sense of positiveness and hopefulness. Optimism based on new goals, improvement, and eradication of distressing symptoms can be conveyed. To get this feeling across to the patient, the worker must first work through his own feelings regarding electrostimulative treatment. For instance, a fearful nurse, or one who thinks of the treatment as awful, or one who blames this treatment for a patient's continued illness, will not be able to be genuinely supportive. Each health worker should avail himself of the opportunity to observe electrostimulative treatment. This will help him clear up his own misconceptions. The rapidity of treatment and the often mild reaction felt by the patient usually comes as a complete surprise.

After the treatment, when the patient is conscious and his physical condition is stable, he is oriented as to where he is and told that the treatment is over. He is aided to walk to a recovery area, and remains there until he has fully recovered from the treatment, his vital signs are stable, and he is able to be released to the care of the accompanying responsible person. That individual must be made aware that the patient usually suffers from transient confusion, and that any directions need to be stated compassionately, concisely and slowly. Directions may have to be repeated often, with time allowed for the patient to respond.

On awakening, patients may not recall where they are or why they are in the hospital. Most express concern about losing their memory, and the confusion and strangeness that they feel. They may express surprise that they have already had the treatment because they usually do not remember receiving it, nor even going to the treatment room. Some do not remember events preceding the treatment. Others remember only that a needle was inserted into their arm. Following treatment, patients are prone to forget much about their stay in the hospital, and familiar objects seem strange to them. When out of the hospital on a day's pass, even their homes may seem odd or unusual. Things the patient knew before his hospitalization may be forgotten, as names, addresses, one's age. Some patients do not remember having made telephone calls, whether they have eaten, or conversations with their physician. This lack of mental clarity, and feelings of vagueness and uncertainty may last for minutes, several hours, or days. Although memory impairment is distressing, it is usually temporary. One cannot predict in advance what a patient will forget or remember. The patient should be told that his memory *will* return, and the confusion will clear. In the meantime, the health worker's physical presence and ability to reorient the patient in whatever way he can will help him immensely. The worker's approach to the patient when he wakens should include information on where the patient is, what has happened, and what is now occurring.

Common physical complaints after treatment are nausea, headache, and muscle stiffness. The health worker should listen carefully to the patient and evaluate each complaint seriously. He should never assume that the patient's complaints are due to the confusion which may follow the treatment, since this attitude not only undermines the patient's confidence but encourages other staff members to doubt the patient's credibility. Many a health worker has, in addition, discovered a more serious problem than that of the initial complaint.

One patient complained of nausea, general weakness, and pain across the chest, which bothered him when he breathed. The alert health worker took the patient's vital signs, put him in an upright position and called the medical doctor. He came immediately, and confirmed the diagnosis of heart attack. However, when complaints are of a minor nature, the patient can usually be reassured that the discomfort is not unusual and medication is available to remedy the temporary distress—aspirin for headache and Compazine for nausea. He can be given a warm bath to relieve muscle stiffness.

In the past, health workers have looked on the patient receiving electrostimulative treatment as not amenable to other therapeutic activity. As soon as electrostimulative therapy was found to be indicated, the patient was viewed as inaccessible to interaction. He was therefore left alone, which only increased his confusion and state of unhappiness. In a sense, he was isolated and as a result his difficulties increased. We know now that he benefits from an active therapeutic approach. When the patient is encouraged to talk about his treatment, he can express his worries, anxieties, and fears. Answering his questions provides clarification, and sharing his concerns helps him to undergo this difficult experience more comfortably.

If the patient does not remember the precipitating conflict after electrostimulative therapy, or tells you how good he feels and that he is ready to go home, it is best not to remind him of what he could not resolve or what troubled him. Let him receive the full benefit from his treatment, after which he will be better able to cope with gradually returning memories of upsetting experiences.

Inclusion in daily activities, occupational therapy, and group therapy decreases the patient's feelings of isolation and rejection, and serves to increase his reality testing. Having the opportunity to talk about his experiences, sharing his feelings and concerns, also allows him to receive support, compassion, and understanding from others who have undergone, or are presently undergoing, the same therapy. Hearing about something from a person who has had direct experience with the procedure and who feels its benefits is of unquestionable value to a patient.

Families of patients undergoing electrostimulative treatment need enlightened knowledge, intelligent answers, and emotional support to help alleviate their own fears for the patient and to cope with their relatives' reactions. In one meeting held for families of newly admitted patients, family members revealed their feelings of fear and guilt. They felt responsible for subjecting their loved ones to this treatment which, they hoped, would provide improvement, although that could not be guaranteed. Suddenly, one person, a well-groomed and seemingly learned gentleman, revealed that he had received a course of treatment during an acute illness years earlier and had been vastly helped. This revelation so reassured the group that the leaders didn't have to utter another word.

Patients and families often ask whether there is a maximum safe number of treatments and whether a patient can have additional or maintenance treatment beyond that number. The answer is that there is *no* maximum number of treatments. The patient receives as many as are needed to produce the desired optimal effect for him (typically 10 or less). Some patients may need maintenance treatments after a series has been completed, and they should be assured that these are available. The patient should also be advised not to work and to allow only a minimum of demands to be made on him during the treatment period. This is especially important if the patient is receiving treatment on an out-patient basis rather than in the controlled environment of the hospital unit.

It is also important to inform both the patient and his family members that although the treatment will relieve his symptoms, it is not a cure-all, nor does it solve all problems and conflicts. However, once the patient is relieved of his immobilizing symptoms, he can begin to work on his difficulties in a more realistic, flexible, and improved manner. To help the patient do this, psychotherapy is strongly encouraged.

THE APPROACH TO THE PERSON RECEIVING ELECTROSTIMULATIVE TREATMENT

Immediate Intervention by the Patient

SELF-MANAGEMENT TECHNIQUES

Follow the pretreatment instructions, reviewing them with the hospital personnel, or, if in an ambulatory setting, with the responsible individual acting as caretaker.

Prepare any necessary medications or clothing in advance.

Make any necessary transportation plans in advance.

Professional or Caretaker Intervention

IMMEDIATE ACTION

Remain with the patient during the night before the treatment. Be certain that the patient follows the instructions, and does not eat or drink after midnight. Plan to remain with the patient before and during the treatment, through the time that he has recovered from the anesthesia.

Help the patient dress appropriately for the treatment (i.e., loose, comfortable, washable outfit.)

Allow sufficient time to answer patient's questions and provide reassurance. Provide clarification when necessary, and correct misperceptions.

Reassure the patient that anyone who is in reasonably good physical health can tolerate the treatment. Tell him that a general physical examination including blood work, urinalysis, and an electrocardiogram will be done beforehand. If anything is found that contraindicates the use of the treatment, the therapy will be withheld. Let the patient know that sometimes physical symptoms result from emotional illness and can be alleviated by electrostimulative treatment.

Remain with the patient before, during, and after the treatment. The physical presence of the health worker is reassuring and necessary on the morning of the treatment. Provide a calm atmosphere; soothing music is allowable. The worker should be familiar with the routine required before the treatment. Tell the patient, "I will be with you during the treatment and will help you until you feel secure and comfortable on your own." Assure the patient that a "hot breakfast will be reserved for after your treatment." This carries the implication that the patient is expected to recover fairly rapidly and will be able to have breakfast after the treatment.

INTERMEDIATE ACTION

Allow the patient to sleep until he awakens after the treatment. On his awakening, reintroduce yourself, with your name and role. Then, reorient the patient slowly to where he is, what he is there for, and what he is to do next. For instance, "You are here at the treatment center where you have had a treatment for your depression. You tolerated it well. I will go with you now to another room, where you may eat a breakfast that has been reserved for you."

Listen to the patient's complaints, and alleviate any uncomfortable effects of the treatment. Give him medication for nausea, headache, or muscle soreness. Advise him that a warm bath or shower is helpful. Give clear directions and repeat when necessary; the confusion from the treatment may prevent the patient from hearing or understanding your directions or explanations. Help him avoid being embarrassed by this. Understand that he will try to mask his confusion by remaining quiet. Initiate conversation with him, but do not probe or put pressure on him to recall details or past events. Assure him that he will recover his memory loss. Explain his inability to recall coming for the treatment or the events leading to arriving there is a desired effect of the treatment. He should not be reminded that he exhibited bizarre behavior or expressed irrational thoughts at the time of his arrival.

Protect the individual from making telephone calls or seeing visitors until he has regained control of himself. This may take several hours.

Do not become defensive or argue with the patient when he blames the treatment for all his difficulties and his inability to accomplish anything. Gently but firmly tell him that the difficulties he had before the treatment created unpleasant and uncomfortable symptoms which necessitated treatment. When he uses the treatment as an excuse for his inability to learn, understand, or pursue goals, he can be told, "You will be able to learn more when you have less anxiety. You will then be able to do more with greater ease." Then use a specific example of improvement: "Before the treatment you weren't interested in doing anything. Now you seem eager to finish the pin you are making in occupational therapy."

LONG-TERM ACTION

Stimulate the person to think about the benefit of some therapy for himself after the treatment. He may say, "Why should I see the doctor? I'm better now." The worker's best approach in this case is to say, "The more one understands about oneself, the better one can handle one's feelings and deal with problems as they arise. This means a more enjoyable daily life. You are surely entitled to that."

Include the individual in all activities. Encourage him to do whatever he is able to do—dancing, walking, or engaging in occupational and recreational therapy. Light activity is preferable on the afternoon of the treatment day; the patient will need extra rest. On alternate days, the patient should join group therapy sessions that stress reorientation and the sharing of feelings and concerns. These meetings will diminish his sense of aloneness and restore confidence in his ability to be with others. This generates a sense of function which the patient previously felt incapable of reaching. It also serves to remind him that others are coping with this experience and have been sustained in it. It will reassure him to know that he is supported in his struggle.

29

The Person With Coronary Heart Disease or a Cerebrovascular Accident

Coronary heart disease is the most frequent cause of death in the United States, while the third most common cause of death is a cerebrovascular accident. In common terms, we hear of the person who has had a "heart attack," while others have had a "stroke" or "brain attack." The two often have many similar components, and both are covered in this chapter.

Although many types of heart disease are serious, this chapter deals mainly with the condition of acute myocardial infarction. In this condition, a portion of the heart (myocardium) is destroyed because of an insufficient supply of blood to the affected area. This occurs when one or more of the coronary arteries which supply blood to the heart muscle are closed or blocked in any way. The sudden onset of this life-threatening illness presents a major crisis to the individual, who previously may have appeared well. He suddenly experiences symptoms which may include severe weakness, excruciating chest pain, rapid pulse, a drop in blood pressure, and profuse sweating. He is aware that something is drastically wrong, and feels an urgent need for help. Life in all its many aspects has been interrupted without warning, and all the patient's thoughts and energies are directed to the process of survival. This is so basic that it is imperative for the staff to realize what this aspect of the illness means to a patient, what some of his possible emotional reactions are, and what psychological factors are important in helping him toward recovery.

When the patient suffers a blockage of the heart muscle, he may be treated immediately with TPA (recumbent tissue plasminogen activator), which will break up the clot and increase the flow of blood to the heart. For others, PTCA (percutaneous transluminal coronary angioplasty, often called balloon angioplasty) involves feeding a balloon into the area of blockage and then expanding it to flatten the atherosclerotic deposit. Artherectomy is another technique to remove the plaque. Stents may be used to be certain that the blood vessel will remain open after having been cleared.

During this initial stage of his illness, the patient may be cared for in a regular hospital unit or in a special unit for coronary care. Usually, he is terrified that he may die. The seriousness of the immediate situation is reinforced by his enforced immobilization, the administration of oxygen and intravenous fluids, and the special medication that is given to help regulate his heartbeat. Constant monitoring on the oscilloscope, with his electrocardiogram observable at all times, adds to the patient's sense of impending doom. This, too, is understandable since he may have difficulty breathing and may be experiencing pain. Again, these difficulties may be magnified by the environment with its elaborate equipment, beepers, and monitors. Often the personnel present a somber appearance as they go about their work. The patient in a cardiac unit may possibly witness the cardiac resuscitation and defibrillation of another patient lying close by. He may also witness a death, since one in ten patients with coronary heart disease will die.

Being a patient with coronary heart disease brings about a drastic change in the individual's routine of daily living. A healthy, independent personality suddenly feels helpless and dependent. This is somewhat reinforced by the patient's isolation from friends and family, and his need to rely on total strangers who know little about him personally. Furthermore, all his activities are restricted, communication via telephone is denied, and visits with friends or relatives are limited to brief periods. The patient is often fed by others initially, and not allowed to bathe or shave himself. Through all this, he is told, ironically, that he must not worry or upset himself. "Let us do the worrying and doing" is a remark commonly heard and easier said than done, for the patient's mind is active. He is bombarded by a multitude of thoughts that center on his fears and anxieties.

Patient care in the coronary unit focuses on immediate attention to life-threatening situations which may arise at any instant. The nurses are the professionals in contact with the patient day and night. They make every effort to keep the individual as comfortable as possible, while maintaining his vital functions at normal or near normal levels. Much of their efforts are preventive. Throughout all this, the patient feels keenly the seriousness of the care being given to him.

The medical-surgical nurses in this setting must be thoroughly familiar with the unit's protocol and routine. They must keep the crises manageable. They must be capable observers of physical signs (i.e., blood pressure, heart rate, pulse quality and rate, urine volume per unit time, warmth or coldness of the skin, diaphoresis, color, and respiratory rate and quality). They must be well versed in the use of cardiac monitoring equipment, cardioverters, defibrillators, and pacemakers. They must be familiar with the procedure of checking central venous pressure and other body-penetrating lines. Indeed, as with most other disciplines, the more they know, the better.

Often, nurses are the patient's first contact on arrival at the hospital. The rapport and confidence they establish initially will serve the patient well during his difficult days of acute illness. It is during the first few days, especially the first and second, that the patient's anxiety and fear are at their height, and must be dealt with by the nurses. Symptoms of anxiety include pain, rigidity, tremors, sweating, restlessness, excessive talkativeness, insomnia, agitation, and weakness. It follows that keeping the anxiety level down is most beneficial to the patient.

The anxiety of a patient can be so high that he is unable to concentrate on or retain explanations regarding care and procedures. Frequent repetition in the days that follow is needed to impart knowledge, reduce anxiety regarding procedures (especially the monitor alarm system), and encourage confidence and trust. Reducing fear is a primary task, as it may be a determinant in escalation of a mild ischemia to a fatal arrhythmia. Medication, such as morphine, may be used in this case not only to alleviate pain but also to reduce anxiety. If a patient should experience cardiac arrest and survive, it goes without saying that the health professionals must help the patient talk about his feelings in order to help him accept the experience. This is a frequent occurrence in the coronary care unit and results in a flurry of activity at the bedside. Intravenous medications are administered; cardiopulmonary resuscitation (CPR) started; and, as quickly as possible, a defibrillator is used to jump-start the heart into action.

Until recently, defibrillation was primarily an ambulance or hospital procedure. Now a new approach may save more lives of those who suffer a cardiac arrest outside a hospital. Until recently, the only hope for those individuals was the early arrival of an ambulance with a staff capable of performing cardiopulmonary resuscitation. In many areas, the ambulance would not arrive in time to save the patient. But now, a newer type of defibrillator may be able to save at least half of the 350,000 people in the United States who die each year of cardiac arrest. The American Heart Association visualizes the placement of the machines in many areas where people may have cardiac problems and the training of nonmedical personnel in their use. The defibrillators could be placed in apartment houses, workplaces, health clubs, airplanes, and even private homes, to be used eventually by family members, doormen, security guards, coaches, and airline personnel. (At this writing, only physicians or those designated by them, may legally operate defibrillators.)

Defibrillation can reorganize the electrical impulses of the heart that occur when the contractions of the heart become disorganized because of a blockage of a blood vessel. Although CPR may be of help, it does not cure the problem. It is imperative that a defibrillator be available within minutes. The longer the time between the arrest and the application of the defibrillator, the less likely the patient is to survive. It must be used before all electrical activity in the heart has stopped.

The newer defibrillators are powered by lithium batteries that last for 5 years. The newest machines are light weight and can be operated by most people. They are capable of analyzing the rhythm of the heart and can determine whether a shock is needed, giving voice instructions if necessary. The process is extremely frightening to the patient, requiring the caregiver to be aware of the patient's emotional needs. Speaking quietly to him, providing reassurance, and letting him know that you are there, even if he does not respond, are important.

The use of a defibrillator by nonmedical individuals present during the emergency may cause those persons great anxiety. If the procedure, no matter how well performed, does not help, volunteers may blame their own inadequacies for the failure. It is important for the professionals who arrive after the attempts have been made to let the volunteers verbalize their feelings. They need to realize that emergency measures are not always successful, even if carried out by medical professionals. Follow-up contact with the volunteers should occur to alleviate any long-term emotional problems, particularly if the patient dies.

Depression is a common occurrence during the third and fourth days after a myocardial infarction. The patient manifests a sad and hopeless mood and is pessimistic. He may weep because he feels that because he is physically unsound, and inactive, he is, therefore, useless. He may begin to verbalize anger by making sarcastic remarks and being critical of the nurses and the way the hospital operates. He may ask, "Why me?" In his anger he may refuse to follow the nurses' suggestions. Some patients may have avoided responsibility as often as possible when they were well. Now the illness provides a secondary gain in the form of permanent relief from obligations. Such a person may develop into what is commonly known as a "cardiac cripple." In contrast, the patient who has had a dynamic, outgoing personality may be unable to face his illness with its threat of future loss, restriction of activities, possible reduction in income, change in his occupation and former habits, as smoking and overeating. He may deny that he ever had a heart attack and threaten to sign out of the hospital, stating that there is really nothing wrong with him. Still another patient may react to his illness by becoming overly cheerful. He takes everything the worker says lightly, attaches little importance to restrictions, and has a good word for everyone with whom he comes into contact. This patient's behavior indicates that he is not accepting the experience for what it is.

The patient may become angry and verbalize his annoyances. Expressions of anger often give the patient the feeling of being in control as well as a feeling of exhilaration. Patients sometimes attempt to fight depression by clinging to the health professional, who provides continuous care. This helpless dependency is similar to a child who must have his parent to protect him from the mysterious outside world. The use of antidepressant medication requires prudence and alertness to possible adverse side effects, such as tachycardia or palpitations. By the same token, cardiovascular disease may be treated with drugs that inadvertently precipitate depression.

The male patient who fears that his illness may cause the loss of his sexual prowess may make suggestive remarks to female nurses, comment on their figures, or openly invite them to have sex with him. He may tell off-color jokes and stories at every opportunity. This behavior can be attributed to denial as well as an attempt to cover up his uncomfortable depressed feelings by using the quick satisfaction of pleasant sexual thoughts.

It behooves the nurses to bear in mind that adjustment to a completely new way of life is difficult for all patients, and impossible for some. A patient may pass the critical period of his illness, begin to feel better quickly, and then be unable or unwilling to follow instructions that limit his way of life. In anticipation of possible refusal by the patient to accept limitations, nurses will do well to learn all they can about his family, occupation, habits, and idiosyncrasies. This will enable the workers to plan an approach that is not only in the patient's best interest, but one that is also meaningful and suited to his total personality.

Nurses will be the ones in most frequent contact with the family. The care providers must understand the confusion, anxiety, and fear of the visitors when approaching the patient. The hurried rush to the hospital, the urgent admission procedures, and then seeing the patient with his many alarm attachments frightens and often bewilders his relatives. Nurses can have a positive influence on the visitors by their calm demeanor and the intelligent explanations they offer. They should provide time for the family to talk about their feelings, a need that cannot be overemphasized. By communicating with the family, nurses obtain information regarding the personal life and habits of the patient. At the same time, professionals may serve as a sounding board for the family to work through some of their own fears, apprehensions, guilt, and anger. Nurses should observe the effect of family members on the patient, and deal with any expressed feelings which may have adverse affects on him, complicating his course of recovery. Family support for the patient may determine whether the treatment is a success or failure.

Nurses who care for the patient with coronary heart disease must be sensitive to their own behavior and reactions. Do they handle themselves with ease, or are they always in a state of rush or uncertainty? Do they speak distinctly, calmly, and with confidence, or are they tense and vague while mumbling their words? Do they react defensively to the patient's anger and criticism, or do they recognize his words as a reaction to his illness? Are they flexible and able to meet the patient's changing needs, or do they always unconsciously strive to satisfy their own needs? The patient observes how anxious the nurses are about his condition, and comes to his own conclusion about the seriousness of his illness.

Staff members go through myriad responses, such as depression, anxiety, cooperation, or hostility. It is not unusual to see the staff work together in tense unison while attempting resuscitative measures, only to lapse into a sullen mood after their efforts have failed. Staff members are not immune to displacement of angry feelings onto one another in an attempt to ward off depressive reactions when a patient dies or is ill beyond their ability to help.

Tests may be ordered to evaluate the extent of heart damage that has occurred. These may include noninvasive echocardiography or an exercise tolerance test, perhaps accompanied by a radioactive thalium uptake to visualize the affected area. A cardiac catheterization with angiography may also be done, with a catheter passed from the femoral artery to the various chambers of the heart. A dye is utilized to demonstrate the location and severity of any coronary artery blockage. Depending on the findings, bypass surgery may be recommended.

Patients scheduled for this surgery are usually very frightened. The heart is viewed as the very core of life, and to have it opened, with blood diverted to a machine during the surgery, is intellectually, emotionally, and physically distressing. Other blood vessels (from the saphenous veins of the legs or the internal mammary artery of the chest) are inserted into the aorta, with the other end grafted to the coronary artery, bypassing the blockage. The hope is that the surgery will result in increased vascularization of the heart, with a decrease in angina and an increase in the quality of life. A cardiac rehabilitation program should be instituted to teach the patient how to control his diet, carry out an exercise program, and improve the way in which he handles stress. Families of the patient need to be included in this planning for the patient's future care.

Those who have undergone coronary artery bypass grafting may worry about their ability to help prevent the need for repeat surgery in the future. About 320,000 patients in the United States require this type of operation, with 10% to 20% destined to have it repeated as the grafted veins fill with cholesterol and clots. Hope is being offered to those willing to control aggressively their levels of low-density lipoprotein cholesterol to under 100 mg/dL by remaining on a regime that includes a low-cholesterol diet, exercise, and drugs such as lovastatin (Mevicor), atorvastatin calcium (Lipitor) and pravastatin sodium (Pravachol) daily. According to a study at the Maryland Medical Research Institute, 31% of the patients will avoid clogging of the new grafts, and 29% will be less likely to require repeat surgery if this plan is used.

For some patients, following any type of regime presents difficulties. It may be regarded as an infringement on their freedom, a dependence on medications that necessitate regular routine blood tests (particularly to determine if there is liver damage caused by the medication), and a sense of being controlled by external forces. They will doubtlessly be told to give up cigarettes, a pleasure that they may not want to deny themselves. There may also be fear connected to the possibility of damage from the very medication that is supposed to help them improve.

Looking at the statistics may make them feel that the odds of prevention are not worth the deprivation of a low-cholesterol diet, or the inconvenience of an exercise program. It is important for the health care personnel to point out the importance of the regime in a way that gives patients choices, so that they feel they are in control of their own destiny. If they have offspring or significant others in their lives, it may help to have patients evaluate their own input into the well-being of those others. If their interest in their influence on others can be recognized as important, they may be able to sublimate their own anger at having to follow the medical plans devised by professionals. In addition, they should be included as plans are formulated, with as much leeway as possible to include their own wishes.

As noted on p. 00, the third most common cause of death in the United States (after heart disease and cancer) is a CVA. All too often, it seems to be a sudden, unexpected occurrence, while in reality it is probably the result of many years of poor health habits. In some instances, the outcome results in immediate death. However, in most cases, patients may suffer from long-term physical or mental deficits, requiring ongoing care that adds to the expense of medical care in this country. Many of the basic problems found in patients with a CVA are similar to those who suffer heart attacks (inability to manage stress, atherosclerosis, hypertension, obesity, etc.). Some clinicians acknowledge the similarities by referring to a CVA as a "brain attack."

There are two different types of CVAs, both commonly called a "stroke." About 80% are *ischemic,* interrupting the blood flow to the brain, and are usually caused by a blood clot preventing blood from flowing through the passage. The remaining 20% are *hemorrhagic,* caused by a rupture of a blood vessel in the brain. Either type results in the loss of nutrients and oxygen to the brain, with the death of the brain cells in the affected areas. Once dead, the cells cannot be replaced and do not regenerate. In some instances, other areas of the brain are able to take over, but usually the patient is left with a deficit in his ability to speak, move, think, or feel. There may be a loss of emotional control, with an effect on personality and mood, or cognitive problems with memory, judgment, problem solving, or a combination of these. Patients may be difficult to care for if their personality angers those providing care, unless the caregivers realize that the patients' actions are out of their control.

Because the body's activity is usually controlled by an area of the brain on the opposite side, a CVA in the left hemisphere of the brain may cause hemiplegia (paralysis) or hemiparesis (weakness) on the right side of the body, and the reverse if the CVA occurred in the right hemisphere. Depending on the area of the brain that has been damaged by the stroke, the patient may suffer different consequences. If the left side of the brain has been affected, patients may be confused, unable to speak or understand speech, be unable to read, write, or solve problems. The confusion may result in disorganization, slow movements, and make them extremely cautious. They will be unable to see items in the right half of their visual field. If the stroke occurred on the right side of the brain, vision will be impaired in the left visual field, and there may be difficulty with spatial perception, causing problems with eating or drinking, reading, or operating a wheelchair. Patients may demonstrate impulsive behavior that could be harmful. Once again, the caregiver must be aware that the patients' actions are beyond their control and should be accepted as such.

Because CVAs are the third leading cause of death in developed countries, affecting about half a million people in the United States each year, it becomes important for us to know how to prevent as many as possible and to bring as many of the survivors as possible to the highest state of recovery. Unfortunately, about one third of the victims will die within a few months, and of those who live, 40% will require institutionalization, 50% will be able to remain at home if assistance is available, and only 10% will resume their preillness level of activity. The cost of maintaining the necessary services for those who have been stricken is more than $23 billion per year including services in hospitals or extended care facilities as well as for those requiring help at home. Medications alone account for $400 million.

As people age, the risk of a stroke increases, with men having 20% higher incidence than women. (Only 28% of strokes occur before the age of 65.) Because memory and cognitive ability are affected by the process, the patient may not be able to recognize the symptoms that are the warning signs of an impending stroke. Individuals who notice weakness in an arm, hand, or leg, or numbness on one side of the body or face should seek help immediately. If there is a sudden dimness or loss of vision, especially that limited to one eye, or sudden difficulty in speaking or understanding, help should be sought right away. If the individual loses his balance, or becomes dizzy, or develops a sudden, excruciating headache, help should be requested immediately. Speed is of the essence because the newer treatments, particularly the newer medications, must be started within the first 6 hours to keep the damage to a minimum.

It is wise to have emergency telephone numbers either programmed into the telephone or taped to the wall near the telephone for those who are at risk for having a CVA. The information should include the name of the physician, family members, and information to be taken to the hospital with the patient including the medications currently prescribed as well as insurance information needed for admission. It would be wise to also have information available about the nearest hospital specializing in acute stroke care.

A transient ischemic attack (TIA), also called a ministroke, is the result of a temporary interruption in the flow of blood to the brain. Although the stroke-like symptoms usually disappear within 24 hours without permanent effects, a TIA should be accepted as a serious warning that a CVA may develop and medical assistance sought immediately.

Prevention is the important key to avoiding serious CVA damage. The existence of narrowed blood vessels, resulting from high levels of cholesterol having formed plaques, must be controlled by adherence to a low cholesterol diet and, if necessary, the use of medication (particularly the statins). Patients with atrial fibrillation are also at risk for a CVA because the atria (two upper chambers of the heart) do not empty completely when the heart contracts. The remaining blood may form a clot (thrombus) as it sits there, placing the patient at risk if part of the clot breaks away and becomes an embolus, traveling through the bloodstream and lodging near the brain, or even in the brain, causing a cerebral infarction. To prevent this, the patient may be placed on warfarin (Coumadin) to inhibit the formation of blood clots. If so, he must be instructed in the signs of hemorrhaging from the anticoagulant effects as well as the need to maintain his dietary level of vitamin K. By increasing the dietary vitamin K excessively, the anticoagulant effect of the Coumadin may be decreased; by lowering the dietary vitamin K, the normal clotting effect afforded by the vitamin will be lost. The professional should be informed of any dietary changes to evaluate the vitamin K level and to adjust the intake to limit complications.

Differing from ischemic strokes are the 20% of all strokes that are hemorrhagic in origin. They are usually associated with hypertension and involve the rupture of a vessel near or in the brain. They can occur in young people and are more likely to result in death. Quick removal of the blood may not only save the patient's life but will help to limit the damage. Severe headaches are usually the first symptom and, if in the subarachnoid space, may cause death within three months. Of those who survive, more than 50% will have neurological damage. Patients with this type of CVA are never given anticoagulants because those drugs would increase the amount of hemorrhaging. It is imperative that an accurate diagnosis be made as to the type of stroke so that proper intervention can be provided.

Individuals who have suffered a CVA are frequently anxious as to the possibility of another stroke. They are aware of the possible bodily or mental damage that can be incurred, and fear the effects of another incident. It is important for caregivers to respect that fear and to use it as a way of having patients follow a preventive regime. It is also imperative to be aware of the feelings of significant others, including young children, who may not verbalize their concerns yet act out in undesirable ways. The professionals should provide honest reassurance and, at the same time, make all aware that they, too, should follow a health program to lessen their own chance of having a stroke.

One of the factors for risk of a CVA is hypertension, which usually is controlled by weight loss, a low-fat (and frequently salt-free) diet that includes fruits and vegetables, no tobacco or caffeine, a limit of one alcoholic beverage a day, exercise, lessening of stress, learning how to deal with unavoidable stress, and medication. As with patients who have cardiac problems, it may be difficult to convince patients to follow the recommended regime. They may resent the loss of control of their lives and refuse to abstain from those forbidden items that they enjoy. Including patients in the planning may make them more amenable to the program.

Depression often lingers on after a stroke and may result in difficulties with rehabilitation. Patients may feel hopeless and helpless, and be unwilling to take part in the necessary exercises and therapies that will improve their status. They may have physical defects that will limit their ability to care for themselves and may see themselves as permanent invalids. Part of their reaction may be due to the realities that they must face in terms of limitations. Some of the depression, however, may be due to medications and will be alleviated if the drugs are changed. Another part of the depression may result from the reluctance of friends or family to visit, or from the patients' loss of status if unable to resume work. Encouraging visits from others, including coworkers, may help make them feel worthwhile again. Introducing new hobbies, or helping them to read (if physically possible) or listen to books or music on tape, may distract them from their gloom.

Patients may be reluctant to be sexually active, seeing themselves as physically unacceptable, or the very involvement in intercourse as being too dangerous and possibly resulting in another CVA. In addition, males may be unable to have an erection or ejaculate. They may need reassurance as to what they are capable of performing and instruction on body positions that will maximize their capabilities. Couple therapy may be instrumental in making each partner more comfortable with the limitations and possibilities imposed by the stroke. Often the reassurance that holding, embracing, and kissing are just as rewarding as actual intercourse may lower the negative concerns sufficiently to help the couple continue in a loving relationship.

THE APPROACH TO THE PERSON WITH CORONARY HEART DISEASE OR CEREBROVASCULAR ACCIDENT

Immediate Intervention by the Patient

SELF-MANAGEMENT TECHNIQUES

Call for help immediately if any symptom of a cardiac or CVA problem arises (e.g., chest, arm, or jaw pain; nausea; perspiration, faintness, palpitations; weakness, numbness, or visual changes). If no one is available, call 911 and ask for an ambulance with a paramedic to be sent immediately. Describe the symptoms. Have the door unlocked, any health insurance papers available for hospital admission, telephone numbers of significant others (including health care provider), a list of medications presently being used, a recent electrocardiogram if available, and a copy of any advance health directive. Those known to be at risk for cardiac emergencies should have as much medical information available as possible, in an easily accessible place. A MediAlert bracelet should be worn at all times. The patient should try to remain calm and as relaxed as possible while waiting for help to arrive.

Professional Intervention

IMMEDIATE ACTION

Carry out emergency medical procedures quickly, efficiently and calmly. Speak to patients in a soft, gentle manner, briefly explaining what is being done. Keep patients warm and as comfortable as possible, exposing as little of the body as necessary to respect their dignity.

If they need to be removed from the home, make certain to take all the necessary personal and medical information with them. Contact the health care provider if possible. If they are taken out of the home, make certain to lock the door as you leave. Keep keys in a safe place with valuables.

Remember that patients may be terrified by the pain and the need for medical intervention. Speak to them frequently and touch them gently.

If significant others are present, offer calm explanations so that their fears or anxiety will not be added to those of the patient.

Be truthful. Give the patient honest and clear answers. Remember, he is usually alert, aware of everything you are doing, and frightened. Respect his intelligence. It is better to acknowledge to him that his illness is serious than to pretend that it's not. The patient will assess your answers and make his own decision as to whether he can rely on you for an honest answer in the future. This will undoubtedly influence your relationship with him.

Assure the patient that measures are being taken to keep him as comfortable as possible. Let him know that the medical and nursing team has everything under control. Mention, "Your breathing will be much easier as you breathe the oxygen and after you receive this medication." Always tell the patient what you are doing to help him. Make sure he understands the unpleasant restrictions that have been ordered—a special diet, limited visitors, and bed rest. These should be explained with emphasis on their helping qualities. "We are enforcing the doctor's orders vigorously because we want you to recover as quickly as possible."

Assure the patient that he is watched and observed at all times. He may ask, "Will I die if I go to sleep?" The nurse can reply, "There is no indication that your condition will change any more while you are asleep than when you are awake. In fact, you will expend less energy asleep than awake." Since many patients fear that they may die while sleeping, assure him that he will be carefully watched even when asleep.

Be supportive during diagnostic procedures. Cardiac catheterization often results in a high level of anxiety for the patient. Although he may be sedated, he must be awake during the test. It will help him cope better if he is distracted by talking about recreational activities or hobbies, or sharing funny stories with him. Keep the environment as stress free as possible.

Be a good listener. Let the patient know you value what he has to say. Be alert to comments that reveal his anxiety or hesitancy in talking to you. If the patient states, "There were so many things I never got to do," or "I've heard that few people survive these things," you can say, "You sound worried, which is certainly understandable. You will gain confidence as time passes and your strength returns."

Provide as restful and pleasant an environment as the unit permits. Clocks and calendars help keep the patient oriented as to the time and date, especially in intensive care units, where lights are on 24 hours a day.

INTERMEDIATE ACTION

Remain with the patient in the emergency room until other professionals take over his care. Explain that you must leave, but that competent health workers are going to provide the necessary care. Tell him what you have done with any of his valuables or information brought with him, and that you have locked the door to his home.

Inform any significant others of what has been done with the patient's valuables. Reassure them about his care before you leave.

Any personnel now responsible for the patient's care should continue the reassurance, calm manner, and gentle touch. The patient may be agitated, wondering if significant others have been informed as to his whereabouts. This is particularly true if the patient is away from his home community, as on a business or pleasure trip. Contact others as he requests, and let him know of your endeavors.

Allow several short sessions for the patient to talk with you rather than one long period. This lessens fatigue and provides consistent attention that increases his feelings of security.

Allow the patient to express his feelings regarding the illness. Let him talk about what it means to him in terms of his daily activities, his occupation, his family life. Patients may attribute weakness to a degenerating heart, when in fact it may be caused by prolonged immobilization. Patient teaching and the initiation of activity in a carefully monitored progressive exercise program is important in preventing him from becoming a cardiac cripple. Often you will find the patient has a distorted view of his limitations that you can clarify. For instance, when the patient says, "This is the end of my sex life," the nurse might reply, "After recovery, the sex life of most patients returns to what it was in the past." It is also important to acknowledge the patient's expressed feelings. "It's understandable that you are depressed now, but as you begin to get better, you will feel less nervous about your physical condition and have more self-confidence." "You will be less perplexed about your limitations as you convalesce, because we will keep repeating all the things you need to know." This last remark also tells the patient you expect him to recover.

Talk to the patient about plans for his transfer to a general care unit. Mention the positive aspects of the move. "You have been improving every day and now you are well enough to leave the coronary care unit." Although the patient wants to leave, he may be fearful that he will not receive equally good care after the move. Nurses should comment on the high quality of the care he will get because the personnel on the general care unit are specially trained in giving cardiac care. Never convey the idea that only the nurse in the coronary care unit can be helpful and knowledgeable, since it is not valid. Remember that such an idea will upset and worry the patient. He may even overreact to the situation and build up enough anxiety to endanger his cardiac status, and land him back in the coronary care unit.

Educate the patient about his medications and any side effects of which he should be aware. Drugs used to lower the risk of a myocardial infarction or a CVA require education of the patient. Heparin, aspirin, or other drugs that help prevent sludging of platelets and clot formation may also cause unwanted hemorrhages. The patient should be warned to check with his prescribing caregiver if he needs dental work or any type of surgery, no matter how minor. He should also be taught to watch for black, tarry stools, frequent unexplained bruises, or any signs of dizziness, or weakness of limbs that may be indicative of a cerebral problem. The information should be presented in a way that will educate the patient but not frighten him to the point where he will not take the medication at all.

Long-Term Action

If this is a first incident, the patient will need to be educated as to his care. The patient needs information as to warning signs and symptoms as well as the actions to be taken.

As the patient progresses toward full recovery, provide an opportunity for him to attend group sessions for patients with coronary heart disease or cerebrovascular accidents. These sessions validate the worth of giving up smoking, sticking to restricted dietary regimens, learning to relax, and working at a slower pace. They also have a beneficial effect by providing a chance for the patient to express feelings and attitudes about his condition.

When a patient is out of imminent danger, he may feel so confident that he denies the presence of illness. This serves to protect him from the implication of what a myocardial infarction or CVA means in terms of the length and quality of his future life. At the same time, it prevents him from cooperating and participating in a therapeutic lifesaving program based on prevention and rehabilitation. Group meetings enable him to become more realistic in assessing his reaction to his physical state.

Use other resources to help the patient work through conflicts that existed before his myocardial infarction or CVA. Because of his vulnerable state, these conflicts may have increased. For example, the patient may have become rigid and controlling. He refuses to have others tell him what to do. He is angry about his helpless state and the enforced restrictions. Let him know that these restrictions are temporary. The need for control may well be a pressure area that will influence his recovery and/or future well-being. Suggest that "Sometimes when people are under a great deal of pressure, their physical health is affected. It helps to know how to deal with these pressures. We have a member on our team who is an expert at talking with people about just that. How would you feel about talking with him?" Deciding whether he wants to be helped gives the patient a sense of autonomy while letting him know that you are concerned about his feelings. Encourage him to know himself so that he can learn what triggers his emotional upsets. Help him find alternative means of solving his difficulties. Don't put a psychiatric label on the patient because he gets upset. He has enough problems already.

Before being discharged from the hospital, the patient should be encouraged to think about times and episodes in which he felt stress. By recognizing his pressure limitations, he can learn to control them. The use of techniques such as biofeedback, exercise, psychotherapy, relaxation, or medication may be helpful in offsetting tension.

Discussion regarding control of diabetes, blood cholesterol and triglyceride levels, obesity, hypertension, and elimination of cigarette smoking should be included in predischarge planning. If the implantation of an artificial pacemaker or coronary surgery is necessary, the staff may need to provide education, support, and reassurance so that the patient will accept the procedure.

The patient will probably be referred to a cardiac or CVA rehabilitation program. Reassure him as to the value of such a program and encourage him to attend as ordered by the care provider.

Evaluate the patient before discharge, making certain of any appointments that he should have. Find out if his living arrangements will be satisfactory (stairs to climb, availability of help if necessary, etc.).

FREQUENTLY PRESCRIBED PSYCHIATRIC DRUGS

Psychiatric drugs frequently prescribed for people with heart disease include the following:

Selective serotonin reuptake inhibitors: fluoxetine (Prozac), sertraline (Zoloft), fluvoxamine (Luvox), paroxetine (Paxil)

30

The Person With Cancer

Cancer is one of the most feared diseases at this point and the second most common cause of death. The initial suspicion that the diagnosis may be made sends chills through most patients, and their relatives or associates. Often the first thought is of life ending in the near future. In fact, for many cancer is now more of a chronic disorder, with episodes of acute flare-ups, that keeps patients and families on edge for many years.

Cancer of the breast is the most common form of cancer in women. Between 5% and 10% of women in the United States can be expected to develop breast cancer. Some women discover for themselves that they have a lump in one of their breasts. Others are unaware of the presence of a lump until it is found on routine physical examination or a mammogram. The reaction to a lump in a breast is often a combination of denial and fear. "No, not me; it just can't be," is the common reaction. Often, the woman waits through the next menstrual cycle in the hope that the lump will disappear. If it has been discovered by a physician, the patient may seek another consultation, hoping for a different finding, one that will result in the statement, "It's okay, you don't need to have the operation."

The possibility of a mastectomy is a frightening prospect. Before this procedure is carried out, a biopsy is done to determine whether or not the lump is cancerous. If it is noncancerous (benign), only the area of the growth is removed, the incision is stitched, and no more need be done. Needless to say, this patient is relieved of much anxiety and fear. But if the mass is cancerous (malignant), then the entire breast, including even uninvolved breast tissue, plus the surrounding axillary nodes and lymphatic vessels may be excised in the hope of removing any and all unseen spreading cancer cells. This surgical procedure is known as radical mastectomy. Some surgeons prefer to perform modifications of this procedure, perhaps excising only the involved area (lumpectomy). However, the decision as to the type of surgery will depend on the stage of the cancer and the judgment of the surgeon in conjunction with the wishes of the woman. The surgery may be followed with a course of radiation therapy or chemotherapy. The same procedures are followed for male patients.

For women, the fear of breast cancer may be overwhelming. Currently, there is controversy over the age at which the first mammogram should be done. Some health professionals believe that it is important for this examination to be carried out on a yearly basis when the patient turns age 40. Other specialists believe that carrying out this procedure before 50 is not worthwhile because the breasts are too fatty to provide correct information. They fear that patients may be subjected to unnecessary biopsies as well as an excessive amount of radiation. Statistically, they reason, the number of cancers that will be discovered is not sufficient to subject so many women to the procedure, unless there is a family history of breast cancer, or the patient is known to carry BRCA 1, the defective gene associated with breast cancer in Jewish women descended from Ashkenazi families from a certain area of eastern Europe.

But others argue that statistics are generalities, whereas patients should be treated as individuals. If even one patient of many is discovered to have treatable breast cancer via an early mammogram, the test has proved its value. One gynecologist demanded that each of her patients have the test at the age of 35, to provide a baseline for her future record. If the result was shown to be negative, it was to be repeated in 2 years. If negative again, the patient could wait until her 40s to have further routine examinations.

In one instance, the patient had no sign of a problem with the first test, but an area showed up on the second. A biopsy demonstrated an interductal cancer, which was removed with a lumpectomy. This was followed by a radiation series. After 5 years, the patient remains cancer free. In another case, the patient had her first mammogram in her mid-40s and was found to have breast cancer that had already metastasized to the lymph glands, requiring more extensive surgery and chemotherapy. One wonders whether this greater involvement could have been prevented had her gynecologist followed the same procedure as the other.

Regardless of the treatment, the woman must be followed carefully in subsequent years to check for involvement in the other breast, or for metastases to other areas of the body. Those who have undergone a mastectomy cannot totally forget the experience: the scar and the missing or reconstructed breast act as permanent reminders.

It is not unusual for a woman to give permission solely for a biopsy. If further surgery is needed, she will then have additional time to prepare herself psychologically and to discuss with her physician the kind of surgery she will undergo. This is a controversial action because a positive biopsy means that the woman will subject herself to anesthesia twice and will also risk the possibility of disseminating the tumor if cells from the biopsy area escape into her blood stream. Nevertheless, more and more women are opting for a role in determining what, if any, treatment should be employed.

Many men are now going through a comparable reaction in relation to a diagnosis of breast or prostate cancer. Breast cancer in men is usually diagnosed by the presence of skin lesions, lumps, or swelling of axillary lymph nodes. A male mastectomy does not have the same emotional impact on males, since their breasts do not carry the sexual connotation for men as for women. However, their fears for future illness and metastases are just as valid.

The use of a blood test, the prostate-specific antigen, now alerts men to the possibility of prostate cancer. The test produces an elevated reading for cancer as well as for benign prostatic hypertrophy. To differentiate, the patient must have a prostate biopsy. As with women who have breast biopsies, men become anxious about the test and its results. If it does prove to be cancer, the patient has a choice of radiation therapy or surgery. The fear of surgery centers on the possible loss of sexual function as well as the possibility of incontinence. Presently, more urologists are proficient at using a surgical technique that spares the nerves, thereby preserving sexual function. In advanced cases, chemotherapy and/or radiation may be required.

If any cancer requires more extensive treatments, patients may have marked changes in their physical status, loss of hair, emaciation from an inability to eat, or distortion of their body image because of steroids or other drugs. They may have difficulty sleeping because of their concerns and suffer from extreme fatigue. Many patients find it difficult to do anything physical. Even getting out of bed and carrying out bathing, mouth hygiene, and hair care may prove too taxing. Some are able to push themselves to the point where they accomplish all the tasks for the day, while others are unable to complete any work at all. Some find that chemotherapy may leave them exhausted on the day of treatment, then all right until the next session. Others find themselves reacting to the treatment even before it begins, imagining the smell and pain associated with the drug being used, and reacting with nausea and tension even before leaving home to go to the place of the treatment. In almost all cases, there is a degree of depression as the patient contemplates the outcome. Increased use of anti-emetic medications prior to chemotherapy has lessened or eliminated the extreme nausea associated with the use of chemotherapy.

Treatment of fatigue is important. Some patients need help in setting priorities, so that they save their energies for whatever they see as necessary. For some, delegating tasks, such as shopping, car pooling, or food preparation may cause them to feel inadequate. If they can be helped to realize that accepting help from others releases them to complete more important tasks, they may feel more comfortable.

Other areas to consider in overcoming fatigue would be the use of a moderate exercise program to maintain stamina and fitness. Patients should also be encouraged to have adequate nutrition, with sufficient quantity and quality of calories to meet their needs. This may require smaller meals taken more frequently, with the possible inclusion of liquid nutritional supplements, and the addition of vitamins and minerals if needed. If anxiety or depression are components in the fatigue, medications and psychotherapy should be ordered to alleviate the distress that cause them. Anemia may also be a factor and can be treated in some cases with medication to intensify red blood cell production.

Cancer can attack any organ of the body. Until recently, the involvement of some organs was tantamount to a death sentence. But as treatment for some malignancies has improved, there have been changes in the odds for survival. In one case, a man with a cancer of the pancreas was given almost no chance of living for more than a few months. He agreed to surgery, followed by a course of experimental medications, and is now, 5 years later, free of the disease. In another case, the use of very strong doses of chemotherapy has allowed a woman to remain well enough to travel to various parts of the world between her appointments with her oncologist. She uses the trips to bolster her desire to live and focuses on her next destination during the hours it takes to complete her painful intravenous treatment.

Some surgical procedures result in the need for an ostomy "bag." The patient who adjusts can lead a normal life, realizing that without the appliance he could not function. Whether it is the urinary bladder, the gastrointestinal tract, or both, the patient can be taught the proper care to keep the area clean and odor free. Ostomy nurses can determine the proper size and shape of the opening. They can also guide the patient into a routine that allows him to get rid of his body's waste products at a time that is convenient for him.

One concern common to many survivors of cancer treatment is whether health insurers will cover the cost of follow-up care. In Florida, a new law assures patients that any insurer who provides coverage for breast cancer treatment must now include mastectomies and breast reconstruction as part of the care. (Additional treatment, such as bone marrow or stem cell transplantation, was not mentioned.) The law is intended to provide patients and their physicians access to appropriate treatment, and to do away with the "drive-by" mastectomies occurring in some ambulatory settings. Some women have had their lumpectomies expanded into mastectomies as a result of the need for removal of additional cancerous tissue discovered during the planned original procedure. In some cases, the patients were sent home from the ambulatory setting as soon as the effects of anesthesia wore off. They were often unprepared emotionally or physically for the more extensive surgery that had occurred.

Prostheses and wigs are now considered as medical necessities rather than cosmetic conveniences and are usually eligible for insurance coverage. Although the concerns about the progress of the cancer are uppermost in the minds of those under treatment, the cost factors weigh heavily, particularly on those who are not insured, or are underinsured. Depression may be due as much to the financial concerns as to the illness itself. In some cases, patients have turned to reverse mortgage plans that pay the owner of property either a lump sum of money or monthly payments to be paid off by the sale of the property after the owner's death. In this way, the family's ongoing expenses, as well as the medical expenses, can be met.

When a major surgical procedure has occurred, and the patient has not been given the necessary emotional support or education on self-care before discharge, there is a risk for a major depression to start. The patient may go home without having seen the operative site, yet be told that it must be cleaned and cared for each day. If the patient has never seen a surgical wound before, is afraid to take the previous dressing off, and is unwilling to look at the area, how will the wound be cared for? The patient may be overwhelmed by the sight of raw tissue and afraid to touch it. Will the area become infected? And, if it does, will the patient recognize the problem before the infection spreads? If the patient is depressed by what is happening, will there be any desire to control the spread of the infection? It is important to make arrangements for a home care nurse to visit as often as necessary to change the dressings and educate the patient.

Regardless of how prepared a woman is for a mastectomy, anxiety, depression, and concerns about sexuality are almost always experienced. The patient has to adjust to coping with the loss of a breast, and will be reminded of her loss every day as she bathes, looks in the mirror, shops for clothes, or makes love. Additionally, she has to adjust to knowing that she has cancer, and the implication of what this means in terms of her future comfort and life span. The worry about the possible spread of the disease, loss of the other breast, or metastasis to other areas of her body is ever present.

The breast is a primary sex symbol in our culture. The breasts have become a source of admiration, overemphasized to the point that they have been equated with a woman's sexual desire, sexual drive, desirability, and even sexual competence. The notion that men are primarily attracted to a female's breasts has also been propagated. Thus, many women have come to believe that the removal of a breast will make one less desirable, less sexual, and less feminine. Believing this, it is no wonder that patients who undergo a radical mastectomy fear they will be rejected by their friends and unloved by their spouses. In their own eyes, they appear irreparably damaged.

The deformity created by a mastectomy is greatly feared. A woman may feel repulsed by the sight of her incisional scar and be unable to make love freely. She does not want anyone to see her body, and even spares her spouse the sight. If she does resume sexual activity, she may never again remove her brassiere or prosthesis. Thus, even the remaining breast is withdrawn from the fondling lover. Self-consciousness may become so strong that the patient wears only clothing that covers her neck and arms, and will not wear a bathing suit because she is sure that everyone on the beach is staring at her.

Additional difficulties involve shopping for clothes, especially in stores where individual dressing rooms may not be available, or where an eager salesperson may increase the risk of the patient's deformity being noticed. Conversely, some clothing manufacturers are now meeting the needs of mastectomy patients with well-fitting, attractive clothes that hide unsightly scars. Unfortunately, many women avoid resumption of sports activities or being in places that include large groups of people because they fear accidental injury to the remaining breast as well as the possibility of rejection.

If a woman is of childbearing age, special significance may be attached to the inability to breast-feed a child. The patient may feel that she is not a fit mother because the child cannot be cuddled to the breast. If she has passed the childbearing age, she may have feelings of inadequacy as a mother and verbalize feelings of guilt because she did not breast-feed when she could have given the baby this nutritional advantage. On occasion, the child that has been breast-fed has been blamed by the woman as being the cause of the cancer because she remembers that he suckled or bit down too hard.

Some husbands experience an adverse reaction to their wives' mastectomies because it brings a fear of being mutilated to the conscious mind. This is associated with the male fear of castration and may result in rejection of the wife, who already feels that she is unappealing. The rejection is often really the spouse's reaction to his own fears and feelings, symbolized by the wife's operation.

If a marriage is already in trouble, the spouse may view surgery with satisfaction because it serves as a release for his anger. Other men may interpret the wife's surgery as a form of punishment for all the wrongs she has inflicted on him. Some men have never matured, and when they married did so because of the extra notice they would receive from others because of this new acquisition. If the wife was just another status symbol to show off to others or to make other men jealous and envious, then the husband may now believe that others will think he is stuck with a worthless, inadequate, and undesirable person. In truth, he thinks of only himself, not of his mate.

Many men do not understand what to do, what to say, or how to behave during the wife's readjustment period. Should he act as if nothing has happened? Should he pamper her? Should he cancel all social obligations? Should he continue love-making? Should he avoid looking at her when they are dressing? Will the wife be an invalid? Will their life style change?

A spouse who reinforces the idea that he married his wife for more than her breasts, while at the same time demonstrating compassion for her loss, can have a significantly positive effect in the patient's recovery. The husband who sees the operative area (a major hurdle for both spouse and patient) while in the hospital can dispel many conscious and unconscious fears. He should also be encouraged to help with his wife's care at home, by changing dressings, massaging the arm on the affected side, and helping with exercises. The husband should be strongly encouraged to initiate sexual intercourse unless his wife is too debilitated or clearly rejects any sexual contact. The persistent spouse who overtly demonstrates his sexual interests in his wife clearly gives her the message that he still finds her sexually attractive, exciting, and feminine. The spouse should be instructed to use sexual positions that provide the least upper trunk pressure (usually male superior). Patients will usually avoid the female superior position, although it avoids any upper torso contact, because it emphasizes the absence of the breast.

The husband should not pressure his wife to undress in front of him, or insist on nudity. Importance should be placed on sharing the heavy load of emotional feelings, reinforcing the wife's feelings that she is still loved, and encouraging an optimistic attitude about their future together. For many couples, the sharing of this traumatic and emotional experience deepens their value of life in general and their relationship in particular.

An aware, knowledgeable, understanding husband can be a vital asset to a patient during an exceedingly stressful time. The husband, if at all possible, should go with his wife to all appointments to the surgeon, radiologist, and oncologist. He should be included in all discussions regarding his wife's care. He should know that if the biopsy is malignant, a mastectomy will be done. His thoughts and feelings should be elicited repeatedly. After all, this is also a stressful and frightening time for him. He has to keep himself together, support his wife emotionally, and sustain the family. Discussion about expected postoperative reactions such as anxieties and depressive reactions is helpful.

The fear and feelings of the patient, both before and after surgery, are usually related to her memories of past experiences. If the woman's childhood and adulthood were healthy and she developed a positive feeling about herself, then she will be able to love herself despite her loss. The family's way of viewing life, as well as their attitude toward the patient, is a significant factor in recovery. Often, the patient's response is related to an ongoing family problem, rather than the immediate surgical situation.

Inability to accept the gravity and urgency of the situation may be recognized in women who delay seeking medical attention, despite the fact that they know there is a growth in the breast. One patient who delayed the operation related experiencing a tremendous sense of relief when it was finally over. She felt she could now move forward, and begin to plan her life, whereas before she was immobilized by doubts, indecision, and fear. More dramatic is the refusal of some women to accept surgery despite the physician's urgent recommendations. The nurse then must provide a great deal of understanding, and emphasize the threat to the patient's life while stressing the potential life-saving results of surgery.

After surgery, a patient's lack of cooperation as well as her overt anger may very well mean that she was ill prepared for the surgery that occurred. Some patients appear either unwilling or disinterested in learning how to rehabilitate themselves. They seem unmotivated, and remain apathetic about learning to care for the incision or going to available exercise classes. They do not want to discuss breast prostheses and refuse to talk with someone who has fully recovered from a similar experience. These patients demonstrate the involvement of the emotions in this type of surgery, and are actually attempting to deny the reality of their situation.

Many women are turning to reconstruction therapy for restoration or augmentation of the removed beast tissue. This is prompted by a woman's desire to feel physically attractive, whole, and feminine. To a lesser extent it is prompted by dissatisfaction with prostheses, and the problems created when the bra frequently moves up on the affected side. There is considerable controversy regarding the safety of implants including the possibility that they may prevent detection of disease, or even cause disease. Some patients are psychologically helped if a consultation with a plastic surgeon is done before surgery, so that they can be assured that enough skin and muscle will be available for breast reconstruction. This can lead to disappointment if the size and spread of the tumor precludes the possibility of future reconstruction. This is often the situation if axillary node involvement is present. A waiting period of at least 2 to 3 years is often advised before undertaking reconstructive surgery. However, other surgeons believe that immediate reconstruction is advisable to lessen the emotional trauma to which the patient is subjected.

Children often become frightened as they see a previously energetic parent suddenly unable to carry out usual activities. They may also view the loss of hair as embarrassing, particularly if it was the mother's crowning glory. The loss of a limb, or a visible scar may also distress a youngster. There is also fear of "what happens to me if my parent dies?" or "will I have the same problem?" That last thought is even more prevalent among children of the same sex, who identify strongly with the parent.

Because chemotherapy and radiation therapy have adverse effects on the immune system, family members who develop any contagious illness will doubtlessly be barred from the patient's room. This may add to the distress of any children in the home, who may interpret this as another instance of being abandoned or discarded. They will need thorough explanations of why they are denied access to the room and reassurance that they are not the cause of any illness that the parent has.

It is important to allow patients with cancer to maintain hope, whether realistic or not. With the passage of time, the hopes that cannot be attained will be relinquished. It is important for the health worker to reinforce realistic hope by suggesting that the treatment methods in use (e.g., chemotherapy, radiation, gene therapy, pain control, or alternative medicine) are under constant scrutiny and upgrading. Even if the physical condition continues to deteriorate, the patient should be encouraged to work toward any goals that are obtainable.

In one instance, a patient realized that all the therapies were not improving his condition. He told his family that he did not fear dying, but that he could not tolerate the severe pain that he described as "engulfing" him. He had a pistol and a few bullets that he had obtained while a soldier during World War II. He told his wife that he wanted to keep the gun in his nightstand but would not use it unless the pain became intolerable. She was extremely upset at his decision but arguing did no good. After a few days, she recognized that he had always been a responsible person, even as a Holocaust prisoner. She told him that she would support him in whatever he decided to do. She then called the psychiatric nurse therapist who had been visiting him each week and told her what was happening. The therapist immediately called the physician to increase the level of pain medication and to have it available in a self-administered intravenous pump.

Once that change was made, the patient brightened considerably. Once again, he was in control of his life. The pain, although not totally gone, was bearable. The drugs were not used without forethought and never resulted in an overdose. In a few weeks, the patient began to refuse most food and slipped into a coma. Just before that happened, he thanked his wife for having supported his decision to have the gun nearby. "The knowledge that I had the power to end it all if I so chose gave me the strength to continue. The fact that I could relieve my pain as I wanted gave me the courage to hold on and let nature take its course." He died peacefully, with his wife and other family members at his side.

In Denver in 1997, a daylong program was planned, featuring patients who had been diagnosed as having breast cancer. The morning program centered on presentations by professionals, with discussions of newer diagnostic techniques as well as newer treatment modalities. A luncheon (low fat, high fiber) was attended by 800 people including many under present treatment for breast cancer. The meal was followed by a fashion show in which all the models were breast cancer survivors. Some models were in their early 30s, but the "star" of the show was an 88-year-young woman who had undergone a mastectomy when in her 40s. A brief history of each model's cancer history was given as she paraded down the fashion runway. The reaction of the audience was intense—some cried, all applauded, and the hope for those presently under treatment was palpable. These women in their up-to-date outfits were not *victims*. They were *survivors,* giving everyone present a positive expectation for the future. The program demonstrated the change in attitude toward those with cancer now as against the feelings just a few years ago.

THE APPROACH TO THE PERSON WITH CANCER

Immediate Intervention by the Patient

SELF-MANAGEMENT TECHNIQUES

The patient should seek medical help on the discovery of any lumps, unusual skin moles or lesions, headaches, visual problems, and so on. Any cancer that is discovered early on has a better chance of being cured. Monthly breast examinations are an important part of an early detection program, as are mammograms.

Professional Intervention

IMMEDIATE ACTION

Answer any questions that the patient may ask as honestly as possible. Prepare the patient for the procedure to be followed. Include information on pain control measures to be used. Describe the appearance of the postoperative site. Describe any self-care that will be needed once the patient is discharged.

Present a positive outlook to the patient, encouraging the belief that the treatment will lead to recovery.

INTERMEDIATE ACTION

Do not force the reluctant patient to view the operative site. Support the patient's right to wait until ready before looking at the incision.

Provide instructions about the self-care of the operative site. The information may have to be repeated several times, depending on the anxiety level of the patient.

Recognize any symptoms of depression. Help the patient accept the need for treatment. Encourage a hopeful attitude for the future.

LONG-TERM ACTION

Involve significant others in discussions about their reactions to the surgery. Provide any necessary information about care needed after surgery. Refer to pertinent groups (e.g., ostomy care) for support and information.

Help the patient make realistic plans for care once home.

31

The Person With Diabetes

A middle-aged woman goes for a routine annual physical examination. During the course of reporting on how she has been all year, she mentions jestingly that she would really like to feel a bit more peppy, just to keep up with her teen-aged children. She states that sometimes she perspires too much and that she has lost weight even though she "eats like a horse." She attributes her weight loss to her active, independent life style. She mentions some minor inconveniences, such as having a small bladder that necessitates running to the bathroom frequently. But then she is always thirsty, so perhaps she should just stop drinking so much. It all sounds quite innocuous to her, but to the physician this attractive lady's complaints register immediately. Her attempts to make light of minor distresses demonstrate some anxiety. At the conclusion of a complete examination, which includes the necessary urinalysis and blood tests, a diagnosis of diabetes is established. When the patient is told this she smiles and displays a mixture of surprise and disbelief. Surely, there is an error. "Me, a diabetic?" The smile quickly gives way to serious concern as it is definitely established that no error has been made.

It is estimated that 16,000 people in the United States have diabetes, but that only 8,000 actually have been diagnosed. The National Institute of Health has endorsed the new guidelines drawn up by an international panel of experts under the sponsorship of the American Diabetes Association that everyone older than 45 be tested every 3 years by initially having a fasting blood sugar test. Previously, the acceptable blood sugar level was 140 mg glucose per deciliter of blood plasma. In June 1997, that level was reduced to

126. Those with levels above that should have further testing, such as a glucose tolerance test.

Diabetes is the sixth leading cause of death, and also contributes to many cases of blindness, heart disease, neuropathy, and poor wound healing that may lead to amputation. Adults usually develop type II diabetes (previously referred to as adult-onset or non–insulin-dependent diabetes), and can usually be treated with diet; exercise; and, if necessary, oral agents rather than injectable insulin. Those at high risk, including American Indians, Asians, Hispanics, Blacks as well as those who are obese, have hypercholesteremia, or a family history of diabetes should start their testing at an earlier age, and more frequently.

The health worker may first encounter the diabetic patient in the physician's office, during a hospital admission for another illness, or when there is an urgent admission for treatment of insulin shock or diabetic coma. What comes to mind is that this relatively common condition can become a rather severe management problem for many patients. Certainly the diabetic patient must adjust to changes in his living patterns. Frequently, premorbid psychological patterns affect the way in which he does this as he tries to keep his illness under control. Sometimes the psychological problems may further aggravate the illness and thus interfere with its stabilization.

Many health workers believe that the more the patient knows and understands about diabetes, the more self-reliant and capable he will become in its management. Thus, the patient is told that his body has a relative deficiency of the hormone insulin, which is necessary for the proper metabolism of glucose (sugar). This results in an inability of the body to make full use of food that has been ingested. When there is too much unused glucose in the body, it spills over into the urine and blood. The patient is informed about a dietary regimen that regulates his intake of simple carbohydrates and calories. He is taught how to test his urine for sugar and acetone. To control the disease, the patient is given the missing substance (insulin), or an oral agent that stimulates insulin-producing cells. If insulin has been ordered, he is taught how to inject it himself.

This all sounds easy. What makes for complications is that often the patient's problems, including premorbid ones, as well as his attitudes and outlook, may adversely affect his ability to make the adjustments necessary for living with his illness. Are there any preventive measures?

Dietary factors and their influence on the development of type II diabetes have been studied in a group of 65,000 healthy women. Those who ate a high-fiber whole grain cereal for breakfast had a 28% lower risk of developing the disease than those who preferred starchy foods (white bread, rice, potatoes, and processed grains). The women who included little fiber, drank lots of cola, and ate a high level of starchy foods were two and a half times at higher risk of developing type II diabetes. Carbohydrates in starchy food are digested and absorbed quickly, resulting in a sudden increase in the blood sugar (glucose) level, with a resultant secretion of insulin by the pancreas. If the pancreas does not have a sufficient quantity of insulin, or the body is not sensitive enough to the amount produced (or a combination of the two), there is a greater risk of developing this form of diabetes. For patients who do develop non–insulin-dependent diabetes, acarbose may be helpful.

Acarbose (Precose) is a newer antidiabetic agent that acts differently from previous hypoglycemic medications. It works by inhibiting the metabolism of carbohydrates. If hypoglycemia occurs, it will not be reversed by most oral sugars. Instead, the patient should take oral glucose in the form of a pill or gel (not sucrose), or milk. He may require dextrose in an intravenous line push, possibly followed by an infusion of D5W. Glucose monitoring is used to keep track of blood levels, with increased monitoring when the patient is under stress, has an infection, or is planning to undergo a surgical procedure. It is also important when diet or medications undergo changes.

Acarbose is employed along with diet and exercise for patients with non–insulin-dependent diabetes. It can be used with other oral hypoglycemics if indicated. The advantage of this new mediation is that there is a smaller increase in blood glucose concentrations after meals, and that it inhibits the metabolism of sucrose to glucose and fructose. It is administered three times daily, to be taken with the first bite at each main meal. It can be used during pregnancy, but not during lactation and not for children because its efficacy and safety has not been established for them at this time.

The health worker frequently encounters a diabetic who denies having the illness; he simply refuses to accept the diagnosis. He sets out to prove that he is the master of his own body, always in control. He will allow nothing to direct his life, nor will he submit himself to a "ridiculous" regimen of injections. He will not be humiliated, lose self-esteem, or be known in any way, shape, or form as someone with a health problem. He refuses to learn to inject himself and fails to stay on any semblance of a diet. He refuses to believe that the consequences of uncontrolled diabetes may be life threatening.

In one case, an elderly man refused to acknowledge the relationship between his mild diabetes and the wound area on his leg. He refused medical treatment for the area, saying that it was "nothing" and that it did not bother him. He refused to follow any dietary restrictions and would not accept the need for surgical intervention. As time went on, the area increased in size and became necrotic. He continued to refuse any medical advice, until he noticed that his leg was becoming purple around the wound.

By the time he got to the doctor, gangrene had set in, and the leg had to be amputated below the knee. The patient still refused to accept the fact that he had diabetes, and demanded that his wife bring treats of ice cream and cake to him in the hospital. He was very angry when the staff discovered what he was doing and argued with them about his diabetic restrictions. He was discharged to his home, with poor healing of the stump noted on subsequent postoperative visits. In time, he was fitted for a prosthesis, but complained that it hurt too much to wear. He was remeasured and refitted for a new prosthesis on four other occasions. Regardless of the fit, he refused to wear the device, preferring to remain in a wheelchair with several attendants meeting his needs. His constant inactivity led to a weight gain of more than 50 pounds within a year. He would not accept any psychotherapy and was diagnosed as being suicidal because of his actions. He finally agreed to take an oral hypoglycemic agent but would not accept any dietary restrictions.

Although the physicians and nurses tried to intervene, the patient refused to change his mode of living. It was evident that his desire to harm himself was his main objective. In time, other areas of his body became necrotic. As deterioration set in, he began to accept his own role in what was happening. He then requested help with diet and hypoglycemic medications. He dismissed the attendants and began a program of self-help. He began to lose some of the excess weight, and started an exercise regime that strengthened his body and helped him to become independent of the wheelchair. He agreed to another fitting of a prosthesis and learned to walk with it.

The nurses and physicians involved in his care were nonjudgmental and supportive as he progressed. As he improved, he told one of them that his main focus had been on "getting even" with his second wife, whom he saw as being uncaring, only interested in his wealth. He said that if the nurses had not continued to accept him, he would not have been able to make the about-face that allowed him to recover. The staff was gratified as he improved but credited their ability to accept him to the involvement of a psychiatric nurse therapist who was able to help them recognize the dysfunctional dynamics displayed by the patient.

Impotence is frequently one of the early signs of diabetes in males. Sometimes it is a psychogenic reaction to the diagnosis, but more often it is due to nerve or vascular defects that are associated with the disorder. Fears of erectile or orgasmic failure add to the stress and may impede performance. In some instances, penile implants may be of help because they enable the individual to perform sexually.

Neuropathy is also involved in female loss of orgasmic capacity. In addition, diabetes often is linked to infections, with an increase in pain and pruritis. Concerns about pregnancy also are frequent. Will pregnancy be possible? Will the fetus and the mother survive? It is helpful to have the couple attend counseling sessions together to gain insight into their sexual problems and to learn ways that will help maintain a loving relationship.

The individual who is basically dependent also presents problems. He may regress further and refuse to have any part in the management or control of his illness. He first becomes immobilized by his disease, and then finds that being cared for meets a deep need and, therefore, is a pleasurable prospect. The fact that he has diabetes may even serve to increase his anxiety, which, in turn, increases his need to be dependent. He may, therefore, exhibit a helplessness, demanding that everything be done for him. When his needs are not met, he may lapse into apathy and depression.

The adult diabetic who is depressed may act on his desire to end his life by going off his diet or neglecting to take his insulin. Or, if the patient feels he is being punished for his misdeeds through his illness, he may become hostile and resentful. He may express his anger and frustration by overeating.

Emotional conflicts and reactions are often activated by the diabetic patient's dietary restrictions. The psychological significance of food is related to support, love, and acceptance. When denied certain foods, the patient may have increased feelings of being unloved, rejected, or unwanted. This can pose particular problems in the already obese individual who overeats to satisfy frustrated drives and to increase his feeling of well-being. The reverse situation is seen in the patient who is unable to eat, or refuses to, when he becomes upset. "You make me unhappy so I just won't eat," is what is unconsciously meant. This behavior may cause a hypoglycemic reaction.

Young diabetics with type I diabetes (previously referred to as juvenile diabetes or insulin-dependent diabetes) may use the disorder as a way of controlling their parents by threatening to disregard their dietary regimen if their request for a new car, for an increase in allowance, or for new clothes is not granted. They may express their anger by undereating, overeating, or failing to take their insulin. Parents themselves may unconsciously resent the trouble or be unable to deal with the guilt of having a diabetic youngster. As a result, they may be either too rigid or too lax in their attention to the child's diet.

Youngsters are often resistant to limitations placed on them by the disorder. If denial is strong, the patient may attempt to prove he can eat anything he desires. This sets the stage for a severe hyperglycemic reaction necessitating hospitalization. Diabetic youngsters often feel that because they are not like everyone else, they aren't worth loving. Special attention and cooperation from parents are essential.

In one case, a 19-year-old girl was admitted to the intensive care unit in a diabetic coma. During recovery, she related that she had had an argument with her parents, who objected strenuously to her dating a boy of dubious character. They had threatened to withhold funds they had promised to help finance her education. She was furious that they did not realize how seriously she felt about her boyfriend and wanted to punish them for not viewing the relationship as she did. She expressed her anger by omitting her insulin and by ingesting several frankfurters, some candy, and a malted milk shake. Her diabetic reaction almost cost her her life.

The health worker must be aware of certain very real and irksome inconveniences that the diabetic faces. The first episode may have followed a viral attack. In addition, emotional stress may have raised the blood glucose level. (In fact, the onset of the disease is itself often related to a stressful period in the patient's life.) When under stress, the patient may develop such psychological symptoms as increased sensitivity, fright, or forgetfulness. He should be encouraged to talk about these feelings and experiences. The health worker can then help him to seek new ways of managing stressful problems before they arise.

The diabetic patient often needs help in seeking and obtaining wholesome satisfactions and pleasures to offset those he is denied. Practicing self-denial is difficult for anyone, so imagine what it is like for the diabetic, who must do this on a continual basis. He also has to learn to deal with feelings of awkwardness or embarrassment if he has to take insulin while on the job, before a social event, or when on a trip. He may have to increase his intake of glucose when participating in sports, and he must be able to test his urine or blood frequently. He is apt to fatigue easily and then develops a sense of frustration when his lack of energy prevents him from doing or accomplishing all he desires. Sometimes this leads him to ignore the whole regimen, and test his limits. Female patients often feel unfeminine and unattractive because they perspire heavily. The patient's self-image may be impaired, and she may blame her inability to attract men, obtain employment, or have friends on the illness.

Whether the diabetic makes a successful adjustment to his illness may depend on the successful working-through of emotional conflicts that existed before the illness and that are now aggravated by it. Concerns regarding future illnesses, fears of becoming incapacitated, doubts about the advisability of having a baby, and worries about dying can be activated. The special meaning of illness must be explored with each and every diabetic patient. The special problems and fears encountered by each patient must be clarified. The health worker should take as much time as needed to uncover the feelings aroused by the illness, to help the patient make a satisfactory adjustment to living with his condition.

THE APPROACH TO THE PERSON WITH DIABETES

Immediate Intervention by the Patient

SELF-MANAGEMENT TECHNIQUES

Recognize the physical target symptoms that are present when hyperglycemia or hypoglycemia are imminent—weakness, sweating, anxiety, hunger, and so on. Differentiate between the two. Use the glucometer for an accurate blood glucose level. Always wear a Medi Alert bracelet or carry a card in the wallet with the diagnosis and a list of the medications that are being used. Seek help immediately.

If on acarbose, carry a supply of glucose tablets or gel for use if hypoglycemic. Carry candy or sugar if hypoglycemia is due to insulin or other hypoglycemic drugs. Have insulin available if hyperglycemia occurs. Take the proper agent if untoward symptoms begin.

Professional Intervention

IMMEDIATE ACTION

Make certain the patient receives immediate care.

Recognize any actions that may have led to the reaction, and be prepared to discuss them later with the patient.

Understand that a patient with diabetes can be a real suicidal risk. The patient may act out his desire to die by not taking insulin or by overeating. Attempt to persuade him to seek relief from his hostility and frustration through acceptable channels. He can take a brisk walk, involve himself in group activities, punch a punching bag, or pound a pillow.

INTERMEDIATE ACTION

Do not argue with the patient regarding his noncompliance or lack of cooperation. Instead, point out that his behavior may be related to an upsetting incident in his life, perhaps precipitated by an argument. Tell him, "It appears that every time your girlfriend and you argue, you overeat," or "It appears that your worry about your work causes you to forget to eat on a regular basis." In other words, help the patient to connect his behavior with the problem that caused it. Then help him develop a plan for new ways of reacting to and handling his problems.

Encourage the diabetic patient to talk about his fears, feelings, and problems. Recognize that his denial of illness is a manifestation of an emotional conflict. Do not react angrily or reprimand him. Instead tell him, "I understand how upset you must be. Other patients have learned to manage successfully with treatment, and, in time, you will also." Explain to the patient that it is important to deal with what exists, even though at times it is painful. Assure him that he will be given every assistance in learning new ways of living. Be aware that the patient's moodiness, fright, or forgetfulness may be related to an unregulated glucose level.

Be empathic regarding the difficulties and hardships the patient encounters in controlling his illness. But stress his rewards and gains in doing so. Maintain an optimistic attitude. Recognize the fact that the patient can continue to lead an adequate and constructive life.

LONG-TERM ACTION

Emphasize the individual's strengths and independent abilities. Allow the patient to do all he can for himself, even though it may seem easier to do things for him. Minimize his dependencies. Instruct him about anything that will make his life easier. Inform him about how to protect his clothing from perspiration odor by wearing absorbent, loose garments, about the use of special soaps that will help prevent infection, and about how to cut his toe-nails and care for his feet correctly.

Encourage the young diabetic to test his own urine and give himself insulin as soon as possible. The more the youngster can do for himself, the less restricted he will feel.

32

The Person Undergoing Renal Dialysis or Transplant

Properly functioning kidney tissue is necessary for life. Inadequate function results in the accumulation of waste products in the blood stream and alteration of the body's chemical balance. This results in a condition called uremia. When uremia is severe and life-threatening, dialysis is generally instituted. Dialysis involves pumping the patient's arterial blood through a coiled tube of thin cellophane-like material. This coiled tube is immersed in a bath of fluid which closely resembles normal blood plasma. Excess waste products that have accumulated in the patient's blood are washed out through the coil membrane into the surrounding bath, resulting in more normal blood plasma. The dialyzed (washed) blood flows from the coil into tubing that leads back to the patient's venous circulation.

Some patients are dialyzed on a short-term basis for acute kidney failure such as may occur in poisonings, shock, burns, severe acute nephritis, or severe injuries. Other patients require long-term dialysis for chronic renal failure when the course and prognosis are uncertain or in preparation or expectation of receiving a renal transplant. A patient on chronic renal dialysis usually has a permanent arteriovenous shunt implanted in an arm or leg to provide ready access to an artery and a vein, both of which are used in the dialyzing procedure. Because the shunts are often external, they may become uncoupled, accidentally or willfully. The patient will then bleed profusely and may die if the tube is not clamped in time.

More recently, surgical preparation of the patient for chronic dialysis has leaned toward creating a permanent arteriovenous connection in the patient's arm or leg. Such an arteriovenous fistula has the advantage of being unexposed (i.e., it is totally beneath the skin). But after it has been created an appreciable period must elapse before it is ready for use. There is also the disadvantage of an increased circulatory and cardiac burden.

The patient in renal failure may have subtle or acute signs that are of psychological significance. However, it is important to realize that the symptoms are probably not related to the patient's emotional stability. Instead, they are related to the presence of toxic products in the blood stream that affect both brain and general nervous system functioning. Often a health worker may mistake the patient's symptoms (rambling, impaired ability to concentrate, complaints of headache, poor attention span, sleepiness, lethargy, twitching or confused state) as being the onset of an acute psychotic episode. In fact, they are the signs of an existing medical emergency. The symptoms disappear as treatment for the kidney failure is initiated and maintained.

Patients undergoing dialysis have a chronic medical condition. Many stresses are encountered by the patient as he adjusts to the treatment program. As happens with other patients who are subject to long-term, unending care, the physical limitations, as well as economic and social adjustments, create problems that have a psychological effect on the patient. It is helpful for the nurse to understand that the patient's behavior is a reaction to these pressures.

The patient's personality before illness and his coping skills when under stress are an important factor in his adjustment to dialysis. Patients who are able to tolerate frustration and can be optimistic regarding their situation are usually more cooperative in meeting the demands imposed by their illness.

The chronic dialysis patient looks forward to a confining life during which he is dependent on a hemodialysis machine to which he is attached for almost an entire day or night two or three times a week. As an alternative, equipment for peritoneal dialysis may be used four times a day, for shorter intervals. This dependency can be resented and feared. It can also create a great deal of anxiety, as it seriously interferes with the individual's ability to perform the work or household duties that he effectively managed before. The fear of losing his job and its income, and no prospect of complete recovery, often lead to a severe depression. A patient's tearfulness, lack of desire to talk, and disinterest in what is going on about him are related to this depression, as are his loss of confidence and self-esteem.

Children who are undergoing dialysis are presently being studied for the differences in the selection of peritoneal or hemodialysis as the treatment modality. Those belonging to minority groups are more likely to receive hemodialysis administered by professionals in a medical setting. White children usually receive peritoneal dialysis at home. The results appear to be better for the latter, usually performed four times a day, with less disruption in their schooling and fewer medical problems. The question is whether there is a professional bias, with the belief that minority children will not receive adequate supervision to carry out the peritoneal procedure properly at home.

Socially, the dialysis patient may not be able to keep up with the pace he previously enjoyed. Friends and family may begin to regard him as totally unable to function, helpless, and ill. Hence, they may unwittingly begin to relate to the patient as if he were incapable of thinking or answering for himself. The loss of self-value often comes about as a result of the patient's regarding himself in the same way that he thinks others regard him. If the patient begins to feel that those around him feel he is worthless, he may begin to believe that it is so. A man may no longer be called on to act as the head of the household, or a woman may no longer be regarded as a competent mother and wife. An adolescent may be avoided by friends and rejected by school clubs because she cannot share in many extracurricular activities. In addition, the physical changes, especially the inability to urinate normally, causes considerable difficulty during adolescence, when the youngster is in the midst of developing a new body image. The sadness and unhappiness manifested in such instances may be so severe that the person may become deeply depressed and feel that death is really preferable to the life he is presently living.

The risk of suicide among such patients is high. The patient can kill himself easily by separating his shunt, which will allow him to bleed to death. Other suicide methods include refusing his dialysis treatment, or ignoring the dietary regimen (usually low protein, high carbohydrate and fat, low sodium and potassium).

Often the patient's emotional difficulty reflects itself in his inability to relate to the hospital staff. He may be a real problem in daily management and be unable to cope with even the simplest daily activities. His need for reassurance may take the form of a demand for constant attention from the staff. Irksome behavior may involve sounding the buzzer frequently and complaining almost continuously about seemingly trivial matters, such as the sheets not being straight or a chair being placed incorrectly. This behavior can become irritating to the staff, particularly if they do not understand that the patient is really saying, in the only way he can at that time, "Don't leave me; I'm afraid; I'm afraid to live; I'm afraid to die."

Some dialysis patients complain of intense nausea. One lady was so nauseated she could not retain any food whatsoever. The staff did not believe that the patient was as nauseated as she complained of being and thought that she was being purposely unpleasant. Their anger and rejection of her created difficulty for the patient. Actually, the patient was nauseated because of her uremic state, but her anxiety and fear increased the already unpleasant symptom. As she eventually became more hopeful, she experienced less nausea.

Dialysis patients are worriers. Why shouldn't they be? They have a lot to worry about. And their worries, furthermore, are not imaginary. They are only too real, because the hardships and the discomforts are real. Patients worry about day-to-day living, a major concern being whether they will be accepted into a long-term treatment program. They wonder if they will ever recover sufficiently to enjoy a trip, the theater, a shopping spree, or even if they will ever leave the hospital alive. One lady had a sister who died from kidney disease at the age of 22, and she naturally questioned her own chances of survival. Patients worry that their spouses will desert them, or that the shunt will be repugnant to others who may view it. They fear that they will run out of money and become impoverished, and that they will be hated for being unable to help with the family plans and routines because of illness, thereby disrupting those plans. One young girl worried constantly about completing high school, having friends, and the possibility of dating, marriage, and pregnancy.

Frequently, patients will appear to deny their situation or illness. Denial often alarms the staff because they feel that the patient who doesn't talk openly and continuously about his problem is surely headed for disaster. This is not necessarily so. Often the patient talks about the weather, shopping, going home, lipstick brands or baseball averages in an attempt to reduce anxiety and the overwhelming unpleasant and uncomfortable thoughts about what is happening. Thus, the individual protects himself and focuses on something that is real to him to hang on to his rapidly decreasing sense of self-control. However, when the patient acts as if he is hearing for the first time what you have told him two hundred times, flagrantly eats the wrong foods, and participates in sports which increase the chances of a shunt separation, his denial must be regarded as a problem.

The patient who needs a transplant is aware that his condition is grave and can be fatal. He knows the misery of being in kidney failure, is fearful of dying, and sees the transplant as the only real hope for prolonging his life. Additionally, the patient sees a chance for a new life without his semipermanent attachment to the dialysis machine. He is grateful if a donor is found but, by the same token, he feels guilty and responsible for the possible shortening of the donor's life. Many patients, fearful of a negative response, avoid approaching relatives who are possible donors. At the same time, relatives may avoid the patient if they suspect that they may be asked to be a donor. They may feel guilty if they refuse yet think that because the donation is only palliative, not curative, it is not worth the risk to themselves.

Potential kidney recipients go through many moods, varying from grief to happiness, as they wait for the news that an acceptable kidney donor has been found. One young patient, on hearing that her father's kidney was not acceptable for transplant, became deeply depressed. She felt that God had forsaken her and that she must be an especially bad girl for him to punish her so terribly. She felt she had been refused a new life and was unloved by her father (God). For a while she refused to talk or look at her father, and accused him of being her enemy. Another patient, who had been told that his sister's kidney was acceptable, was able to lessen his feelings of guilt about the donation by reasoning that his sister was comparatively healthy and that girls don't have to work because they marry and stay home. Thus he felt that one kidney was really sufficient for her.

After transplant surgery, there is always the risk of tissue rejection by the patient's body. Patients realize this, but fear of such rejection is tempered by the knowledge that some transplants last for lengthy periods. However, living with the thought that the possibility of rejection always exists produces a great deal of fear. Although the patient is no longer in need of dialysis, he often questions his own decision to accept a transplant, thinking that perhaps it would have been better to live attached to the machine than to worry so much about the possible failure of the transplanted kidney. Some patients have also expressed the fear of dying as a punishment for accepting someone else's kidney. The patient needs help in coping with the uncertainty as to whether or not he will live. He needs to talk about his personal feelings with a health worker who has come to terms with his own feelings about death.

Family members usually need a great deal of emotional support in handling the stresses created when a family member is undergoing dialysis or transplantation. They may feel useless or guilty if they are unable or unwilling to supply the needed kidney. They may also resent having to meet the many demands of the patient. The burden of personal care, transportation, dietary management, and finances is great, and can become wearing over time.

The quality of the relationships between family members and the patient may undergo subtle changes which may have detrimental effects on all concerned. This is particularly true if feelings of displeasure, resentment, anger, or disappointment are not brought out into the open and discussed. If disagreements and arguments occur, it is imperative for members to talk realistically about what bothers them rather than bottle up their emotions because they are under the impression that such repression spares the patient. Feelings of antagonism are communicated subtly or otherwise, with the patient then feeling that he is unworthy of being included in family matters. He may also misconstrue family conversations, feeling that he is the subject under discussion, even though the actual subject may be as remote as the purchase of a new refrigerator. Talking things over gives the patient the opportunity to discuss his feelings and reveal his concerns and attitudes, and allows for openness, honesty, and improved understanding among all.

If family members are overly protective and continuously try to please and do everything for the patient, they may encourage him to behave like a child. This can also increase the patient's guilt regarding the anger he feels, possibly leading to a severe depression. Finding a middle road is not easy. The family needs help in providing support while, at the same time, encouraging the patient to do whatever he can for himself. This will encourage the patient by demonstrating the family's belief in his capabilities. If the patient is on dialysis in the home, stress is increased due to disruption of normal family life and the increased medical responsibility undertaken by the family. The intelligence and closeness of the relationships between family members and the ability of all to adjust to change and tolerate frustration will have an effect on the degree of success of the treatment.

It is important for health workers to understand the usual emotional reactions of the patient on dialysis so that they can tolerate and cope with the stress. The patient often displaces his own anger onto the staff and may be unappreciative, or even resistant, to the medical regime. His attitude may lead to anger and punitive dictatorial attitudes on the part of the health workers. Occasionally, a staff member will react by becoming oversolicitous and overprotective to offset his own hostile feelings.

THE APPROACH TO THE PERSON UNDERGOING RENAL DIALYSIS OR TRANSPLANTATION

Immediate Intervention by the Patient

SELF-MANAGEMENT TECHNIQUES

Recognize any changes in the physical status that indicate increased kidney problems (retention of fluid in the extremities, headaches, lethargy, twitching; possible changes in mental status, such as confusion, inability to concentrate, poor attention span). Report changes to the care provider immediately.

Professional Intervention

IMMEDIATE ACTION

Recognize that the patient's bizarre behavior may be due to symptoms of uremia. At the same time, recognize the pressures that generate unusual behavior. Help the patient to deal with that behavior, and at the same time attempt to alleviate the underlying pressure and social problems.

Teach the patient what to do in case of an accidental shunt separation. Answer all his questions fully and honestly.

INTERMEDIATE ACTION

Allow time and opportunity for the patient to talk about his serious situation. Do not lie or try to minimize it, as the patient usually learns the truth through his sensitivity to the reactions of those around him. Never deceive the patient. When the patient tells you that he is planning to return to work soon, help him determine what actually can be realistically expected. Tell the patient, "You will be able to return to work eventually, if some adjustments can be made in the number of hours you work per day." Another approach could be, "It is quite possible that you might desire to look into a less strenuous line of work. Have you considered any other vocation?" Or "Many women have been able to earn an adequate salary by working from their homes. Maybe you and I can look into some of the opportunities available." Present an optimistic outlook.

Encourage and support hope. The patient needs to have positive thoughts about his future to cope with the adversity, ongoing discomfort or pain, and concerns about prognosis. Positive attitudes of the health workers can do much to carry patients through difficult times. Staff should reinforce the idea that the patient is entitled to life, regardless of guilt about past misdeeds and wrongs. Offsetting masochistic and depressive behavior patterns by supporting his right to life and by providing hope will enable the patient to summon forth emotional strength needed to face the future and its uncertainties.

Explore the patient's feelings toward having a shunt. Although he may feel negatively about it, he will probably choose to have it when alternatives are presented and understood. Help the patient look at what he *can* achieve even though there are limitations rather than stress what he cannot do. Always try to understand the patient's fear of death and dependency. Your interest and concern in the person may help boost his deteriorating self-image.

Discuss the pros and cons of a transplant with the patient. Patients have few possible alternatives. Therefore, the positive should be emphasized, along with a discussion of what can realistically be expected. Tell the patient, "You can be well for years. Rejection is something that may always have to be reckoned with. If it should occur, it will have to be handled in the best way possible at that time." Emotional difficulties following transplantation are the rule, not the exception. All patients have psychological reactions. Therefore, health workers should help prepare the patient for the usual and anticipated reactions.

Support relatives and allow them to talk about their feelings. This may not alter the patient's condition or the situation, but it is helpful in obtaining temporary relief from intense pent-up feelings. Your warmth, calmness, and sense of hopefulness helps them to feel stronger as they bear their heavy burden. It also boosts family morale.

LONG-TERM ACTION

Be alert for signals that indicate the possibility of suicide. Continue to work with the patient on new solutions to problems that may arise.

Give unending support. Never abandon the patient. Even though it takes time to institute dialysis treatment or to arrange long-term plans for home dialysis, the nurse can still help by listening and stressing the hopeful plans that are under way.

33

The Person With a Dementia of the Alzheimer's Type

As the baby boomers (those reaching their 40s and 50s) become aware of their own memory lapses, they wonder whether they are in danger of developing Alzheimer's or other dementia. They may see parents, friends, associates at work, or nationally known individuals suddenly begin to show signs of cognitive impairment. As they, too, demonstrate some problems with remembering a specific word or fact, they may panic and seek professional evaluation. For some the concern is valid, but for most, the worry is an innocent lapse, what some laughingly refer to as a "senior moment."

Are there differences that can help people distinguish between a lapse and a more serious type of memory loss? In dementia, the memory loss is severer and occurs more frequently. The individual may forget to turn off household appliances, causing food to burn on the stove or clothes to be scorched when being ironed. A memory lapse might be responsible for the accidents, but the individual with the memory lapse will recognize the odor of burning food or cloth, while the person with dementia will not recognize that anything is out of order.

It is wise to have a mental status examination every year after the age of 65 to uncover any problem early, so that available intervention can be instituted. Presently, medications (Cognex, Aricept) are being investigated that appear to slow the process of impairment. Recent experimental studies suggest that new neural cells develop when people are exposed to new activities that stimulate their brains. If these experiments prove to be accurate, people of all ages should become involved in activities with which they are unfamiliar to increase the number of neurons in the brain.

Dementia of the Alzheimer's type is most closely associated with patients older than age 65 and accounts for 50% to 60% of dementia cases. There are several reasons for dementia, with about 20% to 30% resulting from vascular accidents (multistrokes or infarcts), another 5% to 25% from a combination of Alzheimer's and multi-infarcts, and about 5% from other causes, such as senility, syphilis, substance and toxic reactions, AIDS, and neurological degenerative diseases. However, it is the dementia of the Alzheimer's type that presently is receiving the greatest publicity and causes the highest level of consternation. At this time, 4 million Americans are afflicted by this disorder, which has no known cause or cure.

Autopsy studies in Sweden and Finland have demonstrated that almost half of the elderly drivers who died in automobile accidents showed signs of early Alzheimer's disease. They also showed a high incidence of the gene that suggests a greater risk of late-onset Alzheimer's disease. Because many elderly people rely on driving to get around, they are unwilling to give up that activity. In the United States, there were 13 million drivers older than age 70 in 1995, a number that is expected to double by 2020. A psychological test has been devised that detects cognitive impairment in drivers. Although it is unlikely that it will be used for routine testing of elderly drivers, the suggestion has been made that those who have been involved in an auto accident be evaluated to determine whether they should be permitted to continue driving. California now requires that physicians report a diagnosis of dementia to the state. Because an evaluation may then be ordered, patients may avoid seeking the initial assessment for fear of losing the right to drive. Health providers are in a position to help individuals evaluate their right to drive against the danger that they may pose to themselves or others. Those with severe dementia do not really pose a problem because they are usually unable to drive (or possibly even find the car).

As people age, their cognitive abilities begin to diminish, and the dementia associated with Alzheimer's disease may occur, usually in stages, over a period of 3 to 20 years. Often the first phase is signaled by forgetfulness, with mild cognitive deficits that include an inability to recall familiar names or where articles were left. (It is not uncommon for "normal" individuals to misplace keys, but it would not be normal to have left them in the refrigerator.) At this point, the decline is so mild that it frequently goes undetected at work or in social situations. As the disorder progresses, confusion may set in, with an increase in cognitive decline. The individual may be unable to find his way to a familiar location, such as the theater around the corner, and be unable to maintain his competence at work. There may be problems in remembering names or new information as well as an inability to concentrate.

In time, the cognitive abilities decline even further, with obvious memory deficits. The person may not recall his own important life events (where he went to school, exciting trips taken with loved ones), and may be unable to perform complex tasks that were once easily undertaken. There may be a sharp decline in his response to events around him, such as noticing that the green traffic light has changed to red. At this stage, he may deny the presence of any deficits but may withdraw from any challenges that he used to enjoy, such as doing crossword puzzles or participating in card games.

At the point where actual dementia sets in, there is a moderately severe decline in cognitive functioning. The individual needs assistance in many of the activities of daily living. He may demonstrate disorientation as to time, dates, and place, but is still aware of his need for toileting and can feed himself. He may not be able to dress himself completely, perhaps trying to place pajama pants over his head or underwear over his street clothes. As further decline occurs, a severe cognitive deficit is obvious. He becomes completely dependent on others to survive. He may be unable to recognize his spouse, parents, or children, and may remain unaware of the events occurring around him.

At the last stage of dementia, there is a severe decline in cognitive functioning, marked by an inability to communicate verbally or to walk without assistance. Patients may not remember how to chew or swallow their food, causing them to lose weight, perhaps even choking as they eat. They may not recognize their need to go to the bathroom and become incontinent. It is at this point that a caregiver may seek institutionalization for the patient. For many family members, the decline in a loved one's abilities has been painful, but with the patient incapable of recognizing anyone, and unable to care for himself in any way, it may be too difficult to maintain him at home.

Some of the symptoms to watch for in dementia are aphasia (deterioration of language), apraxia (difficulty with motor activities), and agnosia (failure to recognize objects) as well as difficulty in executive functioning (failure to think abstractly, plan, execute, monitor, and stop the sequence). The loss of neurons is one reason for the decrease in memory with the loss of recognition of people and objects. The resultant confusion and inability to carry out the activities of daily living puts a burden not only on the patient but also on the caregiver. The patient may not remember how to carry out daily hygiene activities—bathing, brushing teeth, hair care, toileting, or dressing. A patient may fight attempts to assure his personal cleanliness, and may refuse to bathe or change his clothing. This may be due to embarrassment at undressing in front of others, which may be lessened by draping a large beach towel over him during the undressing and bathing processes. Bath water should be readied in advance, with its temperature carefully checked because the patient may be unable to recognize the potential for being burned if it is too hot. The patient may fight to wear the same clothes each day, perhaps because they are loose, soft, and comfortable. It may be necessary to sponge bathe the patient and have several identical outfits available to allow clothing changes without fussing.

The provider may feel frustrated at having to repeat suggestions several times, and often needs to be reminded that the patient may no longer understand the words being spoken. The patient may be more alert and capable at certain times of the day, yet unable to function at all at other times. The caregiver needs support and understanding as the deterioration continues. Most blame themselves for the lack of improvement, making it important for professionals to help them realize that the course of the disease is unremitting. The caretaker will need time away, if only for a short period, to regain the energy needed to care for the patient.

The search for helpful medication continues. Some believe that the use of estrogens or anti-inflammatories may stay the course, if only for a short time. Vitamins have also been tried. However, at this writing, only two drugs have been approved by the Food and Drug Administration specifically for treatment of Alzheimer's. Both drugs inhibit the disintegration of acetylcholine, which is needed by nerve cells to communicate with each other. Although neither drug prevents Alzheimer's from progressing, each helps ease mild to moderate symptoms. Aricept (donepezel) acts on only the acetylcholine in the brain and, therefore, has fewer side effects than Cognex (tacrine), which can affect related chemicals throughout the body and may also cause liver abnormalities. Aricept requires only one pill daily, while Cognex must be taken four times a day, which may pose a problem if the patient is uncooperative or has difficulty in swallowing. Neither drug is effective for all patients, and the effectiveness of each can be expected to decline in time.

Most patients are maintained at home unless they become totally unmanageable or violent. They may no longer recognize a spouse, other family members, or friends. Day care may be available, with group activities that stimulate them. This has the secondary gain of giving the caretaker time away from the situation. If patients require institutionalization, visits from family and friends may help them keep some contact with their own world. However, even moments after visitors have left, patients may be unable to recall their having been there.

Because the patient is not expected to recover, some thought should be given to advance proxy planning for the time when self-determination may not be possible concerning the extent of medical intervention in a crisis situation. (Legally acceptable advance directive decisions have been executed by only about 20% of all Americans. The other 80% are subjected to the will of others should an emergency arise.) Interested parties (usually family members) should designate a surrogate decision maker, who will work with the professional health providers to determine the level of care to be offered. In most instances, patients with Alzheimer's die from secondary complications, such as aspiration, infections, or injuries from falls or burns. Treatment can range from aggressive care in intensive care units to palliative care as in a hospice situation, depending on the desires of the surrogate decision maker.

Nurses may be called on to help in the determination of the most suitable care, and to provide support to the surrogate decision maker. Should the patient be resuscitated? Should there be nasogastric or gastrostomy feedings? Should infections or other medical conditions be treated aggressively? The more advanced the planing, the easier it will be to incorporate the plans into the nursing care appropriately. The patient should receive the most humane care possible, with consideration given to safety, prevention of exacerbating any disability or discomfort, and preservation of dignity. The physical and psychological well-being of the patient should be a major consideration as long as the patient lives.

The health provider's role extends from the patient to the family. It is almost impossible to anticipate how long the patient will survive once severe deterioration sets in. Some families choose to transfer the patient to a hospice when death seems near. However, the rapid growth of such care as well as the increase in Medicare costs for it (presently $2 billion a year) has led to the government stipulation that hospice care be available only during the last six months of life. In fact, 29% of the patients die within 2 weeks of entering a hospice. Conversely, the excellence of nursing care may lead to a prolonged hospice stay.

Regardless of the time, the family needs emotional support as the patient disintegrates. Most of all, the surrogate decision maker needs to know that any decisions concerning resuscitation or aggressive care can be reversed should it be desired. Family and friends will benefit by seeing how well the patient is cared for by the nursing staff. Conferences that include the surrogate decision maker, any interested family members or friends, and staff can be used to explain the reasons for the care being given and to bolster the surrogate's decisions about that care.

Staff members may differ in their concepts of the level of care to be offered. It is important for staff to settle their differences by coming to a consensus through sharing their thoughts. Each may be reacting to previous personal experiences, as well as religious, ethical, or moral beliefs that may differ from those of the other professional involved in the care. The beliefs of the patient and his significant others must be examined so that a consensus can be reached by the staff that will be in the best interests of the patient and acceptable to all who are involved.

THE APPROACH TO THE PERSON WITH DEMENTIA OF THE ALZHEIMER'S TYPE

Immediate Intervention by the Patient

SELF-MANAGEMENT TECHNIQUES

Recognize the signs of increasing confusion, and lessen the stimulation that may have caused it. Keep the patient in a quiet, calm atmosphere, without demanding that he do anything that will anger him. Have additional help available if the patient is likely to become violent.

Remove and hide car keys if the patient wants to drive.

Remove any materials that may result in harm to the patient or others, such as lethal weapons, toxic substances, pills (prescribed or other) as well as alcohol.

Remove stove handles, lock bathroom and kitchen drawers and cabinets, put plugs in electrical outlets, put a buzzer on outside doors so that they will make noise and alert the caregiver to their being opened.

Remove bathroom door locks, but keep the door closed to prevent the patient from entering, opening the faucets and forgetting to turn them off, resulting in an overflow of water.

Professional Intervention

IMMEDIATE ACTION

Initiate the approach. "You seem unwilling to take your bath today. Perhaps you would enjoy a sponge bath and a change of clothing. We have an outfit identical to the one that you are wearing now."

Be certain that the patient maintains adequate food and fluid intake. Be aware of any dental problems that may interfere with eating. Check temperature of all food and fluids to prevent him from burning his mouth.

Be aware of signals that the patient requires toileting. The patient may not be able to verbalize his need. He may pull at his pants, start to tug at the zipper, or rub his hands on the pubic area. It may be necessary to toilet him at regular intervals to train his bladder and prevent accidents.

Pay attention to daily hygiene including mouth and hair care. It is helpful to put the toothpaste on the toothbrush and to remind the patient not to swallow the residue. Help will probably be needed to brush and comb the hair, insert dentures, or attach other prostheses.

INTERMEDIATE ACTION

Engage in activities that the patient enjoys. The patient may respond to music, dancing, or painting. His attention span may be short, requiring that activities be changed frequently.

Involve significant others in planning patient care. Family members and close friends may be disturbed as the patient deteriorates. Understanding the rationale behind treatments, medications, and activities will help them encourage the patient to whatever extent possible.

Try to understand the reason for the patient's actions. If the patient is wandering, is he trying to find a rest room, or does he want to go home or to work? Is he wearing an identification bracelet so that he can be returned home if he leaves the property? Is the wandering a sign that he needs exercise or is bored by a lack of activity? Is the refusal to wear a denture a sign that it is uncomfortable and needs an adjustment?

Get the individual's full attention when speaking to him. If he is unaware that you are trying to engage him in conversation, touch him gently and establish eye contact.

Do not use a negative approach. Instead of saying, "Don't go into the street," use a positive statement, such as, "Stay on the sidewalk."

LONG-TERM ACTION

Engage the patient in physical activities that provide fun for him and the caretaker. This will lessen stress, provide an outlet for excess energy, and improve his sleep patterns. Mental activities should be kept on the level that allows the patient to succeed and gain a sense of accomplishment. Basic, simple household chores are usually acceptable to the patient and make him feel that he is helpful.

Support the caregiver by reassurance and prevention of burnout. Suggest involvement in a support group and acceptance of help from others. Encourage time away as needed to maintain some semblance of serenity.

Encourage the caregiver to focus on what the patient can do rather on the lost abilities. Help the caretaker realize that anger, guilt, and sadness are normal components of exerting so much energy in providing round-the-clock care, particularly if the patient is unable to express any appreciation.

Maintain the patient's dignity. The patient's appearance (cleanliness, and neatness of self and clothing) will affect those who visit. If he appears slovenly, they may question the level of care that he is receiving.

Tend to the patient's health needs according to his own or the surrogate's directives. If the patient develops a physical problem, check to know the level of intervention that should be instituted. The advance proxy should provide that information clearly.

Teach the caregiver some basic techniques in behavior modification. The patient cannot be expected to change his behavior or understand why he is asked to do certain things. It is easier for the caregiver to validate the patient's perceptions, and follow his lead so that he dos not feel belittled or embarrassed. For example, if he insists on placing clothing on the floor rather than in drawers, compliment him on the neat piles rather than fighting with him about the placement. The clothes can be put away properly while he is engaged in another activity or asleep.

Help the family; friends; and, above all, the surrogate to accept the inevitable. Help them recognize that their interest in the patient has helped him through a very difficult period of his life. Give them as much positive feedback as possible. Point out all the positive aspects of his life that you can, so that their memories can focus on them.

FREQUENTLY PRESCRIBED PSYCHIATRIC DRUGS

Drugs frequently prescribed for Alzheimer's disease include the following:

Donepezil (Aricept), tacrine (Cognex)

34

The Person Who Is Homebound With a Chronic or Presently Incurable Illness

Hospital stays are limited by many factors. Finances are a prime concern for many patients, with insurance payments often confined to a specific number of days for a specific diagnosis. As a result, those suffering from a chronic illness may not be able to remain in the hospital for a prolonged period. The patient may not be eligible for placement in any other facility and may have to be treated at home.

Some people rejoice at the thought of a family member being returned home for recuperation or long-term (or terminal) care. However, there are instances when this will result in hardships. Professional care may not be available at all, or for an inadequate amount of time. The burden then falls on family or friends to provide care that may be beyond their physical or emotional capacities.

Those with chronic disorders may require help for the rest of their lives. The initial enthusiasm shown by those responsible for providing care may wane as the patient's needs continue over months or years. The providers may feel trapped as they have to bathe, feed, and become involved in treatments that may be difficult or time-consuming. Others who have volunteered their services may have additional outside commitments, and be unwilling or unable to help when their turns arrive.

Chronic illness usually leads to changes in the patient's personality. When hospitalized, and receiving care from strangers, the patient may keep his negative feelings under control. At home, old conflicts may feed into his behavior. The man who sees his wife as being the controller may refuse to accept her ministrations, even if they are what the doctor ordered. The woman who sees her adult children as incompetent may question whatever is being done for her while in their care.

Long-term care at home for a person with a chronic problem may become more difficult as time goes on and the patient's condition deteriorates. Typical of this situation is the patient with diabetes. The initial home care may involve blood testing for glucose levels several times a day, with dietary adjustments as needed. Supervision of skin care may be required to prevent breaks in the skin or pressure sores. If any areas of the skin do break down, they may take a long time to heal because of the diabetes. They may even require debridement, or hospitalization for grafting. This may lead to self-recriminations by the caregivers or anger on the part of the patient.

The patient may develop a diabetic neuropathy, resulting in an inability to feel pain. He may burn himself; be unable to button or zipper his clothes; or, if unable to feel the floor beneath his feet, may fall. This, in turn, may lead to a fracture. Once again, healing time is prolonged. Other problems resulting from the diabetes may be a diabetic retinopathy with a loss of visual acuity or blindness, cardiac and vascular problems with the possibility of gangrenous limbs, and kidney disease. As each problem arises, the caregiver may become more overwhelmed and more frustrated. There may be overt anger at the situation as well as at the professionals who may be viewed as uncaring or even incompetent when the patient's condition continues to disintegrate.

The patient may have to be readmitted to the hospital at intervals for treatments or surgery. Although he may have followed the medical directives, his condition may continue to deteriorate. He may verbalize dissatisfaction with everything in the hospital situation. His faith in the professionals may diminish and he may become hopeless about his condition. Regardless, he may continue to fight for his life, wanting to get better. The staff should realize that he may displace his anger about his condition on them, and not take any of his insults personally.

For most people with diabetes, there is the fear that they will eventually have to face the amputation of a limb. Once again, because of the underlying disease process, the stump may not heal well, and a prosthetic appliance may be difficult to fit. If both legs are amputated, the patient becomes dependent on those around him for even the simplest activities of daily living.

If kidney failure becomes a problem, the patient may be faced with hemodialysis or peritoneal dialysis. In either case, the patient may go to an outpatient ambulatory facility, or be taught to carry out the treatment at home. If home treatment is chosen, the supplies are usually available without cost through the hospital in charge of his care. Once again, the patient will need a great deal of emotional support as he undergoes lifesaving treatments anywhere from several times a week to several times a day. He may insist on carrying out his own care as long as he can because that will give him the feeling of being in control of his own life to some extent.

If the patient is being cared for at home, the person acting as his caregiver may need as much emotional support as the patient, particularly if that person is the spouse. There are many emotions tied up with being the responsible helper: fear of inadvertently doing something harmful, fear that there will be more complications, fear that the patient will die, fear of becoming incapacitated and thus unable to help the patient, anger at having the whole responsibility, or anger that other volunteers are no longer there. Arrangements should be made to provide relief for the caregiver, allowing her to have time away to give her the chance to renew her own strength.

AIDS is another disease that has not offered much hope until recently to those who are infected. The individual can become infected with HIV and remain symptom-free for a long time. Once the antibodies for HIV have been detected in the blood, it may take 8 to 10 years for AIDS to develop. AIDS-related complex may become apparent, with night sweats, weight loss, and opportunistic infections as the most frequent symptoms. Death may occur in 18 months. Most AIDS patients are helped through their illness by friends, health professionals, and family. Their support system is important in keeping their hopes up and prolonging their lives.

The patient must receive the latest information on medications in an effort to keep the infection under control. At this writing, the use of protease inhibitors has brought the levels of antibodies down to almost imperceptible levels for some patients. However, this does not mean that the patient has been cured. He must recognize the need to practice safe sex or abstinence to protect others. The federal AIDS treatment guidelines issued in June 1997, call for a three-drug combination: two nucleoside reverse transcriptase inhibitors (like AZT) and one protease inhibitor (like indinavir) to suppress the disease.

Many people who suspect that they may have been infected refuse to be tested, fearing the stigma; possible loss of a job; refusal of insurance companies to grant health coverage; and, above all, loss of loving relationships. Usually the patient is overcome with feelings of anger, anxiety, and depression as the thought of physical deterioration and a shortened life set in. Significant others may worry about their ability to care for him as the illness progresses. They may also suffer from depression as they anticipate his loss. There is need for professional counseling regarding the illness and its ramifications. The client may object to changing his sexual or drug habits, particularly if he feels well, thereby placing his contacts at risk.

Even with testing, some cases of AIDS go undetected because of the inability of the enzyme immunoassay tests to recognize variations of the HIV virus types. Presently, the Centers for Disease Control are working with test kit manufacturers to update their product so that all the HIV-1 variants can be picked up. Variations are known to occur in the virus according to the geographical area of origin and may also be complicated by existing as a hybrid of two variations. The disease is pandemic, found in all areas of the world. As it emerges in a new area, it is quickly disseminated through sexual intercourse (frequently anal between homosexual men) or through the use of contaminated syringes (usually by drug users), escalating as it passes from one infected person to another. By 1995, the incidence was increasing among heterosexuals through intercourse or drug usage. Women then accounted for 18% of AIDS cases, while the percentage of homosexual men decreased to 45%. There has been an increase in adolescents and young adults, who now account for 18% of those affected with the disease. At the same time, adults older than the age of 50, who are not receiving sufficient education about condoms, now account for 11% of the AIDS cases, as a result of unprotected heterosexual intercourse.

Presently, many patients with AIDS are cared for at home by significant others, returning to the hospital only for resolution of severe or emergency problems. Gay and lesbian organizations have strong support networks available for care of the homebound. Many homosexual sufferers choose to die at home where they can be surrounded by their accepting friends, fearful of being in a perhaps hostile hospital atmosphere.

Professionals called in to help with care for a patient with AIDS should be fully supportive, making certain that necessary equipment is obtained, and that the caregivers know how to provide the needed care. Although the professional may not be a member of the gay community, it is important to accept the patient as he is, without appearing judgmental. His care should be of the same high quality that would be afforded to a "straight" patient.

One group with an unexpected increase in AIDS has been the elderly. Years ago, a woman who became a widow usually retired to a quiet life, and was sexually abstinent. As the life span increased, and women were more able to lead an active life style, they began to return to the dating scene. Some remarried, but others, often for financial reasons, did not seek marriage, but rather satisfactory relationships, often including sex. Many are very naive about the dangers of sexually transmitted diseases, and do not think in terms of safe sex and condom use. Their partners are usually older, and may refuse to use a condom, fearing that it will interfere with attaining an erection.

Although the elderly lady may be a great-grandmother, she should have questions about her sex life included in her routine physical examination. Sex education may be needed to protect her from being infected with any of the sexually transmitted diseases. Health providers have to be aware of their own reaction to the elderly enjoying an active sex life, and should try not to demonstrate any embarrassment or amusement, nor be judgmental while discussing this area of the health examination.

The increase in AIDS among women, particularly in Africa, has led to another problem. For many years, women on that continent have been told of the advantages of breast feeding their newborn infants as a way of improving the babies' chances of survival. The use of formula feeding there has been discouraged because of the lack of safe water and facilities to sterilize the bottles and their contents. These educational programs have been successful, with most women breast feeding. However, studies during the past few years have shown that HIV is transmitted through breast milk. Now women have to be reeducated as to the method of feeding their infants to protect them from becoming infected with this dreaded virus. The women who must switch to bottle feeding must also learn techniques to prevent diarrhea and other illnesses of the newborns caused by environmental deficits.

Many women are reluctant to change from breast to bottle, fearing that they will then be recognized as being infected with HIV. Excuses for the change are invented if necessary, so that family and friends will not suspect the truth. One woman blamed her change on asthma, while others said they were unable to eat a proper diet, and their babies were ill as a result. The United Nations has become involved, with one of the first thoughts being to have wet nurses (women who were postdelivery and lactating) to nurse the babies of those positive for HIV. The problem that surfaced was the inability to know whether those women might become infected while nursing. The solution now under advisement is an attempt to get producers of formulas to distribute prepared formula in presterilized bottles, at low cost so that the infants can be fed safely.

Health care workers are often involved in counseling patients who have been tested for the HIV virus. This has legal ramifications because even those who have tested negative for the virus may actually have been infected. Adding to the legal pitfall is the fact that those patients who are seropositive may or may not eventually develop AIDS. Incorrect counseling may leave the provider open to liability.

It is impossible to cover every risk of liability. However, the professional can reduce the risk by providing all the available pertinent information, using a checklist to be certain that nothing has been omitted. This requires a constant updating of knowledge about the HIV virus as well as AIDS. It also includes an ability to advise the patient about safe sexual practices, with the suggestion that all sexual or needle-sharing contacts be advised of the patient's status.

One legal area that has not been completely defined is that of the legal responsibility of the counselor if the patient refuses to notify contacts he may have infected with the HIV virus. This involves the issue of confidentiality versus the duty to warn an individual of potential harm. The best solution, of course, is to convince the patient of his obligation to provide his contacts with the information about their exposure so that they can seek medical attention as quickly as possible. If the patient refuses that option, it is helpful for the care provider to be aware of the law in the state in which he practices. It is also advisable to seek direction from administrators in the agency or from a lawyer if in private practice. As unacceptable as it may be to the dedicated practitioner, legal protection is a necessity in this instance.

Legal maneuvers have been used to prevent health care workers from refusing to provide care, or in some instances from even wearing gowns, masks, or gloves in an effort to protect themselves. The dependence on these mechanical barriers, which were once commonplace in protecting health workers from then untreatable infectious diseases (tuberculosis, polio), is looked on by some as an insult to the psyche of the AIDS patient. (The psyches of other patients who need to be protected from opportunistic infections, and are, therefore, on reverse isolation with everyone gowned and masked, have not met with resistance.)

When these protective devices are taken away from the staff, coupled with the likelihood that the patient will die of his disease, its sequelae, or an opportunistic infection, it is easy to understand why care providers may be reluctant to become involved. Ongoing education of the staff is imperative to lessen any incorrect or irrational fears of contracting the disease. At the same time, protection against contamination should be provided in accordance with the latest medical information.

Some disorders that were acute and fatal in the past (amyotrophic lateral sclerosis, kidney failure, etc.) may no longer result in immediate death but rather in a chronic state of illness. It may be necessary to provide care on a continuing, perhaps constant, basis, with no present possibility of a cure. This may resemble a state of suspended animation, with the individual surviving but incapable of functioning normally. Patients and families vary considerably in their reactions—and so do health care workers.

All too often, patients who are physically incapacitated are treated as though their mental faculties are also lost. Rather than encouraging the patient to use his mental and physical capabilities to the fullest possible extent, those around him may do everything for him to get things done quickly. They may not afford him the opportunity to speak if his speech is impaired or to carry out activities of daily living (bathing, dressing, feeding) if he requires inordinate amounts of time and supervision to do so. He may then become reluctant to participate in his own care, recognizing the impatience of those around him. He will then probably become increasingly dependent on others as time goes by.

Placing the patient in any type of setting away from home doubtlessly relieves the family situation to some extent. The lessened responsibility for the patient's physical care will certainly ease that aspect of concern. However, there may be an increase of guilt feelings as the family ponders whether the placement is speeding the patient's mental deterioration. There may also be guilt about the sense of relief that comes when the individual is no longer physically present, or because no one has to be available to anticipate and meet his needs.

THE APPROACH TO THE PERSON WITH DEMENTIA OF THE ALZHEIMER'S TYPE

Immediate Intervention by the Patient

SELF-MANAGEMENT TECHNIQUES

The patient should be given every opportunity for self-care. Information about the most recent treatment advances concerning the illness or disability should be made available and discussed with him. If he desires to enter an experimental protocol, all the known facts should be presented, so that he can make an informed decision before joining. Recognize any changes in physical status and report it to the care provider as soon as possible. This is particularly important if the patient is on any experimental, immune, or other therapy that may have life-threatening consequences.

Professional Intervention

IMMEDIATE ACTION

Accept the patient's anger. He may express anger or act out as his hope of recovery or improved health disintegrates. Do not personalize verbal attacks he may direct toward you. Remember, he is angry at the situation and may regard you as the personification of everything negative that is connected with it.

Health workers should be aware of the latest medical information concerning the specific illness. All too often, staff members may have outdated ideas about treatment, survival statistics, or even pain control.

Health workers should evaluate the ability of the caregiver who will be in the home. Some may mean well but need guidance in how to provide the necessary care.

Be certain that food and fluid intake are adequate but not excessive. Give the patient as much choice as possible about his diet.

Help the patient and the caregiver verbalize their feelings. Often home care leads to isolation, particularly if the patient has been homebound for a long time. Visitors may come less frequently, resulting in a feeling that no one is interested in what is happening.

INTERMEDIATE ACTION

Encourage activities that the patient enjoys. Encourage visits from friends, family, and colleagues.

Provide appropriate resources for the patient and his significant others. Referrals to agencies directly involved with the specific illness may open avenues for physical, financial, or emotional aid. Depression is often a factor that compounds the reaction to the physical illness, requiring referral to an appropriate psychiatric resource (nurse, social worker, psychologist, or psychiatrist) for the patient and his significant others.

Reinforce independence by having the patient do as much of his own care as possible. Plan sufficient time so that the patient does not feel rushed.

Provide support for the caregiver. Regardless of the correctness of the care, some patients have conditions that result in continuing disintegration. This is discouraging, to say the least. Help the provider with any feelings of guilt. Arrange for relief at regular intervals.

LONG-TERM ACTION

Help the patient live to his fullest potential. Activities should be encouraged, particularly during times of remission. These should include returning to work or participation in social, educational, or other areas.

Do not abandon the patient, particularly during an exacerbation of the illness. He needs to know that you care.

Help the patient accept his limitations. The patient may be unable to provide as much self-care as he would like. The underlying issue may be the need to control his environment. Help him find other ways to exert control by consulting with him on times for treatment and the place where it can be carried out, dietary requests, clothing to be worn, and activities for the day.

Help the patient and the caregiver accept rehospitalization as needed. The fact that the patient requires additional care is not a negative reflection on the care given at home.

Plan appropriate supervisory visits by professionals to check on the individual's physical and mental status. If deterioration occurs, have plans for additional care, either in the home or a residential facility that has been chosen in advance. Preplanning will give the patient a sense that he is in control of his own destiny.

35

The Person With a Terminal Illness

Perhaps no patient affects the emotional core of health care workers more deeply than the patient with a terminal illness. The dying patient is in constant fear of losing his right to life, liberty, and happiness. The finality of the loss of one's identity, one's being as he has come to know it, may seem like an overwhelming insult to the mind and body for some. For others, it may be welcomed as an end to their suffering.

The experience of dying belongs solely to the patient in the moment-to-moment happening. Regardless of the disease he may have, the terminal patient loses ground gradually, day by day, hour by hour. Sometimes he appears to improve markedly shortly before death, giving his family and friends hope that he will recover.

The patient may or may not have been told his diagnosis and may or may not know the truth about his condition. How much he knows depends on whether he expresses a desire to know. Often the family may make the decision to "protect" their loved one from knowing the truth. Many times the physician himself is not comfortable handling the subject. In one instance, the doctor could not bear revealing the unfavorable diagnosis to the patient or family while facing them. He used the telephone as his intermediary, and the effect on the person who received the call was devastating.

Regardless of what they are told, most terminally ill patients sense that something is not right. In fact, they know that things are drastically wrong. One such patient said, "I feel like I am in the midst of a personal disaster." The patient is aware that he is not getting better. He does not perceive slight improvements or gains. He recognizes, consciously or unconsciously, that his life is coming to an end. He must cope, in some way, with what is happening to him. Most people have an awareness of their own mortality but dismiss thoughts of it as unimportant in the here and now. Essentially, if one dwelt on his anticipated death, he could not function in everyday life.

Most people are reluctant to talk about their own death, or to become involved in an advance directive or planning in the event that illness leaves them unable to make decisions. Even medical professionals are lax about this form of planning. Nurses may explain the need for, and wisdom of, advance directives to patients and their families, yet do not carry out any plans for themselves.

A study of 20 terminally ill patients at Beth Israel Hospital in New York demonstrated the difficulty and discomfort felt by families who had to determine what their loved ones would have chosen as final treatment for themselves. Many family members expressed anger at their physicians and other staff members for not discussing the available choices with them in advance. They were grateful to those professionals who helped them think through the situation, most finally arriving at a "Do not resuscitate" decision. Yet, even after agonizing about the patients' situation, many staff members did not prepare advance directives for themselves.

Those wise enough to have a health care proxy before the need for it arises spare their families the grief and guilt of making end-of-life decisions for others. In one case, two daughters with opposing views found themselves at odds when their 89-year-old mother fell while at the home of the younger sibling, resulting in a broken shoulder.

The mother was admitted to the hospital for a closed reduction of her shoulder. She suffered a series of setbacks during the recovery period including an infection at the operative site; followed by a coronary occlusion; then a perforated stress ulcer; and, finally, toxic side effects from her cardiac medication. She had to be placed on a life support system, with an endotracheal tube attached to a ventilator. At this point, the mother was barely responsive.

The younger daughter, who lived in New York, requested that the older sister come there from her home in California because the outcome looked bleak. Not only did the older sibling refuse to come to see her mother but refused to take part in any health care decisions for their mother. She unfairly blamed the younger sister for the mother's fall and stated that she realized that a decision would have to be made about maintaining the mother on the life support equipment. The older sister believed that removing the system would be tantamount to murder, whereas the younger one felt that the equipment was prolonging the dying process and causing the mother extreme agony. If the mother were to continue living, she would have been totally dependent on others for her care, with poor quality of whatever life was left.

The younger sister sought medical and legal advice as well as counseling. After a few days, and before a final decision was reached, the mother died while on the respirator. The younger sister accompanied her mother's body to California for burial, but the sisters have been unable to restore their previous close relationship. If an advance directive had been available, the sisters would have known what their mother preferred for her care, and the agony of facing painful choices would have been avoided.

In another case, an 83-year-old father suffering from emphysema, and cardiac and kidney problems was placed on a respirator. Several weeks before, he had shared with his older daughter his wish to "pack it in," his way of saying that he was ready to die. His physical condition left him too weak to join in any activities. An inveterate chain smoker, he even had to stop smoking (though he did manage to sneak a few cigarettes each day) and had to move to a geriatric nursing facility. The physicians wanted him to have a permanent tracheotomy, and he refused, stating that attachment to oxygen on a permanent basis was unacceptable to him.

His daughter believed that his decision should be honored. The doctors said that his condition left them no choice and were set on doing the surgery the next day. At that point, the daughter called another physician who was sympathetic. To prevent the unwanted surgery from occurring, the daughter signed her father out of the hospital against medical advice and had him taken by ambulance to the hospital where the second physician was holding a bed for him. Other family members assembled there, and all had a pleasant visit with him. He died peacefully and quietly the next day, after thanking his daughter for intervening. The daughter had no regrets, saying, "I would have felt terrible guilt if I had been unable to stop a plan that was unacceptable to him." Because the family knew of his wishes, they all agreed that he should not be subjected to surgery to which he was vehemently opposed.

There was, however, one error made. Nothing had been put in writing before the doctors stated their intention regarding the permanent tracheotomy. If the patient's wish had been placed in an advance directive, the hospital would not have had the power to force him to accept the surgical procedure. The more individuals think through what they want, and put it in writing, the easier it will be to carry out their wishes.

Dr. Elisabeth Kübler-Ross, who has written much on the subject of death, has noted that the experience of dying progresses through several stages. At first, the patient *denies* what is happening and refuses to believe the diagnosis. He may seek other medical consultations, hoping that another physician will offer a more acceptable opinion. Once belief occurs, the patient may show great *anger.* Life is too cruel! He then tries to *bargain* for more time, usually making promises to his God in exchange for living to see some happy family event. *Depression* may then set in, as the patient realizes that his illness is in its terminal stages. (However, he has, in truth, been depressed even before this knowledge.) Finally, the patient is able to *accept* his fate and finds peace within himself. He can then separate himself from everyone and spends an increasing amount of time sleeping.

When a patient is informed of his prognosis, he may become so upset and bewildered that he is actually unable to hear or fully comprehend what he is being told. He may appear to be calm, and this may be interpreted as meaning that he has heard and understood. Later, he appears never to have been told for he heard only what he wanted to hear. The full meaning may be too shattering to accept, and the patient will ask the same questions over and over.

When a patient does not want to believe that he has heard the truth, he denies it. This mechanism is frequently encountered in terminal patients. It becomes apparent when the patient believes that he is improving and expects to get well rapidly. He may rationalize by telling others that he is being treated for a lesser condition, or that the doctors must be incompetent because they can't come up with adequate treatment for him, or they haven't yet made up their minds as to what is wrong. Even when a patient admits verbally that he has a terminal illness, has apparently accepted it, and speaks openly about it, some denial is observed in his behavior. One patient stated, "I know I have a malignant cancer, but I am lucky that it was caught in time for a cure." This was not what the patient had been told but what she had to believe. The coexistence of acceptance and denial is not unusual, and inconsistencies in the patient's verbalizations are most apparent to the staff.

Some illnesses cause severe pain, with patients believing death would be more preferable than the pain undergone on an almost constant basis. Medical professionals are often reluctant to provide the patient with a sufficient quantity of pain medication, fearing that the patient will become addicted. When patients are inadequately medicated, they become even more conscious of their pain and the intervals between the doses of relief-giving medication.

If patients are responding to the inadequate amount or timing of the medication, the nurse can help by being creative. With the provider's approval, it may be helpful to give the patient half the dose at half the interval. In that way, the patient will receive sufficient medication to alleviate the severe pain but not have to wait for what seems as an inordinate amount of time for the next dose.

Another solution would be to introduce a self-administered intravenous pump. This allows patients to have the medication when needed, in a preset dose, thereby controlling their own intake of the medication. By pressing a button, the medication (usually a narcotic) can be administered through the intravenous solution running into the arm. The knowledge that they can supply their own relief is comforting and does away with their need to watch the clock anxiously to determine the time for the next dose of medicine. (When the patient is able to take the medication orally, he may be entrusted with a supply of pills and told to take one as needed. Another method would be to apply a transdermal patch to release the medication continuously.) Studies have proved that patients in control of their own medication schedule actually use *less* medication than those forced to abide by a rigid time schedule. They do not feel the need to take the medication when they can tolerate the pain because they know that additional medication will be available when needed.

The human desire to survive, to prolong life, is strong. The professional worker has no right to decide for the patient the course by which he should live out his remaining days. The spark of hope that he may need, even though in reality there is no hope, should not be destroyed. One patient revealed her mixture of reality and hope by saying, "You know, I always thought that if anyone told me I had cancer I'd kill myself. Now that I know, I see I really want to live after all, and hope that with the new drugs, I'll be able to." Another patient stated, "I had a feeling that I had a fatal disease, but it took me weeks to get used to the idea. Even though it seemed like I was doing all right on the surface, underneath I couldn't believe it. Now I think I should plan ahead anyway. After all, you never know."

Some patients seek alternative therapies when they do not believe that the conventional methods of treatment will be of help to them, or relieve their pain sufficiently. In some instances, insurance companies are willing to pay for the alternative plans, which may include acupuncture, relaxation techniques, special diets, or other forms of homeopathic approaches. Some of these methods are now accepted as an addition to traditional care, giving patients greater input and choices of care.

Should an unproven, illegal, possibly harmful drug be prescribed as treatment for patients who anecdotally report positively on its worth? There are patients and physicians who agree that marijuana, or Cannabis sativa, is a helpful adjunct in the control of AIDS-wasting syndrome, nausea resulting from chemotherapy, glaucoma, chronic pain, spasticity, arthritis, multiple sclerosis, epilepsy, and migraine headaches. Its active ingredient, THC (delta-9-tetrahydrocannabinol) acts by binding to certain receptors in the brain, disrupting the reception and processing of sensory information in the hippocampus, where learning, memory, and sensory experiences are controlled. The smoking or ingestion of the dried, shredded flowers and leaves of this hemp plant has been credited with appetite enhancement, relieving the nausea associated with chemotherapy and the reduction of intraocular pressure.

Are its effects greater in the natural state than in the synthetic forms? At present, the federal government has started a review of the marijuana literature and is supporting research in an effort to isolate compounds in the drug that may be of medical benefit. One such available synthetic pill form of marijuana contains the active ingredient, Marinol. However, users report that greater relief is obtained more quickly while inhaling lesser amounts of the natural drug, and that fewer side effects (including aggressive behavior) occur when smoking in contrast to using the synthetic oral pill form. Some have questioned the banning of marijuana for medical purposes by the federal government, which has classified it as a Schedule I drug (i.e., an illegal drug with a potential for abuse).

Several states have passed laws recently, allowing physicians to prescribe marijuana legally for certain medical use. At the same time, the federal government has threatened to revoke the federal license to prescribe controlled substances of any physicians who disobey the federal law, and to bar their involvement in Medicare and Medicaid programs. Because federal law supersedes that of the states, the physicians would place their practices in jeopardy if they decided to follow the more lenient state laws. The same would probably be true for nurses with prescriptive privileges.

Objections to the legalization of marijuana, even for medical purposes, are based on fears that it may lead to addiction not only to Cannabis, but to other more dangerous drugs. In addition, there have been studies by the National Institute of Drug Addiction that nerve cells in the brain can be damaged or destroyed by chronic exposure to the active ingredient (THC) in marijuana. Some components of marijuana are suspected of being carcinogenic, and

capable of causing lung damage, with as few as three joints a day being equal
to the damage that can be caused by 15 cigarettes.

Patients who are terminally ill frequently may find themselves abandoned
by family, friends, and coworkers who are unable to tolerate the disintegration that they see. One prominent physician with a glioblastoma was emotionally pained by the lack of visits during his 13-month illness. He was an
unusual man, in that when others did have the courage to visit, they were
immediately comforted by his warmth, interest in their lives, and the ease that
they felt when talking to him. When close friends took him out for a day's
excursion, even though his vision was blurred, and he demonstrated memory
loss, slowness in gait and speech, and some disorientation, he was later able
to tell his wife about the wonderful day. He described how meaningful it was
to him to have friends who valued his friendship enough to be with him for
the day despite knowing that he would soon succumb to his invasive and virulent tumor.

Sometimes a patient is isolated by the caretaker as a way to be certain that
he is not given information about the seriousness of his illness. This may be
due to the caretaker's denial of the actual extent of deterioration, or the mis-
guided belief that only she can provide proper care. In time, that person may
become exhausted by all the responsibility, and resentful that others are
unavailable and do not volunteer to help. Meanwhile, the provider may not
recognize her own role in pushing others away. When this occurs, the patient
is often prevented from verbalizing his feelings or rectifying relationships that
he needs to repair. This increases the turmoil felt by the patient as he feels life
slipping away. Even though he and the person providing the care are constantly together, their inability to speak meaningfully to each other precludes
any true closeness.

The dying patient may well feel neglected and uncared for, as it seems that
he must wait for everything—for the doctor to visit, for his family to come,
for the nurse to respond to his buzzer, for the meal tray to be removed. Even
the patient who isn't told his prognosis senses it and finds out the truth
sooner or later. He picks up clues from the family, friends, or hospital workers. He is sensitive to false reassurance and gaiety. Some patients become very
dependent and angry about being dependent. Consequently, they become
hostile toward others.

A terminally ill patient feels deeply wounded. He does not want to be
deserted. At times he feels rejected. He fears pain, or becoming ugly,
unwanted, and unloved. He does not want to be considered repulsive and be

avoided by others. He needs human contacts more than ever. To be alone during the long hours of his final journey is intolerable. He appreciates genuine gestures of warmth, sincerity, and closeness, even having someone just sit silently, sharing the moment by holding his hand. He may become obnoxious and angry and lash out with unjust and irrational remarks for no apparent reason. He needs to be understood and befriended with compassion. He needs the chance to talk about his feelings and worries, and the reassurance that his pain will be controlled.

Some patients refrain from speaking openly about their situation. Because of the imminence of death, patients often solve problems and difficulties that ordinarily would require a great deal of concentrated therapy. Whether or not he has been told his diagnosis, the patient knows that he is very sick. He will usually welcome the chance to tell you what he thinks he has, if he is asked. He may cry uncontrollably. Feelings of pain and discomfort are shared readily. Death may be mentioned in symbolic language, using disguised terms. The word "death" does not have to be used in answering questions or talking about deep concerns. Many times irrational fears and guilt associated with death can be alleviated and anxiety reduced by talking about the patient's feelings.

The patient's family may respond to his poor prognosis with anger. As he moves into the acceptance stage, they must be helped to know that he is accepting his dying and is gradually drifting away from them all. They need to be reassured that their behavior is not the cause of his speaking less frequently and dozing in their presence.

The time spent with individuals who are dying can be valuable if used well. The significant others have the opportunity to communicate thoughts and feelings that will bring them closer to the patient, resulting in a more harmonious relationship. Prior conflicts, past misdeeds, suppressed love, can all be discussed and worked through in therapy in a matter of days, where it might have taken years without the motivation of limited time. Whether at home, in a nursing care facility, a hospice, or a hospital, the patient and the significant others will need a great deal of support during this time. Care providers should not interject their own values or beliefs and should refrain from being judgmental about any decisions that are made by those acting in the patient's behalf. Above all, there should not be statements accusing the family or designated surrogate of harming the patient because their feelings differ from that of the caregiver. If there is reason to suspect that the motives are questionable, they should be brought to the attention of medical or legal authorities.

Some individuals may have a near-death experience during the terminal phase of their illness. They may describe meetings and conversations with dead family members, and find great consolation in the event. They often discuss going through a tunnel that has a bright light at the end, or of seeing their bodies on the operating table during surgery, with staff members talking about the lack of a heartbeat or respiration. They may describe in vivid detail occurrences in the room at the time that they were perceived as being dead and the return to life with the application of resuscitation techniques. It is important for the staff to listen to these patients and not to deny the possibility of the experience. The patients may later talk of the inner peace felt during the occurrence, and of the newly gained lack of fear of dying including the belief that they will find friends and relatives awaiting them in that other place.

Children who are terminally ill impose a deep responsibility on their parents or guardians, particularly if a decision is made to terminate treatment against medical advice. In one instance, a 15-year-old who had received two kidney transplants and years of antirejection drugs decided that the pain and lifestyle restrictions had reached the point where he no longer wished to continue. Without consulting his physicians or parents, he secretly discontinued taking the drugs. When his actions were discovered, the case was referred to the courts. An order was then issued for him to return to the hospital for treatment, stating that his parents were guilty of medical abuse for not forcing him to remain on the medical regime. The charges were made despite the fact that the parents were always very loving, considerate, and available to him.

An ambulance and several policemen were dispatched to the home without advance notice to the family. The teenager, screaming, kicking, and even biting the ambulance staff was strapped to a stretcher and carted off to the hospital. The court was notified that the patient still refused to allow treatment and that he had been deprived of visits from his family. After a hearing, the judge agreed that the 15-year-old emotionally stable youngster, having been through years of treatment, had the right to refuse any further medical involvement. He was then released to his parents and returned home to live out his remaining time in relative comfort. One has to wonder about the tactics used by the medical and legal professionals in this situation.

By the same token, elderly patients are sometimes forced to undergo painful surgical procedures that will not return the individual to a better lifestyle. If the person has not made his wishes for care known in advance, the likelihood is that procedures to keep him alive will be instituted with or without his acquiescence.

As stated earlier, those who have written advance directives will not have them honored unless the health care providers are aware of their existence. If the directive is unavailable, or the instructions not explicit enough to guide the caregiver, the desires are usually ignored. Many patients with strong feelings about their final care may not believe that they are dying or may change their minds about what they want to be done as death approaches. It has been suggested that the patient and health care provider should be able to communicate honestly with each other while designing the care plan, and include contingency plans to cover any changes that might be desired at a later date.

Children who are dying, or those with loved ones who are dying, need the opportunity to vent their anguish and to be included in explanations of what is occurring. All too often, adults feel that it is too painful—both for themselves or for the children—to discuss the events with the youngsters. The exclusion of the children increases the sense of abandonment that they feel as the death process continues, and they become distrustful of all those who are unable to share the truth with them. It is important to share facts in a way that they can understand, and not to dwell on any gory details, nor increase their anxiety and fears.

Many diseases that would have resulted in death in the past are now treatable to the extent that they become chronic, forcing the family to come to terms with a member who may be very ill at some points and reasonably well at others. Overpreparation for death may cause other family members to deny that anything is wrong and result in anger that shows up as difficult behavior. A child witnessing several near-death episodes may experience bad dreams, eating disturbances, fears of people or social events, poor grades in school, avoidance of responsibilities at home, unprovoked physical or verbal attacks on relatives or playmates, or develop somatic complaints concerning himself that are without a physical basis. Some of this behavior may be so unacceptable as to cause adults to punish the child rather than to understand the underlying problem. This does not mean that the child should be permitted to continue his rampage because that will probably result in feelings of guilt. Instead, the parent or interested other should listen, spend more time with the child, be truthful about plans if the situation worsens, and help him participate in positive activities surrounding the illness. For example, helping him make little gifts, writing letters to the patient, or recording a story about daily happenings at home or in school may increase the ties to the ill individual by stressing positive rather than negative aspects of life.

It is not uncommon for health workers to lose hope in the face of a patient's extensive treatment and to withdraw in an effort to protect themselves from the idea that they are adding to a patient's torture. Staff members may question additional treatments that do not reverse the disease process immediately or that cause additional pain. Often other health workers voice anger at the physician, projecting and displacing onto him their own sense of inadequacy.

It may be difficult for health care providers to realize that most patients will endure discomfort and hardship if there is even the slimmest chance that life can be extended or the illness halted, if only for a short time. The staff can be assisted to view their own negative reactions to ongoing treatments as part of their sense of impotence when the patient continues to deteriorate or dies. They need to be helped to tolerate the situation rather than act out their anger by sabotaging the patient's treatment. By accepting what is happening they can help the patient cope with unpleasant or painful treatments that may bring the gift of a longer life.

Of course, there are times when, despite medication, treatment, and expert medical and nursing care, the inevitable must be accepted, and the health worker then recognizes his inability to "save" the patient. Often, his frustration is painful. His ability to cope with his sense of failure is lessened, thereby evoking a sense of impotence that results in feelings of extreme uselessness and haplessness, causing him to withdraw from the patient long before death. This premature termination of the relationship cheats the patient of an important source of support as he nears death.

Some patients choose to end their suffering by rejecting heroic treatment measures that will prolong their lives but will not lead to a useful state of living. Others may refuse standard care, such as intravenous or tube feedings that they see as prolonging the dying process. There are legal disagreements as to whether these wishes should be honored, particularly if they have been discussed before the patient has lost the ability to express his desires.

Hospitals may ask the patient to determine how he wants to be treated if incapacitated and in a terminal state, without hope of recovering. This may be incorporated into the admitting procedure, with a written declaration of the patient's wishes. It is hoped that this may do away with the need for court cases to determine the patient's right to refuse treatment or to die with dignity.

The family may disagree with the patient's decision. They may need professional help to understand that the expressed desire is not a rejection of them but rather a thoughtful evaluation of the situation. The patient realizes that there is nothing presently available to return him to a level of functioning that is acceptable to him. Therefore, he has chosen to let the dying process continue rather than prolonging his agony.

THE APPROACH TO THE PERSON WITH A TERMINAL ILLNESS

Immediate Intervention by the Patient

SELF-MANAGEMENT TECHNIQUES

Help the patient verbalize how he wants to be treated should he become incapacitated and in a terminal state either now or in the future. If possible, his thoughts should be put in writing so that there will be no question later about their validity.

Professional Intervention

IMMEDIATE ACTION

Make the patient comfortable. Do what you can to preserve his feelings of usefulness by encouraging him to perform whatever tasks he is able to carry out in connection with his care. Do not force him to talk if he doesn't want to, but be alert to signs that indicate his desire to talk and then provide opportunities for him to do so. Do not point out inconsistencies or contradictions when the patient talks. Recognize his need to deal with fear by confronting it at times and avoiding it at other times. Remember, the patient's defenses are allowing him to collect himself, so do not destroy them. Help him to resolve unfinished business or plans if he asks for this kind of assistance.

Accept the patient's anger. Do not react in such a way as to increase his sense of loneliness or to make him feel humiliated or guilty for having feelings of anger. Do not personalize it. Remember, he is angry at the situation, not you.

INTERMEDIATE ACTION

Whenever possible, the staff member who feels most at ease with the patient and his family should be selected to work with the dying patient. This will make it easier for both patient and family to ventilate their feelings.

Offer yourself as a willing listener. Share his grief verbally or nonverbally. Let the patient know you understand the seriousness of his situation. Say, "This must be a difficult time for you." Do not avoid him. He interprets avoidance as a rejection of himself, not as your inability to deal with death.

LONG-TERM ACTION

Do not abandon the patient. Even when there is no possibility of a remission of his disease, approach him frequently, if only briefly. Never dampen his hopefulness. Respond with concern for his problems, no matter how trivial they may appear. Say, "This seems important to you. Let's see if we can settle it together."

Respect the patient's individuality and protect his right to die with dignity even if his desires conflict with your own convictions.

PART FIVE

Working With Different Age Groups

36

Crisis Intervention in the Life Cycle

A crisis is a situation in which the usual balance in living is disturbed, and for which problem-solving techniques used previously are inadequate. Patients may view their difficulties as being insurmountable. Under ordinary circumstances, they may have been able to cope well, but the additional pressure of a crisis situation may have immobilized them. They must now find new ways to solve the problem to return to a state of equilibrium. Successful solutions may be based on past life experiences that turned out well. Unsuccessful attempts may bring back memories of other failures that are in some way symbolized by the present conflict. Individuals can expect to continue in a state of disequilibrium until they can devise a solution that allows them to cope adequately with the present situation. Intervention by professionals may be needed for this.

Health workers often find that the patient's actual problems may not be related to those that are presented for treatment. Feelings may be vented about something totally unassociated with the real problem. For example, a teenager may lament her imperfect profile, blaming it for her lack of boyfriends, while it is her argumentative, imperious manner that is the real culprit that drives boys away. The therapist can help her explore the personality factors playing a part in alienating others. A determination of the real factors can lead to the formulation of helpful solutions.

MATURATIONAL CRISIS

Crises occur throughout life as part of the growth process. These maturational crises may be dealt with in a variety of ways, depending on the individual's method of formulating and understanding problems, and the coping
mechanisms that are used. If problems are viewed as insoluble because the
established problem-solving techniques are faulty, the person will probably
feel overwhelmed, perhaps becoming tense, anxious, even depressed. Some
may develop somatic complaints, regress in behavior, or perhaps withdraw
into an unreal world to escape the problem. Working with a therapist to formulate the problem correctly and find a suitable solution should restore the
patient to a state of equilibrium that is *higher* than the initial level of functioning. However, there are times when that level may only *equal,* or even be
lower than that before the crisis. More help will be needed until a satisfactory
state of equilibrium is established.

Crises tend to last from 1 to 6 weeks. They may end by being resolved,
redefined, or avoided through a change in the original goals. If none of these
techniques has been successful, disequilibrium continues. When this happens,
tensions rise, anxiety continues, and the patient may exhibit physical or
behavioral symptoms that interfere with functioning.

Maturational crises start with birth. The birth process may be more haz-
ardous for some than others, depending upon the intrauterine environment,
genetic factors, and the relative proportions of the maternal pelvis and the
neonate. The infant who reaches gestational maturity, has no defects, and
goes through the birth process easily is better able to adapt to the external
world. The child who is born prematurely, or has a birth defect, certainly
faces a crisis as soon as he is born. He may have to be separated from the
mother immediately and sent to an intensive care unit. He is then cared for
by professionals who meet his physical needs but who may be unaware of his
important emotional needs, or may be incapable of meeting them. A lung,
heart, or kidney abnormality may preclude his being removed from the iso-
lette for cuddling. A cleft lip or palate may prevent his sucking needs from
being met. (He may need to be fed with a syringe. His elbows may have to
be placed in restraints to prevent him from bending his arm to place his
thumb in his mouth.)

How do parents usually react to extreme prematurity, defective organs, or
severe illness in their newborn child? When there is a possibility that the child

will not survive, they tend to hold themselves back from any emotional attachment to him. In a sense, they prepare themselves for his possible death by starting their "grief work" while he is alive. They may have a feeling of failure for having produced an imperfect child. They may have feelings of guilt for real or imagined reasons. For example, mothers who, during pregnancy, used substances that have been proven responsible for birth defects (e.g., cigarettes, alcohol, some medications) often feel personally responsible for what has happened.

Parents who have not been given a reason for a neonatal defect often look upon what has happened as a penalty. Women who have terminated previous pregnancies and men who have had extramarital affairs may look on the child's deformity or death as punishment for what they now consider past misdeeds. Staff members can be of great assistance by helping parents verbalize these feelings, and by reassuring them if their actions were not connected to the present problem. The parents may also need genetic counseling before another pregnancy is attempted, to determine whether subsequent pregnancies will have similar outcomes.

If the neonate survives, the parents usually start to become emotionally involved. Their interest in the baby is reawakened, and they attempt to assume a parental role. They become aware of the baby's special needs and learn how to administer any special care. However, if future hospitalizations are needed, or surgery is anticipated, there may be continued interference with parenting. Fear of losing the baby continues until the problem is corrected or the baby dies.

When a baby dies, parents sometimes find that their outlets for expressing grief are limited. Hospital staff members are often too busy working out their own sense of failure about the death to help the parents. Staff members may try to "cheer up" the mother, but succeed only in isolating her further in her grief. Often husband and wife find it difficult to talk to each other about the death—each wants to protect the other from being wounded again. Staff members can be of greatest help when they acknowledge the death and encourage the parents to talk about it. Unreasonable guilt can often be examined and put to rest at this time, before it has a chance to cause major familial problems. The couple should be encouraged to talk to each other, regardless of the pain, because this helps each to ease his own burden while communicating on a more meaningful level with the other. The husband-wife relationship can be strengthened at this time if the staff does judicious counseling. Unless grief for the loss of this baby is worked through, future attempts at parenting with other children will be hampered.

Following successful delivery, usually the next crisis that occurs is weaning. This process, whether from bottle or breast, can be traumatic if it is done before the baby is ready for it, or if it is accomplished too quickly. If the baby's need to suck is not met adequately during feeding time because he is being weaned, he will have to find other ways of satisfying his oral drive. He may suck his thumb, fingers, tongue, lips, or pacifier. (At a later age, he may bite his fingernails as one reaction to the previous inadequate meeting of his oral needs.)

Those who work in postpartum areas can guide parents into an understanding of how weaning should be carried out. Many times, parents consider it a triumph when they succeed in weaning the child to a cup at an early age, regardless of the baby's need for more sucking. Knowledge about this infant need may help parents relax and let nature take its rightful course. The cup should be substituted for the bottle or the breast for only one feeding a day at the start. When the baby has adjusted to this, another feeding is changed. Progressively, as subsequent adjustments are made by the infant, the rest of the substitutions are made. The baby, not the parent, must set the pace. The baby may sense the approval or disapproval of the parents as he meets *their* goals.

A similar crisis often occurs during the time of toilet training. The eliminative process becomes the focus of family concern and possibly results in frustration for all. If the infant cannot let go of his urine or feces on command, his actions may be interpreted by the parents as a sign of insolence or stubbornness. The lines of battle may be drawn for months or years, until the child has enough control over his own functions to perform on the toilet. Regression, with wetting or soiling by the child at a later date, may be met with anger. Enuresis (bed wetting) or encopresis (soiling with feces) often causes severe problems within the household, for which parents may seek professional help. They often feel a sense of shame when the child continues to wet at night, and usually will not permit him to visit friends overnight, or go to sleepaway camp, for fear that others will discover their secret.

Children who continue to wet or soil themselves by school age may become targets of taunting by their schoolmates. Increased pressure by parents or others to have him remain dry and clean may have the opposite effect. The child becomes even less able to attain the parental goal set for him. Health workers can ease the situation by helping the parents to lessen the stresses of the child's daily living. They should emphasize the child's need for autonomy in as many areas as possible—including that of his excretory functions. The child's schoolteacher should also be advised of the problem, and should permit the child to go to the bathroom whenever he feels the urge to do so. In school, as at home, pressures should be eased as much as possible.

Starting school, in and of itself, constitutes a crisis. Children usually rely on previously learned techniques of making new friends as they find themselves among strangers. If they have been overly protected, and have not had this opportunity before, they may have to experiment with ways to approach the teacher or other students. They may imitate parental behavior, or remember a story or television program that showed such meetings. If children are outgoing (though not aggressive), are able to make themselves understood, and are pleasant in appearance and manner, they can usually fit in with the group. Conversely, children with incomprehensible speech, or those with a noticeable physical defect or who are overly passive or aggressive may find themselves outcasts, not included in the activities of the others. A skilled teacher should be able to integrate the child into class functions, while modifying any unacceptable behavior of the classmates or the child.

School or community nurses may recognize psychological problems exhibited by children while engaged with them in screening programs. Procedures can then be instituted with the teacher or families to help the child cope. If forming friendships appears to be a problem, the nurse may be able to convince the parents to include a new acquaintance in tempting family activities, thus stimulating the child to be more comfortable with outsiders.

Hospitalization of a young child, regardless of the reason for it, always creates a crisis situation. Separation from the family (particularly the mother) and the home can be very traumatic. A child's first reaction may be one of protest—he cries, screams, clings to his mother, even vomits. If the parent cannot remain with him, he may continue to cry until an overwhelming sense of despair sets in, and he quiets down because he has given up. He develops a sense of detachment and in his passivity is viewed as a "good" patient. He sits quietly, doing whatever he is told, believing that he has been deserted by those whom he loved and trusted.

Hospital rules may prevent parents from remaining with children on a full-time basis because their presence "upsets" the *hospital* routine. Hospital personnel often ignore the fact that such a regulation upsets the *child's* routine. Workers who keep the whole child as the focus of their care will certainly encourage parents to remain with young children for as much of the time as possible, for they will recognize the need of the child to have the parent available and the need of the parent to be with the child. Whenever possible, a parent should be permitted to sleep in the room with the child. If that is not possible, the visiting schedule should be flexible. Parents should be coached to tell the child when they are leaving, and when they will return. If the child cannot tell time, the parent should relate his return to hospital activity: "I will be back when you are eating breakfast." Placing a note to this effect at the bedside enables the staff to corroborate and reinforce the information for the child.

Beginning adolescence is another time when maturational crises occur. Growth patterns at this age, including the acquisition of secondary sexual characteristics, may disturb the individual's sense of identity. Neither child nor adult, the adolescent finds his goals changing, the demands upon him increasing. He must make many decisions for the future—whether to continue his education, what his vocational talents are, which friendships to continue, and how to withstand parental or peer pressures which do not coincide with his own desires. He wants complete autonomy on one hand, while continuing his dependency state on the other. He wants complete independence at times, but feels safer when parental limitations are set for him. Health workers can help parents accept this duality of behavior by explaining the need of the adolescent to try his wings while still within the security of the home.

If hospitalization occurs at this time, every effort should be made by the staff to provide as much autonomy for the patient as possible, within set limits. Insofar as is feasible, the adolescent should choose his own diet, determine his own care and the extent of his involvement with others, share a room with others in his age range, have appropriate activities available, be aware of limitations placed upon him, and be held to set limitations in all these areas.

Advance knowledge of sexual changes and drives should be available to both boys and girls. Unless menstruation has been discussed in advance, the first appearance of blood may be a fearsome episode for a girl. In the same way, his first nocturnal emission can be very upsetting to an unprepared boy. Health workers are frequently asked to present sex education programs to adolescents. Those who accept must be certain that the information they give is correct, and that the presentation itself encourages healthy attitudes toward sex and sexuality.

Many youngsters today become involved in sexual activity at a very young age, even in their pre-teens. Adolescent pregnancies have reached the highest rate ever, resulting in children raising children. Certainly abstinence would be the preventive measure of choice, but it may not be a realistic option in some situations. For this reason, many school systems offer information on contraceptive measures while encouraging the students not to engage in sexual activity before they are capable of accepting responsibility for their actions.

It is important to help young people understand that the juvenile mother may not have the opportunity to enjoy her own youth, or to complete her education. She then may not be employable, resulting in a reliance on welfare payments. In addition, when children become parents, they usually lack the skills for competency in parenting.

The crisis of parenthood may be further complicated if the mother has been abused when growing up, and, not knowing any other way, may in turn abuse her children. Young mothers often feel overwhelmed by their role, perhaps turning to drugs, including alcohol, for solace. They may utilize any monies available to them for support of a drug habit, rather than for infant care. They may not know how to get necessary services for themselves or their children, placing the children at risk of not receiving proper immunization or other health care. All of these topics deserve to be included in sex education classes as a way of encouraging the young to think about the consequences of their actions.

In addition to the problems brought about by parenthood at too young an age, the problems of sexually transmitted diseases must be addressed in educational programs. Young people often feel that they are invulnerable, and will not become infected. For some, initiation into sexual activity is considered a rite of passage, and a desire to do what "everyone" else is doing may lead to acts of unprotected sexual activity with the danger of disease, perhaps even AIDS. Education may help youngsters realize the folly of such actions.

The older adolescent may leave home for college, and find himself once more in crisis. If he has been given the freedom to make his own decisions while at home, he will probably be less overwhelmed by all the responsibility that he must accept in this new situation. If he has always been told what to wear, when to eat and what, where, and how to study, he may find decision making very difficult. He may go wild with his newfound freedom, or be afraid to venture out of his room alone. Once more he is called on to make friends among strangers. The individual whose early childhood attempts were successful may have no difficulties. If those early attempts were *not* successful, then he may be afraid of rejection and hesitate to involve himself with others. When parents have provided youngsters with opportunities to make decisions for themselves, the chances are that decision making will not be a problem for the youth away from home. A youngster who is given the responsibility for choosing his own future at college and is allowed to enroll in courses of his own choice rather than those selected by his parents, will have an easier time in establishing his own identity.

The high rate of suicide among college students is an indication of their inability to cope with the many problems that are present on the campus. Most college officials note keen competition among students for marks, particularly among those who plan to attend professional graduate schools. If the student finds the competition too strenuous, or feels that his parents are demanding too high a level of performance, severe depression may set in. He may decide to drop out of school "to find myself," or may turn to such avenues of escape as drugs, somatic complaints, homosexual or heterosexual love affairs, or the creation of a fantasy world. As a last resort, he may attempt suicide.

Crisis intervention centers are available on many campuses, manned by professionals or trained lay people, to provide an immediate outlet for students with emotions that are too difficult to handle alone. When such a center is not at hand, the personnel in the student health service may be called upon to provide emergency service. Workers must have the ability to listen without imposing their own values, while helping students to think their problems through.

Entering the job market is often another time of crisis. The availability of jobs for which the applicant has been prepared is a major factor in attaining a desirable position. Perhaps the market for one's skills no longer exists, and other types of work are unappealing. Then a feeling of worthlessness may set in. When a person's skills are very specific, and he cannot alter them, he may not be able to find any work that is satisfactory. The college-graduate applicant may find that his superior education is no guarantee that he will be rewarded with a worthwhile job opportunity.

Selection of a job within one's area of competence may be made difficult by self-set standards. For example, the newly graduated chemical engineer may refuse to work for any company connected with products that are harmful to the environment, but if the only job that is available is in such a company, he may find it necessary to sacrifice his ideals.

Although satisfaction with one's work is important, that factor may have to be set aside for higher wages or a job more in line with one's abilities. Some people prefer to be in creative work but do not have the innate capabilities required for such jobs. They may have to accept less stimulating work in an administrative or secretarial capacity, and then they may feel frustrated by the lack of opportunity to be creative. If previous life experiences have encouraged creativity in hobbies or avocations, this need may be met. If, however, the person's creative talent has only been job-connected, the substitute situation will not provide any inner satisfaction. He then builds up tensions that may lead to accidents on the job, somatic complaints, or depression. This individual needs help in determining priorities—do the assets of the job situation outweigh the deficits, or should another job be sought?

Soon another crisis looms. Conventional marriage, although disregarded by many, still attracts a large number of couples. Reasons for marriage vary. The health worker who is present during the premarital physical is often able to pick up reasons why the contemplated marriage might not be a stable one. The prospective bride or groom may be using marriage to escape from an unpleasant home situation. Others may feel that this is their "last chance" for marriage. Still others may marry only to have children or to legitimatize them, or to be supported financially, or because "everybody else" is getting married. Premarital counseling in such instances may prevent a lifetime of unhappiness.

Alternative life styles have become more prevalent in the past few years, causing their own crises. A monogamous couple may be composed of homosexual rather than heterosexual members. They may have children through adoption, or a woman may become pregnant to afford her lesbian partner the opportunity to join her in raising a child without necessitating an adoption procedure. In other cases, singles have adopted children or single women have become pregnant through sexual intercourse or artificial insemination, not wanting to be involved in a marital relationship, but desiring the experience of parenthood.

Homosexual liaisons involving either sex may culminate in stable, long-term relationships, equivalent to heterosexual marriages. For some, a ceremony that states the permanency of the relationship is used to inform the community that each partner is committed permanently to the other. Support from family and friends is as helpful to homosexual couples as it is to heterosexuals. Some communities permit adoptions by homosexual couples, who may then seek help in solving any child-rearing problems that arise. Nurses should examine their own feelings about homosexuality and not be judgmental when input is sought by those couples.

The next maturational crisis comes with pregnancy, which may be wanted, unwanted, planned, or unplanned. The wanted, planned pregnancy tends to be less upsetting than that which is not only unplanned but unwanted. The parents may blame each other in the latter case, and may vent their feelings on each other. They may feel trapped, and attempt to terminate the pregnancy. Even when such termination is done properly and legally, emotional problems about the right to end the life of another may ensue.

Conversely, even the wanted, planned pregnancy leads to some emotional turmoil. The sudden realization by the parents that they will be primarily responsible for another human being, and that the responsibility is theirs around the clock, is often frightening. They may not have had role models available to learn how to be a parent and may worry about assuming this new role. Antepartum nurses have the opportunity to help prepare couples for parenthood. They should listen to what expectant mothers say or ask during their visits, and work with them to solve problems and overcome anxieties. This is as important as checking weights, blood pressures, and urines. If classes are given to prepare couples for childbirth, the nurse has the chance to watch husband-wife interactions. She is in a position to pick up unhealthy patterns, and to help the couple find acceptable ways of working out problems.

Husbands who have been prepared to help their wives through labor and delivery often describe the experience as "the most thrilling of my life." Wives feel a closeness to their husbands, and may comment, "I could not have done it without him." Yet even under these circumstances, mothers often speak about their feelings of unreality after delivery ("Is it really *my* baby? How could this have come out of me?") and the lack of a sense of motherliness. They are also usually beset by overwhelming fatigue, and may even have episodes of emotional lability, crying and laughing without control. Unless the postpartum nurse has explained the normality of such behavior in advance, the mother may suspect that she is "going crazy," and both husband and wife will worry about it unnecessarily.

Although crying episodes are normal after delivery, insomnia should arouse concern in the postpartum staff. Total lack of sleep may be the first sign of postpartum depression, and the patient should be watched closely for any other signs of depression. Immediate intervention is one way of preventing prolonged illness. The primiparous mother may be so overly concerned about her ability to care for both her newborn and her husband that she becomes immobilized. Multiparas worry about how the new child will fit into the established pattern of the household, and need reassurance that it is a solvable problem.

Today, the new mother is usually limited to a 2-day hospital stay following an uncomplicated delivery. This may not afford the hospital nurses sufficient time to evaluate the patient's emotional status. The short hospitalization may not even provide enough time to acquaint the mother with techniques to encourage breast feeding if desired. Community-based nurses should be able to follow up after discharge, referring the mother to a lactation nurse if needed as well as to a psychiatric nurse if the mother or family shows evidence of emotional dysfunction.

Women may find themselves in a crisis situation when deciding whether to remain at home with the newborn or to continue working. In today's world, many women value their careers and professions to the same extent as do their mates, and are unwilling to give up their work and remain homebound for child rearing. At the same time, they do not want to miss the exciting experiences of parenting—the first time a baby rolls over, the first unassisted step, the first spoken word.

Some mothers try to do it all by being "superwomen," carrying out all the domestic chores and as many of the child-rearing tasks as possible, while working on a full- or part-time basis. They may exhaust themselves to the extent that child, family relationships, home, and work become overwhelming, with no pleasure to be found in any aspect of life. Child care facilities or mother substitutes for the working hours may be inadequate or available only on an irregular basis, affecting the child's sense of security.

Conversely, not working may cause the woman to feel deprived of the status she had while employed, and bored with repetitive and unsatisfying tasks within the home. The dichotomy of wanting to be involved in two demanding, different life experiences at the same time and feeling inadequate in one or both may lead to depression that may not be recognized at its inception.

Nurses caring for mothers during the postpartum period, or those involved in well-baby care, would do well to spend time evaluating the mother's adjustment to her new role. In some communities, groups are available for new mothers to talk about their feelings, thus lessening their sense of isolation or of being "different." A recommendation for psychiatric counseling is in order for any mother who appears to need more than the informal groups.

All too soon, the children have grown, and the "empty nest" syndrome becomes the scene of the next crisis. A woman who has spent her years "mothering," and has developed no outside interests, may suddenly feel unwanted and unneeded. Her reason for living is over—her task is finished. She has been so busy with her children that her relationship with her husband has disintegrated. To prevent this eventuality, women should be coaxed to develop outside interests *before* all the children leave. This can be done by health workers who prepare women for physical examinations, or who are present when women bring their chliren in for checkups. The importance of strengthening the husband-wife relationship should also be stressed throughout the years of child rearing.

The times of menopause and the male climacteric may also be times of crisis. Self-doubts become prevalent as each partner realizes that the days of procreation are nearing an end. Retirement often coincides with this time, perhaps bringing a sense of failure because of unfulfilled dreams. If the individual has had a meaningful life, with a degree of success, the disappointments are usually limited. New interests, even new careers, may be explored, bringing a new sense of accomplishment and rewards.

If, however, life has been a series of frustrations and compromises, it may be difficult to accept the fact that it is approaching the end. One may have to face old age without a mate, and with a narrowing circle of friends as people die. One's children move away, become busy with their own families and pursuits, so plans must be made for the elderly who live alone or for whom self-care is no longer feasible. As life nears its end, elderly people may regress to a state of child-like dependence, even when trying to maintain their own autonomy, just as they did in adolescence.

Health workers can encourage activities appropriate for the older person's physical and mental status. Senior citizens should be aware of community agencies which make such activities available, and use them as an opportunity for new friendships. Physical problems must be considered, and arrangements made for securing proper medical attention. During the time when such care is given, the health worker should assess the patient's abilities and encourage him to live up to his physical and mental potential. The more active he is, the slower the aging process is likely to be, and the more satisfaction he is likely to derive from his life. Life expectancy has increased to the point where "old age" is now said to start at 75 years of age. Consideration must be given to making the additional years meaningful so that people can *live* the later years of their lives rather than deteriorate, waiting for life to end.

A life style that has become more frequent, and seemingly insoluble, is that of homelessness. There are disagreements as to who should be considered homeless—those without a place to sleep, those who change addresses frequently, those who live in shelters or on the streets over a period of time, or those who do not have a conventional home available.

Since the homeless are often afraid (or unable) to spend time in one place, they tend to move around, making it impossible to count them accurately. Some live in their cars, or find abandoned housing that they take over. In some instances, communities place them in single rooms or motels, without adequate facilities for cooking or bathing. Figures as to their numbers range from 300,000 to three million.

The homeless may avoid shelters, fearing that they may be assaulted or robbed there. They may be fearful of being committed to an institution, of being arrested, or of having their children taken from them. The average age of people on the street is 35, with almost a quarter of them women. About 20% of the population is composed of single women with their children.

Some outreach programs have been developed to provide care to the homeless. These facilities are primarily utilized by women with children. Health care necessities such as physical examinations, emergency treatment, immunization, medication, and some meals are provided. Perhaps the most helpful part of these programs is the counseling, particularly for mothers, many of whom are adolescents, in parenting techniques. Because many of the mothers have come from abusive homes, with poor parental role models, they tend to abuse their children. Many of the mothers are on drugs, have born drug-addicted children with short attention spans who tend to be listless or hyperactive. The babies are often difficult to engage, unresponsive to being cuddled, giving the mothers a feeling of being rejected. The mothers, in turn, ar unable to provide love for their children, and may hit them for misbehavior, in imitation of their own upbringing. The mothers need a great deal of approval for anything that they do correctly in order to boost their badly deficient egos.

Health care providers working with the homeless often feel overwhelmed as they meet with dirty, odorous, disheveled, lice-infested, argumentative, distrustful and frequently unappreciative clients. All too often, the patient ignores health care suggestions, failing to show up for medical appointments, while demanding that his needs be met immediately when he does come. Many are unable to withstand the frustration of having to wait until the provider has finished seeing another patient, bursting into the room to demand instant attention. It is obvious that it takes a very special type of person to work in these circumstances.

Adequate statistics have not been compiled to assess how many of the homeless are also mentally ill. Because there are inadequate numbers of centers for residential treatment, many of the mentally ill have to fend for themselves. Housing may be unavailable or inconvenient, resulting in their living on the streets or in shelters. They may be unable to find food for themselves, and may have their mental status further impaired by starvation or dehydration. Many mumble to themselves or scream or make threatening gestures as a way to scare off others who may try to get close. Those who are on medications may not take them because of forgetfulness, whereas others may overdose, not remembering that they have taken the dose earlier.

It is important for health care providers to form their own support system when working with the homeless. Families, friends, and even peers may express feelings of revulsion when told of this kind of work. They often cannot understand why anyone would want to work with this type of client.

The providers may find themselves angry at a health care system that does not sustain those who are the weakest among us. They may also feel guilty as they leave their clients and return to their own homes in acceptable areas. Some express outrage at their own impotency, at not being able to solve all the social and medical problems that face our society. The providers should be encouraged to have their own needs met without a sense of guilt, and to look to each for support in their situations as a way of reinforcing their own healthy equilibrium.

In the mid-1990s, unsettled work situations resulted in a new breed of homeless people. Some had been living well, without financial concerns. Suddenly, often without any warning, the breadwinners lost their jobs, finding themselves unable to find work or, if they did, unable to earn salaries comparable to the previous one.

If the family had been living up to (or even beyond) its means, the home may have been lost for nonpayment of mortgage or rent. What had been a stable situation drastically changed. The family may have had to seek shelter through a public assistance program or had to rely on others for financial help. In some instances, they were too proud to ask for help, and resorted to living in a car, using public facilities to meet their personal hygiene needs, and receiving food through local agencies. The sense of desperation was so acute for some that they became severely depressed and unable to cope.

It is important to recognize these families, to help them overcome their reluctance to accept assistance, and to make certain that they and any children receive the care that they require. It is imperative that they be informed of available psychiatric help to prevent further emotional deterioration. All health personnel who work with them should be aware of any potential for suicide if family members appear hopeless and helpless. Those are prime symptoms shown by people who have given up any hope for the future and who no longer want to go on living.

Workers may not agree with the various alternative life styles to be found today. They may even feel discomfort or embarrassment in situations far removed from their own. Some workers are unable to accept the fact that although the client has chosen to lead a "different" type of life, he will still face crises for which he may seek help. Regardless of personal feelings, it is important to provide nonjudgmental, supportive, therapeutic care in order to help clients reach and maintain the highest possible level of mental health.

Divorced couples also face alternatives to previous life styles. Mother or father may be awarded sole or joint custody of their children. At times, the ex-spouses arrange to live near one another, sharing custody by either exchanging abodes or having the children spend part of their time in one household, and the rest of the time in the other. Regardless of the arrangement, children need the reassurance of knowing that both parents love them and will not "divorce" them. The parents may need counseling about ways to control their anger concerning the ex-spouse or help in understanding the destructiveness of involving their children when seeking information about activities of the spouse. The children frequently need counseling to resolve issues of loyalty to each parent, anger at either or both, and even guilt if they see themselves responsible for the breakup of the marriage.

In the past, many unhappily married couples believed that divorce would be less traumatic for children than living in a hostile household. As a result, divorce rates escalated to 43% of all marriages. However, more recent studies have demonstrated that divorce is more destructive to children than previously realized.

The effects of divorce, with the anger that may continue through the years, affect offspring not only when they are young, but into their adult years. Depending on the circumstances leading to the divorce, the children may grow up to distrust the opposite sex. They may fear investing their love in a relationship that may disintegrate in the future. If they do marry, they may constantly be on the lookout for signs of infidelity or financial dishonesty. They may be reluctant to develop closeness with their own children, fearing that the relationship will be destroyed if they lose their children through a future divorce of their own.

Remarriage may lead to the melding of two families, with competition between both sets of children for parental attention. Each parent has a responsibility for the welfare of children from his or her previous marriage as well as a commitment to this new "blended" family. The children may be angry at the lessening of attention from their own parent, who now not only has to deal with two sets of children, but the new marital relationship as well. Each child may be angry at any negative criticism received from the parent's new partner and may act out dysfunctionally in response. Blended families should be encouraged to seek professional counseling to prevent or resolve any difficulties.

37

The Young Child

The focus of pediatric care has shifted from the purely physical to the integrated holistic view of the child who requires care not only for his body but for his emotional and mental development as well. Until recently, most of the health efforts were centered on the early childhood routines of immunizations, nutrition, and proper proportions of sleep, play, and elimination. Although all of these are still considered important (particularly immunization), there is a growing awareness that the emotional environment and mental stimulation of children are also to be considered.

Families today vary in their size, structure and components. Single parents (usually a mother) head most households now living in poverty, unable to provide regular health care or other needed services. These include almost 25% of those families with children under 3 years of age. Many of these youngsters spend their days in unsafe day care facilities, with care provided by undertrained workers. Nor are only those from poor homes subjected to inadequate care. With 56% of mothers whose children are under 4 years of age now in the workforce, many children spend their days, from early morning into the evening, in situations that are less than desirable. Presently, there are no federally specified child care standards, educational requirements, mental health testing, nor licensure for those who claim expertise in child care. The parent who leaves a child with a care provider may believe that the individual is caring, based on what is seen when the parent is present. However, that trust may be misplaced when the parent is absent, as shown in several media-highlighted stories of providers who have been cruel to their charges.

Yet most parents work because of the children. Grandparents, who used to be the mainstay of substitute caregivers, are often themselves in the workforce, or live too far away to be of help.

Presently, there are more than 15 million children in the United States below 4 years of age. If the environments in which they grow do not provide the stability, emotional caring and mental stimulation for their proper growth, there may be multiple problems in their later lives. Do their caretakers recognize the need that infants have for stimulation, for being held, cuddled, spoken, and sung to? Do they know how to respond to the touching by the infant, or do they become angry when the infant pulls their hair, or spits up on their clean clothing? And what of the exhausted parent, who arrives home after a difficult day of work? How much energy is there for the child who wants to play, or is perhaps unhappy, and unable to be soothed? If the parent is alone, unable to control a temper that may be precariously at the breaking point, or even married but unhappy for the moment (or longer), how safe is the child, physically and emotionally?

Child care experts are less inclined to set standards for the ages at which certain maturational tasks should occur. There is recognition that some perfectly normal children will develop more quickly or more slowly than others. When their neurological and muscular coordination finally work together, children usually catch up to their peers. That does not mean that basic considerations should be ignored. The child who does not respond to sounds or voices may have a hearing deficit, or be autistic. Certainly this should be considered. However, the parent who is anxious because the child is not as fluent in making sounds or words, or not as physically coordinated as the child of the neighbor down the street, needs help in recognizing the child as an individual, with his own growth patterns to be honored.

The efforts to provide female children with opportunities equal to those long enjoyed by their male counterparts has led to greater awareness of the need to place less emphasis on physical attractiveness, and more on the chance to develop skills and interests. Children in a two-parent household are often cared for by either parent carrying out the basic daily schedule because mothers may have workloads equal to the father. In some instances, mothers travel, and are away from home because of job commitments, with fathers providing the care, cooking meals, feeding, bathing the children, and becoming involved with school activities, parent-teacher association meetings, and homework or the child's social schedule. Children in this type of environment tend to regard either parent as available for their needs and have the chance to see each parent in various roles. Either parent may be the caregiver, and either parent can be in a work-related role. Boys and girls no longer have to remain with the stereotypes so common for parents in years gone by.

However, some child care experts are now beginning to question the wisdom of both parents being so involved in their work patterns that there is little time for relaxation and play in the family. The pendulum, having swung so far in the direction of equal opportunity for parental exhaustion, may soon try to find a medium where both parents can pursue their work interests but maintain the family structure in a gratifying way. Health care specialists often are in the same predicament, trying to elevate their work role by continuing their education, even as they do the mundane household and child-rearing tasks at home. Understanding parental pressures becomes easier for health care providers as they, too, become overinvolved in the multiple tasks of daily family life.

Mothers tend to be the role models for their daughters, whereas fathers do the same for their sons. It will be interesting to see if future generations find new ways to set up their roles and whether the inclusion of fathers in daily tasks will make their sons more aware of the ways in which they can increase their role within the family. Girls, seeing their mothers as more than the family nurturer, may also seek careers that require increased education and time demands rarely seen in the past. Will they opt for this, or will they revert to staying at home to raise their children?

THE CHILD WHO REQUIRES HOSPITALIZATION

Patients of all ages have some difficulty in accepting and adjusting to a period of hospitalization. The child—because of his limited reasoning ability—has an even harder time. He cannot fully comprehend the reasons why he is in the hospital. He wonders why he must undergo procedures that are often painful and scary, and why people who are in no way related to him are handling and poking him when all he wants is to be with his parents.

The child can never be fully prepared for hospitalization. For him it simply means being away from his home and separated from his parents, grandparents, siblings, and friends. He may be there because of a condition of sudden onset that threatened his life, or he may be there for elective surgery. Often, the pediatric patient's stay in the hospital is fairly short, but some children with chronic or terminal illnesses will spend many weeks or months in the hospital. A child who is uncomfortable and in distress may accept hospitalization more easily than one who is unaware that he has a problem. If he has been in an accident and requires immediate treatment, it may be impossible to provide an adequate explanation. It then becomes important to spend time with the child afterwards, to review what has happened and why certain procedures were done.

Because children have limited experience with illness, and are less able than adults to handle frustration, anything that can be done ahead of time to prepare them for events to come is generally helpful. Simple, matter-of-fact explanations of what is going to occur, where, and who will be there, allay anxiety. In cases of elective admission, the child's fears and apprehensions can be lessened by giving him a tour of the pediatric unit, and letting him see the sleeping and playing accommodations and having him meet some of the patients. In the prehospital visit, the child should be made aware of the pleasant features of hospitalization, such as continuous parenting, toys, playroom, books, as well as the pertinent unpleasant features, such as medications, tests, and treatments. To reinforce understanding, some hospitals have prepared booklets which describe almost everything that a child will experience. Allowing the child to have a part in planning for his hospitalization helps him feel he has some control over what is happening. It is always better to be truthful about what is to happen than to have the child draw conclusions, which are usually far worse than the reality. When there has been no preadmission visit, it is important for the staff to display genuine interest in the new patient and spend time with him. When the child feels up to it, just telling him about the unit is better than nothing and may help dispel much fear regarding what might be behind certain curtains or doors.

A child's logic is not the same as an adult's. He has his fantasy world—his inner psychological world—to which he responds, and this may differ from what is actually happening as the adult sees it. For instance, a child cannot understand that it is helpful for him to be in the hospital and that what is being done to him is really necessary. He cannot foresee that regaining his health and being well is worth going through an unpleasant experience. Rather, he may feel that what you say is good for him is really terrible. He may very well feel that the hospital is a prison and that he has been put there because he was "bad." He may worry about being punished for snitching those dimes, eating the forbidden candy, pushing his little brother downstairs, wishing something bad would happen to his mother, or for having masturbated. A child can easily feel that he must certainly be the very worst person alive for all this to be happening to him. He is sure his parents are angry with him. Why else would they have left him here? He hears no familiar voices. His brothers and sisters may not be allowed to visit. He can't go out to play, and no pets may be permitted. Practically speaking, personnel on the unit cannot replace the continuous care and presence of family members. Is it any wonder that he feels resentful toward the doctor, the nurse, and others who, he rightfully feels, are keeping him where he doesn't want to be and who are doing some very unpleasant things to him?

Hospital policies have relaxed increasingly in recent years to permit continuous presence of parents. This is particularly important for a child who fears separation from his mother and wants the attention, emotional comfort, and security she can provide. Sometimes hospital routines are disrupted by the presence of family members on the unit. However, that is a small price to pay for the valuable physical and emotional care his family provides for the child.

A child's sense of trust is strongly influenced by what his relationships with adults have been in the past. If his parents have lied to him repeatedly, even though they felt they were protecting him at the time, he will be less likely to accept what others tell him. Previous hospitalizations and experiences with medical personnel will also influence his expectations. For instance, the smiling professional who pats the child complacently, says, "Everything is just fine," and then orders unpleasant restrictions and tests lays the foundation for suspicion during future encounters.

The child who is ill at home, like the adult, fears what he does not know, has not seen, or does not understand. However, the child knows less, has seen less, and understands less than adults. By making the unknown known to him, and increasing the child's understanding, there should be a beneficial and soothing effect. Pretending to give a doll a hypodermic or intravenous injection; being allowed to play with an oxygen mask; being asked to hold cotton, tape, applicators, or tubes or ointment; helping prepare one's special feeding; seeing pictures of other children in situations similar to his own all help to make the experience concerned with illness more understandable and, therefore, more bearable.

The child brings all of his fears with him when ill. These fears—real or imagined—may be due to previous experiences, or they may be based on bits of conversation overheard at home. For example, he may have heard his mother talk about a neighbor who was ill and then died, and conclude that this, then, is what is in store for him. Perhaps his grandmother had a heart condition and died from it. The child may feel that this is the natural outcome for all those who have heart trouble. Or he may believe that his broken leg is a punishment for disobeying his parents who had told him not to climb trees. These partially comprehended situations instill very real fears in a child because he has not yet learned to reason logically. Thus, the child views any illness as a threat to his being.

In addition to the stress of his physical illness, the ill child who must be isolated within the home may require care to be given by a professional. This separates him from his usual caregivers, his parents, who are in the home but not totally available to him.

The young child does not like to feel helpless. Being removed from the care of his parents on whom he is necessarily dependent increases this feeling, particularly when he cannot accept what others are doing to him. He is not consulted about plans that are made for him. He feels that he is at the mercy of others, confined, and trapped. He responds by protesting in the only ways he understands—he cries, shoves, hits, kicks, and throws things. He may refuse to eat, become withdrawn, avoid looking at the worker or responding to any approach, and refuse the toy offered to him. He is angry, resentful, unhappy. He wants his parents to be available constantly but when they are present, his happiness at seeing them gives way to his unhappiness, and he may cry and cling to them or remain silent and ignore them. All too often, such behavior is interpreted by others as an indication that "the poor child is so upset by his parents that he would really be better off without them." On the contrary, crying and silence are both pleas for affection and support, for help and hope, as well as outlets for tension and anger.

Parents' reactions to their children stem from their own background. They see their child's "bad" behavior as a reflection of how poorly they have brought him up, and this makes them feel inadequate. Spontaneously, their anxiety levels rise and they may berate, admonish, and threaten the child, which only makes him feel worse and increases his fear. The health worker who is not judgmental in such instances can do much to help parents change the situation by encouraging them to give the child extra attention and to demonstrate their affection for him.

Some children are so undemanding, accepting, and uncomplaining that they are seen as perfect, lovable little models of adults. Because they do not pose management problems, their emotional needs tend to be overlooked by their caretakers. However, these children are the ones who often need more attention than those who are noisy and demanding. They may be extremely inhibited and unable to demonstrate any aggressive behavior. They may believe their illness is a punishment and that they will be released only if they behave perfectly. Often they submit to everything without a murmur out of fear of what will happen to them if they do not.

Reactions to separation vary in light of each child's previous experiences with his parents. It is not uncommon for a child to engage in regressive behavior—including bed wetting, refusing to eat, and using "baby talk"—as reactions to the stress. Health workers should understand and accept such regressive behavior for what it really is.

Children have limited ability to cope with frustration. During their early years, they demand immediate satisfaction and seek pleasure naturally and instinctively. Since the child's ego is not yet developed, he cannot deal with the adaptations required of him and his reactions may seem irrational and emotional to adults. The healthier the child's development has been, the more secure he is, and the more consistency he has experienced, the better able he will be to deal with his present frustration. However, he may manifest his inability to deal with it by having a tantrum, hitting his head, sucking his thumb, throwing up food, and assaulting others. At such time, he worker allows the child to release his tension but protects him and others from injury. An attempt to help the child face the situation by acknowledging his predicament, rather than offering excuses, is helpful. The worker can share his feeling and show him that he is accepted by providing substitutes for any family love he feels is missing. This can be done by holding, cuddling, talking, and participating in an activity with him. At the same time, the health worker must begin to introduce the child to healthier ways of satisfying his wishes and obtaining attention. Pointing out how other children are able to obtain satisfaction will induce him to perform in a like manner in order to gain acceptance.

All children fear being unloved, uncared for, or abandoned. Any separation or illness increases this fear. The health worker must understand that being isolated for any length of time is almost impossible for the child to endure and, because he does not yet have a sense of time, it seems to be lasting forever. A child does not understand the meaning of "Wait just a moment," "I will be over in a little while," or "I'll be there in a short time." Minutes seem like eternity. The notion of the future, soon, or later are too abstract for the young child. It is more helpful to respond to his questions by referring to the present.

Sometimes a child's reactions are based on unconscious conflicts, as when unhappiness is carried over from a previous experience. Fortunately, most children are quick to express their feelings. It is important to listen to them in order to pick up clues to hidden but real meanings in their reactions. Often what a child reacts to is not obvious to the adult, but bear in mind that all behavior has meaning and that the child's behavior is his best way of expressing himself. Thus do not fall into the trap of accusing a child of malingering or purposely "carrying on," or of being a "phony." He is not, and what is more, he does not comprehend most of his own reasons for his behavior.

It is important for the health worker to take into consideration the relationship between the child and his parents and the parents' attitudes and demands which affect the child during his illness. The worker will benefit if he can develop a good relationship with the parents by providing support, counsel, and information regarding health practices and the child's care.

Parents require help in dealing with their own reactions to the child's illness. If a child is fatally ill parents will react with shock, disbelief, and denial. Advances in treatment of incurable illness often extend the period of dying, but may necessitate frequent, repeated hospitalizations. This causes much anxiety and anguish for the grieving family. It is not unusual to find family members displacing their anger about their tragedy onto the health professionals, God, or each other. Health professionals must be careful not to personalize the parents' criticism, but to meet it with understanding and support and to accept their difficult behavior as a symptom of distress in a trying situation.

A child's chronic illness is often too painful a burden for friends or others outside the family to share. Family members are often avoided by outsiders, who seek to protect themselves from the thought that this could also happen to them. As a result, the expression of grief is limited to the family unit. The health worker is often the only outside person strong enough to allow the family the opportunity to vent their feelings.

Children do remember what happens to them. Too often the illness experience is embedded in the mind so deeply that it becomes the basis for a lifelong emotional problem. The health worker should make every effort to alleviate pain and decrease frustration. Only people who genuinely enjoy being with, caring for, and communicating with children, should work with them. Professionals should also be able to work with the parents, who may become overprotective when a child's illness is chronic. This can result in preventing the child from enjoying and developing his ability to the fullest that his life will allow.

A child's reaction to any loss that he suffers results in a variety of responses which offer clues as to the depth of his feelings. The precipitating event may be the loss of a body part, lack of availability of his parents, or separation from his siblings and playmates. His responses may fluctuate from a sad mood to irritability, or he may provoke others by hostile actions, voice numerous complaints of aches and pains, or chastise himself for being "bad." One child with severe burns was overheard frequently sobbing and repeating, "I'm a bad boy." He had been burned during an apartment house fire and believed this must have been a punishment for misbehaving in school.

The nurse should learn as much as possible about the child from his parents, especially facts about his feeding and toilet habits, since they carry so much significance. She may have to set aside some of the rules during episodes of hospitalization and provide a less disciplined atmosphere in order to lessen the child's anxiety and increase his feeling of security. A child may fear punishment if he does not eat, humiliation if he wets the bed. The stress of separation from home and family often causes regression to an earlier type of problem and may induce enough anxiety to cause bedwetting. The nurse should assure the child that he will not be punished or rejected for this regression. By avoiding attitudes that reinforce fear and anxiety, and by expressing warmth and tenderness, the nurse can help reduce the child's feeling of self-devaluation. Such attitudes can also help reduce a child's fear of retribution based on previous experience in his home—an important point, since the anxiety such fear causes can adversely affect the outcome of the illness.

An explanation by the nurse of procedures that will be carried out will help reduce the parents' own anxiety. It will also help them prepare the child for whatever is to come, and deal with his reactions to it. Keeping them as informed as possible, anticipating some of their concerns, and providing adequate explanations for what is worrying them can be very helpful to the child's parents.

PROBLEMS OF SEXUAL ABUSE

Children who become victims of sexual abuse are often too frightened to tell their elders what has happened. They may be threatened with further violence, or even death, if they disclose what has happened. In some cases, they are told that a parent or other loved person will be harmed or killed if the story is revealed. If the abuse has been part of an incestuous relationship (usually father and daughter), the child may be afraid to tell even the mother because the story may not be believed, or the family may disintegrate if the authorities are notified. The child may also be afraid that reporting the events to anyone may cause the father to withdraw his "love" from her. If the mother discovers the situation on her own, she may be reluctant to report the father to the police because his arrest might result in the end to his earnings as well as the loss of their relationship. If the mother is without work skills, she may view the loss of his income as a catastrophic blow, and not know where to turn for help.

Girls who do tell of their experience usually find help available. The perpetrator—usually a family member, trusted family friend, teacher, health or religious professional, or possibly a stranger—is blamed by all who discover what happened. He is sought by the authorities with the help of those familiar with the child and punished for his act. The child is evaluated and helped to recover through therapeutic efforts of professionals. If the therapy is successful, the child should reach adulthood with a minimum of sequelae. If, however, the therapy is inadequate, the child may have years of psychological problems, seemingly unrelated to the underlying cause. There may be multiple visits to health providers for physical, psychological, or somatic complaints that do not respond to treatment. There may be fears of any close relationship in the future and distrust of people in general. There may be self-loathing, with blaming of herself for what happened, even though she may realize that she was too young, too frail, too immature, or too distraught to protest.

In one case, a woman in her 40s had a history of many visits to her physician, without resolution of her complaints, which centered on difficulty in swallowing, digestive discomfort, shortness of breath, and palpitations as well as marital and family problems. Eventually, the physician referred her to a nurse therapist, who took a detailed history, asking whether anyone had ever abused her as she was growing up. At first, she denied that anything had occurred. During the next session, she suddenly asked, "Why did you ask that question?" She then broke down in sobs and told the story of her father coming into her bedroom from the time that she was 6 years old, involving her sexually, while telling her how much he loved her. He also said that he did not want anyone else to know—that it would be their secret. He would leave her bed before morning and ignore her during the day. When she began to menstruate, his visits abruptly ended. She became depressed, unable to understand why he no longer wanted to "love" her. At that point, she told her older sister what had happened. The sister then told her that the father had come to her once, also when she was about 6 years old, but that she had thrown him out of her room, threatening to tell the mother. He never accosted her again. That information overwhelmed the patient, who felt doubly betrayed—for having been abused and for having believed that she was the only one her father truly loved. Within a few days, she began to have physical symptoms that required professional intervention. As one symptom subsided, another took over. And so it went through the years until the real basis for her problems came to light. Once she was able to connect her symptoms to having been abused, she was able to deal with her emotional problems in a less destructive way.

Males who have been abused tend to have a more difficult time and are, in a sense, blamed for their having been abused. First, they are thought to have been inadequate in not fighting off the aggressor, and, second, they are expected to keep their feelings to themselves, and not tell all or complain. This often results in years of dysfunctional behavior. In one case, a teenager was sexually abused by a stranger, and although he was involved in therapy immediately, his behavior demonstrated his anger and inability to move on to any resolution. In later years, he became involved in taking and selling drugs. His school performance continued to be on a high level, and he graduated from a professional school. Although he had his own private practice, he was found to be cheating his clients and involved in illegal situations. He eventually lost his license, was divorced by his wife, lost any custody of his children, and served time in jail. He was unable to relate his behavior patterns to the adolescent abuse and is still dysfunctional.

THE APPROACH TO THE YOUNG CHILD

Immediate Intervention by the Patient

SELF-MANAGEMENT TECHNIQUES

Encourage the youngster to become comfortable under the circumstances of impending care to be given by others, or painful care to be given by parents. The presence of transitional objects (e.g., doll or blanket) may increase his comfort. Help his parents or guardians realize his need for their support, and discourage their demeaning any regressive behavior.

Professional Intervention

IMMEDIATE ACTION

Establish a friendly relationship with the child. Talk with him, especially when his parents are not present. Speak to him as you would to a friend, respecting his unique feelings, desires, and needs. Do not use "baby talk" or speak as if he doesn't matter. Be aware of what you say to others when within his hearing. Go along with his way of doing things providing it does not interfere with his therapy. Do not be critical. Accept the child for himself and show an interest in his interests.

Understand how difficult it is for a child to wait. Try to take care of his physical needs as quickly as you can.

Do not assume that because of your greater knowledge of behavior that you are better for the child than his own parents. If you do, you are meeting your own needs to be a mother or father. If a child of your own is hospitalized, assume the role of the parent, not health worker.

INTERMEDIATE ACTION

Be flexible. Be prepared to change plans, as the child's condition may change rapidly. Daily plans are best, and provide the most satisfaction, especially when a child has a long-term illness. Flexibility is particularly essential when working with children. Give the child advance warning of any tests or procedures, so that he can complete his activities beforehand.

Provide outlets for the child's hostile feelings. Let him hit a doll, pound clay, cut paper, or draw pictures depicting his experience. Allow adequate play time. Provide dolls, doll house, table, chairs, unbreakables, push-and-pull toys, drawing paper, watercolors, crayons. Encourage drawing because free drawing may disclose his inner feelings.

Arrange for a storytelling time. Do not use stories that depict horror, hurt, sorrow. Encourage the child to make up stories because they may give the worker insight into the child's fears or a difficult family situation.

Give the child a choice only when you know you can respect his decisions. Do not ask him if he wants a treatment when you know he will be made to have it even if he says no. Let him help with procedures when possible.

Encourage the parents to ask questions, and answer them truthfully no matter how upsetting the facts may be. This does not preclude helping to alleviate their feelings of guilt by explaining: "It is well known that the best precautions in the world cannot prevent this condition." "Children break legs and have other accidents, whether parents are there or not." "A child's curiosity and zest for pleasure is primary, therefore, he doesn't think about the dangers involved in what he wants to do."

Recognize that the child sees any limitations (food, fluids, activity) as punishment. Being examined may also be viewed by a child as a form of punishment—a way of checking up on him. Remember that the child will not thank you for your wonderful care. Tolerate his behavior when he pushes you away and says, "I hate you," but continue to approach him and show genuine concern.

Do not approach a pediatric patient when you are overly anxious about something. He will pick up additional insecurity from you.

Do not overwhelm the child with facts and explanations. Instead, encourage communication using whatever materials (drawings, pictures, equipment) necessary to help him understand what is happening. Answer questions as they are asked, on a level that he will understand. Children fear pain and worry about harm to their bodies. Give reassuring, brief explanations regarding what is happening. Remember that avoiding the subject does not lessen anxieties, but leads to fantasies that are usually much more frightening than reality.

Help the child deal with problems as they arise. Keep him informed, in simple terms, of what is taking place. Be truthful. Recognize the fears and fantasies that he may have. Offer honest explanations and genuine reassurances that offset inaccurate beliefs.

LONG-TERM ACTION

Come to terms with your feelings toward your own parents. If you don't, you may react to the child's parents as you would to your own.

Health workers should be aware of their own feelings and reactions to the child whose condition does not improve. Often a very sick child is avoided just when he needs the worker's presence. Instead of deserting the child, all the resources that are available should be brought in. This includes social workers, psychologists, and various special therapists. If the child's physical condition permits, close cooperation should be maintained with the school to help the child maintain his grade school level.

38

The Postpartum Woman

Many people cling tenaciously to unrealistic notions of what marriage and parenthood are all about. They dream of romances between wholesome girls and boys who will love each other forever. Each will be aware of the other's needs, and be supportive. Finances and in-laws will never cause arguments, nor will any other problems arise. The wedding and honeymoon will be the beginning of an idyllic life together, which will be even more perfect after the arrival of each child. The bride and groom dream of matrimony and parenthood as devoid of difficulties. Love will conquer all!

If this has been one's expectation, consider the disappointment when the festivities of courtship and honeymoon are over and the realties of everyday living begin. With added responsibilities, psychological adaptations to a new mate, social pressures, and adjustments to their families of origin, both partners are apt to feel discouraged and disillusioned. Usually those who have sufficient ego strength and who have had a fairly healthy upbringing can weather the difficulties and work out a reasonable solution. They may make some compromises, but a new understanding of self and situation evolves.

The fact that most women learn to cope with marriage and motherhood may obscure the fact that it is not unusual for a woman *not* to be able to cope with the added stresses and strains that marriage, pregnancy, and motherhood impose. For such women, a pyramiding of various factors may result in a serious emotional problem following a pregnancy. One should anticipate the possibility of postpartum illness in any woman who previously has not adapted well to extra pressures in life, who is having difficulty in her marital relationship, who experienced a serious trauma in early childhood, or who has a poor self-image. At times, pregnancy itself may activate an upset in one who has had a previous psychiatric illness. This is especially true if the person never fully resolved all her conflicts during the earlier period of treatment. In cases in which overt psychiatric problems were present before pregnancy, there may be a lessening of symptoms during the pregnancy. However, the original problems often reappear during the puerperium. Pregnancy may also activate repressed feelings about sex. Many women still have feelings of shame regarding intercourse. Pregnancy produces obvious evidence of a sexual relationship and may force these repressed sexual feelings into conscious awareness.

Emotional difficulties during pregnancy and following delivery are considered by some researchers to result primarily from physiological changes in the body accompanying pregnancy, parturition (delivery), and the postpartum state. There is much evidence to support such a concept because it is known that changes do occur in thyroid, adrenal, and pituitary hormones during these times. Conversely, it is also evident that postpartum emotional disturbances usually occur in those with a background of long-standing emotional problems.

A period of postpartum "blues" is fairly common within the first few weeks after delivery. In addition to the hormonal changes, there are subtle social changes for the new mother. Up to the time of delivery, *her* health status has been the center of focus. However, once the baby has been born interest shifts to *his* welfare, *his* eating, sleeping, and defecation patterns. Some mothers are unable to cope with the shift of attention from themselves to this new person, to whom they often lack a sense of attachment. They frequently resent the intrusion of this demanding infant who does not recognize maternal needs for peace, quiet, and, above all, a good night's sleep. Once the attachment process begins, the "blues" usually disappear. However, the vulnerability to unconscious and conscious stresses is greater at this time, and symptoms of deeper emotional illness may appear, requiring immediate intervention.

Orientation programs for new jobs or new roles are standard practice in industry. Yet parenthood, a vitally important role, is often learned as on-the-job-training, without professional input. How much more therapeutic it is to use anticipatory guidance, including information and special help regarding the baby's care, and to give assistance in the adaptation to becoming a mother. Antepartum and postpartum classes are helpful for both parents as a way of providing support and as a vehicle for anticipating situations that may lead to physical or emotional difficulties.

In our Western culture, we tend to think that pregnancy, childbirth, and the bearing of a new baby are happy times for all. We sanction this ideal and give our approval to those who give "proper" responses. For example, we want to believe that every mother really wanted to be pregnant and that she is proud of her changing physical appearance. We also want to believe that the mother is really immersed in planning the infant's care, that she is fixing up the baby's room, taking child psychology courses, and shopping for the layette. If all this is so, we smile, pat her shoulder, talk about baby names, and even say that she will be a "good" mother. Conversely, a woman who is unfortunate enough to feel otherwise has no eager or sympathetic listener. If she complains that she is not really ready to have a baby, or that she can't stand herself in maternity clothes, or that she doesn't know how to take care of a baby and fears doing so, she is turned off quickly. She may feel that she still needs mothering, that she still needs someone to take care of *her*. Even her smallest verbal indication that she is unhappy may provoke responses that let her know her remarks are unacceptable. "How could you feel that way?" "It's wrong to say what you're saying." "You'll see; you'll feel differently when the baby is born." "Don't complain. After all you got yourself into this. You have no one else to blame." These responses tell the woman she is not supposed to have negative feelings, that she may incur punishment if she doesn't rid herself of them, that things will be better afterwards (although "after" may be what she fears the most), and that she is to blame for her predicament and thus deserves to suffer. Instead of the help she may be crying for, the woman who expresses her unhappy feelings finds that she has an additional problem. She now feels that she is "bad," thus increasing her guilt feelings about her thoughts, which are uncontrollable. Also, she may think that no one will be able to understand her feelings and, therefore, she tries to protect herself from any possibility of rejection, humiliation, and ostracism. Hence, even though she may want to seek help, she is afraid to do so.

The new mother encounters increased anxiety and fear about caring for the infant and all the implied responsibilities. If she is reticent or has misgivings regarding the baby's care, she may begin to feel that perhaps she doesn't love her infant as she thinks she should. The crying, frequent feedings, and diaper changing are demands she may have difficulty in meeting. If the woman is not feeling physically and emotionally well, she usually cannot assess what is really bothering her. In the hospital, an alert nurse may observe that her sleeplessness, fatigue, and emotional lability are out of the ordinary, more than the usual postpartum "blues." The nurse may also observe that the patient is in an overly cheerful state, overly talkative, and that she engages in excess activity that accomplishes little. Most women experience a sense of unreality following delivery. It is difficult to believe that *this* baby was in the uterus. It is normal for the mother to be devoid of feelings of "motherliness," but she may misinterpret this as a sign that she will not be a "good" mother. She may be plagued by excessive fatigue as she wakens during the night to make certain that the newborn is all right. She may even have dreams of infanticide, with subsequent guilt feelings.

The new mother who is breast feeding may have difficulty in getting the baby to suck. She may feel frustrated and angry, and fear that her milk is poisoning the infant, or that the infant will be smothered by her breast. The many chores, including having to be up at night for feedings, decrease the amount of sleep she gets and increase her feeling of being disorganized. At the same time, she may feel inadequate as a housekeeper if her standards are unreasonably high. She may be unable to keep her home in the same tidy condition as before the baby's birth and feel that she will never catch up with the housework.

If the woman has recently moved to a new location, she may begin to feel overwhelmed by everything and be unable to cope with her rising anxiety. In addition to having no one nearby for support, her family may be having financial difficulties. The woman may have given up a job with its second income, which had made her life easier. Now there is an added mouth to feed and less money. If her husband's salary is not adequate, she may not be able to afford even temporary help, let alone a housekeeper.

Today, many women plan to return to work within weeks or months after the delivery. Some do so for economic reasons, while others must return because of career commitments. For some, the thought of being at home with the baby may escalate fears of being an inadequate mother, or of being bored. The woman who does return to work may need guidance in setting priorities re household or work tasks as opposed to child-rearing and family tasks. She may also need to learn how to delegate responsibilities at home and at work to save her energy for meaningful activities.

Many mothers feel guilty or sad when at work, particularly if the child is ill, or when new developmental accomplishments occur (baby's first tooth, first step, first word). If possible, the mother should plan uninterrupted time with the child on homecoming to recommit her feelings and thoughts to the family rather than work.

Many women feel trapped in the home while taking care of small infants and bored with the entire process. A woman who has held a fairly good job feels little status arising from her skills as a homemaker. Perhaps she went into marriage and pregnancy expecting sudden inner fulfillment, or anticipated that having a child would add new meaning to her life. Perhaps she wanted to prove to herself that she could produce a child, or that she was still young. She may have thought that the child would serve as a stabilizer for a rocky marriage—usually an erroneous idea. Instead of finding happiness in her new mother role, she may become depressed to the point where professional intervention is necessary.

She may begin to feel hostile toward her mate in general, and the baby in particular, for causing all these problems. Hostile feelings may be intensified if the marital relationship was poor from the start. The husband may be insensitive and self-demanding, or he may just be the target for his wife's unhappiness. He may be blamed for the entire situation as her guilt regarding sexual relations increases and her feelings of inadequacy come into the open. Impulses, thoughts, and desires may focus on the wish that her husband would die and/or the possibility of killing the baby. These thoughts create so much anxiety that often the patient cannot distinguish between what she did or did not do. Her thoughts and emotions are in conflict with what she believes should be appropriate for a new mother. She is considered psychiatrically ill if the problem becomes great enough to interfere with her ability to function effectively and satisfactorily for her own and her family's sake.

The course of the illness may assume one of two directions. In one, the mother may begin to feel more hostile and act on some of her pressing impulses and repressed urges. In the other, she feels she has failed as a mother, withdraws from the infant, and is overly depressed. Whichever form the illness takes, the onset usually appears suddenly following the birth of the baby.

At times the patient may be in a completely uncontrollable manic state. She may swear and shout profanities. One patient raced through the psychiatric unit, taking off all her clothes, yelling, "I am a virgin, I am a virgin." Another continually sang, laughed, and cried to keep herself awake because she had a dream that the baby would die if she slept.

Again, depending on the course the illness takes, the patient may either lose all her sexual inhibitions or become completely uninterested in sex. Understandably, it is the relationship between sex and reproduction that makes sex so much a part of one's thoughts during the illness. Among the sexual difficulties described by women are an inability to feel responsive or to reach orgasm. Often the woman has a difficult time admitting these sexual problems to herself or others, particularly if she wants to project a "femme fatale" image. Previous love affairs are remembered as failures because they did not culminate in marriage. Guilt, fear, and shame associated with intercourse are not uncommon, but usually are not confided to the spouse for fear he will laugh, ridicule, or accuse her of being half a woman. During the patient's illness, inhibitions are weakened, and a barrage of sexual ideas, words, and actions are apt to be heard. One patient started simulating intercourse, cursing the fantasized partner at the same time.

If the illness is of a depressive nature, sexual drive will be decreased or completely absent. Here the woman may feel guilt and shame about intercourse. She may fear another pregnancy, or perhaps she is too exhausted to participate in sex. A patient whose pregnancy terminates with the death of the infant may experience similar difficulties. In addition, she tends to blame herself for past misdeeds, seeing the death as a punishment for the real or fantasized behavior.

Emotional illnesses that develop following delivery are characterized by extreme fatigue and sleeplessness; extreme emotional lability with tearfulness at the slightest provocation; overconcern with minor aches and pains; expression of fears related to handling the baby; and inability to mobilize oneself. Delusions regarding oneself and others in the environment are not uncommon, and may include doubt regarding the husband's continued love, fear of his unfaithfulness, and the possibility of being deserted.

THE APPROACH TO THE POSTPARTUM WOMAN

Immediate Intervention of the Patient

SELF-MANAGEMENT TECHNIQUES

If the postpartum woman develops signs of a psychosis, help her realize that hospitalization may be necessary for her own safety and that of her infant. It is important for the staff to listen to and chart any information provided by the patient or family about her behavior and actions before admission. Record any information about the baby so that the patient will not be given conflicting information about where the baby is and who the caretakers are.

Professional Intervention

IMMEDIATE ACTION

If the patient exhibits any signs of psychosis, watch her carefully for any suicidal ideation. The patient may attempt to end her life in response to feeling inadequate as a mother, or because of a real or imagined problem with the baby's father.

Do not argue with the mother when she describes hallucinations or delusions. Tell her, "You feel this way because of your illness. As you feel more comfortable and get needed rest, these thoughts will subside and be less bothersome." Help her to understand that her dreams did not really happen.

Do not appear shocked by ideas expressed in bizarre forms. Suggestive or seductive movement or remarks, or abusive and vulgar language are the result of a lowering of the patient's inhibitions, and the nurse should understand this.

Give full attention when the individual talks about her symptoms. Do not slough them off as unimportant. Tell her that her symptoms can be relieved with treatment and medication. Emphasize the steps that have been taken in that direction—providing her with a quiet room, warm baths, activities to release tension, medication to help relieve discomfort, or warm milk before sleep. Stress the availability of a support system (e.g., spouse, relatives, friends, and professional health workers).

Arrange for frequent and consistent one-to-one interactions. Two or three staff members should take turns with the woman during the day, and provide continuous care while avoiding excess strain and fatigue of any one staff member.

Inform the patient of any medication and treatment she will be given. Stress their benefit to her in terms of alleviating depression, reducing her anxiety level, allowing a good sleep, and bolstering her nutrition.

INTERMEDIATE ACTION

Reassure the patient that her present feelings will be relieved as she improves. Tell her, "Some of these feelings are due to your illness." Don't give her cause to believe that she is not being a responsible and devoted mother. Accept her expression of her angry feelings toward her baby and husband but do not dwell on them. At this time she needs complete relief from thinking about the baby. Direct her into concrete and simple tasks (e.g., stamping envelopes, typing, clay modeling, or recreational activities).

Listen to what the patient has to say. Offer a warm, concerned, understanding relationship. Avoid questioning her or probing for information with which to round out the history. She cannot discuss her experiences at this time; besides, uncovering them may lead to an increase in her disturbance. Avoid reminding the patient of what she has said that was either irrational or inappropriate. No doubt she has already forgotten what she said previously and reminding her may cause a severe exacerbation of her symptoms.

Set reasonable limits. Help the patient to appreciate limitations and controls to avoid embarrassment to herself. Present reality to her. Deal with impulsive acts as necessary (e.g., if the patient starts taking off her clothes at an inappropriate place say, "You are taking your clothes off in a public place. Now I will help you return to your room so you can dress." Then assist the patient to do so.).

If the patient becomes uncooperative, obtain adequate help, and then take stern action. If she is unable to follow directions for her treatment and management, explain what you are going to do, the reasons why, and then act promptly. "You are being given these medications to make it easier for you to sleep."

If the patient asks about her baby, answer truthfully. Present her with the reality of the situation in a kind, firm manner, saying, "Yes, you have a baby. He is fine and being cared for." If she is fearful of harming her baby, accept her fears calmly. Tell her that her baby will be well taken care of until she feels less anxious and can resume that care herself. If the doctor has imposed limited visits because of the patient's anger toward her infant and husband, tell her, "As your condition improves, the visits will be increased."

LONG-TERM ACTION

As the patient improves, discuss plans for her immediate future. Help her to plan for extra help when she goes home. Instruct her about how to secure financial assistance and how to use the services of the public health or visiting nurse.

If the patient's pregnancy ended with death of the infant, share her grief. (See approach for depression following loss, pp. 71–76.)

FREQUENTLY PRESCRIBED PSYCHIATRIC DRUGS

Psychiatric drugs frequently prescribed during lactation include the following:

   Tricyclics: Nortriptyline (Pamelor), desipramine (Norpramin)
   Selective serotonin reuptake inhibitors: sertraline (Zoloft)
   Mood stabilizers (for manic-depressive disorder): valproate (Depakote)

Electrostimulative therapy can be given a week after delivery for treatment of severe depression or mania.

39

The Adolescent

The adolescent is a vacillating combination of dependent child and independent adult. Even as he yearns for freedom to make his own decisions, he clings to the security of parental authority. He fights for autonomy and adult responsibility, yet is grateful for limitations that protect him from situations for which he is not ready.

The "growing up" years are often referred to as the best years of one's life. This may be true for some, but for most people it is true only in retrospect. In reality it is a turbulent period of doubt, insecurity, mixed feelings, and struggles, all intermingled with joys and sorrows. A glance at the years from ages thirteen through nineteen will show how tremendous are the emotional, social, and behavioral changes demanded of the adolescent. This period may present severe problems, depending on the particular healthiness or unhealthiness of the individual and his family.

The adolescent may frequently find himself unable to satisfy the overwhelming and divergent demands of self, family, school, and peer group. At these times of crisis, he needs to relate to individuals he feels he can trust, so that he can discuss, dissect, understand, and resolve new as well as daily problems that arise. Prevention or early intervention in adolescent difficulties is needed, regardless of whether the problems are of organic or purely emotional origin.

Adolescents are prone to intense feelings of love in which another person becomes the object of adulation. Usually the love object is someone who is secretly admired, older, and possesses wisdom, a special skill, or provides a unique service. It is not unusual for the health worker to become a love object while the adolescent is receiving counseling for problems. The youngster usually fantasizes about various aspects of the relationship, embellishing it far beyond the real situation. Often the adolescent interprets a kind comment or action by the love object as an intense sexual interest.

The adolescent may not talk about his feelings to the individual, but may act them out by making special requests, writing affectionate notes, or talking to a peer about his secret desires. He may even allude to a planned time for physical intimacy with the idolized person. The adolescent's strivings are an unconscious attempt to feel loved and needed by an important and idealized individual, who may be a teacher, movie star, health worker, or sports hero. Health workers who find themselves the object of such feelings should recognize the meaning and importance to the youngster and accept the flattery and affection in a sincere, genuine manner. This reassures the patient that his feelings are being taken seriously. At the same time, the reality of the relationship must be gently presented, in a manner that reaffirms the adolescent's status as an appealing, intelligent person.

Every encouragement should be given to the development of appropriate relationships by the adolescent with others, through providing frequent visiting periods with those (particularly peers) who can supply his unmet needs for friendship and a mutually reciprocal relationship.

Until recently, the adolescent problem years were, for the most part, ignored or glossed over. Parents and others expected that they would be lived through, with all their funny, awkward, and, from the adult view, minor dilemmas. Yet some of the problems of this age group seem earthshattering to the adolescent. He may be going through an identity crisis, not knowing who he is or what he wants to be. Social events may be marred by a face full of pimples; gym may be consistently missed by a female youngster because of painful menstruation. Adults compare these problems with their own—making a decent living wage, for example, or keeping the house in order. By comparison, adolescents may seem trouble free. The adult is often so busy with his own pursuits and problems that he doesn't have time or patience to listen, nor does he seem to understand when he does listen.

Today we know that time does not always erase the awful effects of mishandling of youngsters who have difficulties but receive little help during adolescence. They feel lost if they are not treated with dignity and respect or if they receive little compassionate understanding and are seemingly misunderstood, discredited, and judged critically on the basis of appearance and behavior only. If professionals intend to intervene, they must begin to comprehend the adolescent's viewpoint. How does he feel about the world he lives in? What pressure does he feel, and what conflicts does he face? Workers must recognize that the child brings to adolescence all of his childhood insecurities, anxieties, and needs. Similarly, his previous conditioning will manifest itself in his reaction to struggles and problems that arise when he is subjected to the stresses of illness. This is particularly true when his freedom is restricted, when he is completely immobilized, or when he has to cope with health-oriented authority figures. It is, therefore, important for care providers to apply what is known about adolescents when dealing with them both in the community and in the hospital.

The adolescent's concerns about his schoolwork, career goals, involvement in drug use or sexual activity need to be recognized, with guidance and counseling made available. An appreciation of the special needs of these youngsters by health workers is a basic factor in establishing a therapeutic relationship. For example, a sense of deprivation may engulf the adolescent as he is separated from friends, close family, and pets during any hospital stay. Helping him deal with the impact of this temporary isolation is crucial. The health worker should encourage rational thinking by pointing out the realities of his situation. For example, a lack of visitors should not be interpreted as meaning that the whole world is against him or that no one cares about him.

As adolescent girls experience changes in their physical appearance, they often incur attention and teasing, particularly from boys. In the same vein, boys are often teased about their high-pitched voices or their lack of height. Boys may begin to have nocturnal emissions. Both sexes become aware of new feelings and sensations and of the new interest of others. It is as though the changing body has caused others to take note of a new and meaningful person. Much emphasis is put on increased awareness of sexual feelings and impulses. The adolescent is often in conflict between the wish to fulfill his desires and the restrictions and prohibitions imposed by family or society. As his sexual drive and awareness is at a peak, he finds himself frustrated on the one hand and fighting for self-control on the other.

Adolescence often involves a loss of old childhood friendships and a seeking of new relationships. New peer group loyalties become intense and are a mode of seeking support from friends, while loosening dependency ties to one's family. The peer group serves to diminish the feeling of being alone.

Some adolescents involve themselves in romances. If this meaningful social relationship ends, the adolescent who is also alienated from his parents may feel that he actually has no one to whom he may turn and, in his loneliness, becomes very vulnerable.

The adolescent feels the need to establish a personal identity. In his search to find himself, he begins to be assertive. His quest for autonomy is often interpreted by the family as being a threat to them—a contradiction and condemnation of parental standards and demands, and a hostile reaction purposefully intended to hurt them. Instead, that need to find his identity is actually a maturational crisis, relevant to the adolescent phase of development. As a consequence, disruptions occur in what was once looked upon as a peaceful family existence. The adolescent sees his behavior as reasonable, justified, and meaningful. He sees himself as being able to make decisions concerning his own well-being, including the choice of foods, clothing, hair style, and friends. He may disassociate himself from his family and align himself with causes, groups, and even daring activities. In doing so, he often must deal with opposing parental reactions, which he views as interference with the establishment of his independence. Indeed, this assumption is often correct, because some parents threaten withdrawal of financial or emotional support, and even physical abuse if their adolescent children do not comply with their demands. His parents' reactions have a deep effect on the adolescent's development of his autonomous self. The dilemma between the drive for independence and the still-present dependency gives rise to conflicts which generate much anxiety and uncertainty.

Conflicting attitudes between parents regarding each other's roles in the family will affect the adolescent, resulting in further confusion about his own identity. For instance, if the mother believes in permissiveness and the father is a rigid authoritarian, the mother may undermine an already difficult relationship between adolescent and father by creating situations in an underhanded way that enable the youngster to obtain more freedom behind his father's back. The message the adolescent then receives is that women must use subterfuge and dishonesty to have an ongoing relationship with men. If the adolescent is a boy, he may become suspicious of the motives of all women with whom he has relationships in the future. If the adolescent is a girl, she may adopt these same coping mechanisms for herself. All the while, the adolescent may feel that something is not quite right, and becomes increasingly uncertain of himself, as well as angry at his parents.

Parents are often stunned by the sudden changes in their child. They do not realize that a total lack of teen-aged rebellion could be a sign of regression. Normal adolescent behavior may include a derogatory attitude, unusual dress, foul language, and opposition to parental control of activities. These are ways of being an individual and asserting oneself. However, such behavior gives rise to much anxiety when parents do not trust their children to act without parental direction. Even those who claim they do often respond to their children's actions defensively. They see the adolescent's behavior as a blatant contradiction and "put-down" of themselves. They often unfairly interpret it as a war that has been declared, a competition between themselves and their offspring. Their anxiety is so heightened that they perceive only the negative characteristics of the behavior and ignore the positive ones. Parents ridicule, condemn, and tear down their youngsters in response to their own intrapsychic defensive operations. All of this adversely affects the youngster's development of his ego identity.

The family situation through childhood has an important bearing on adolescent behavior. If parents have always communicated with massive threats, the adolescent may respond by severely inhibiting his actions. This may result in so many restrictions on himself that dependency and a need for approval remain problems all his life. The adolescent in such a situation may displace his hostility from his parents to society in general. In families in which parents have been inconsistent, unconcerned, and have given little attention or discipline to their children, the adolescent may have difficulty in making decisions, have poor self-control, and find it difficult to accept any authority. Still another reaction may be found in youngsters who have been raised in an excessively strict home. Here the adolescent may rebel against any moral restrictions, and consequently develop conflicts caused by guilt feelings.

When parents shout, frequently become upset, and cannot control their anger, their child may act out in similar ways as he matures. That is, he may well displace his anger onto others. Conversely, when the parents are generally fearful and resistant to change, they may discourage any free expression of self, or dissuade the adolescent from venturing into meaningful though difficult new undertakings. This may lead to a severe conflict in which the adolescent wants to be independent, but at the same time is fearful of assuming responsibility. Children who are overly protected and smothered with love are shielded from most responsibilities and prevented from participating in decision making. As they become aware of their lack of experience in coping with ordinary daily problems, they become resentful, angry, and depressed. In a sense, they feel grossly short-changed. Their anxiety is so high that they are unable to function, often drop out of school, or fail to show up for work, and do very little but hang around the house.

Adolescence is a time of experimentation. The adolescent may want to try marijuana, amphetamines, cocaine, LSD, cigarettes, and alcohol. In many instances the abuse of drugs is connected to depressive symptoms. In turn, the depression can precipitate suicidal thoughts and suicidal attempts. Because adolescence is a time of adjustment, change, and stress, the youngster may be affected by periods of depression for which he seeks relief. Drug use can often lead to exaggeration of the problem and to the false conclusion that it is unsolvable.

Jenna, age 19, had been unhappy since her parents' divorce. Despite reassurance from her parents that they cared, their preoccupation with their own lives left her feeling unloved and unappreciated. She began to spend more time alone and often would use alcohol to numb her pain.

When her father noticed an increase in her moodiness, he lectured her, pointing out that she had all the material things she could possibly want and, therefore, had no reason to complain. In a fit of unhappiness, she expressed a desire to die. Her father, feeling frustrated and angry, responded by saying sarcastically, "Well, do a good job and blow your brains out." The next day, Jenna did just that by taking her father's gun and shooting a bullet through her brain.

The health worker needs to be alert to symptoms of depression exhibited by the adolescent (i.e., angry outbursts, sudden irritability, fluctuation in mood, or tearfulness). These symptoms can be precipitated by relationship problems, difficulties in school, and sometimes family problems (divorce).

When a youngster goes through puberty, sexual drives, aggressive inclinations, and childhood conflicts are intensified. In addition, the adolescent must cope with changes in his world, possibly attending a distant school, separation from former friends and family as well as the possibility of entering into intimate relationships. These changes may result in a roller coaster of moods, such as despair, confusion, conflict, loneliness, anger, emptiness, and uncertainties about future goals and values. Most adolescents experience some turbulence as they strive to become independent. Few adolescents are in a chronic state of upheaval. Most do maintain satisfying friendships and positive relationships with parents, siblings, teachers, and friends. Symptoms of dysfunction that persist and linger are serious signs of distress, and generally not a passing phase.

Illness in the adolescent may cause psychiatric symptoms as the youngster worries about his self-image including any change in the appearance of his body. Coping with illness and treatment can be difficult. The adolescent requires a great deal of information and explanation before medical procedures occur. If the adolescent is hospitalized, the deprivation suffered by separation from family or friends adds to his discomfort and resulting anger. Supportive interventions, such as reassurance, encouragement, persuasion, and positive advice, are essential.

Adolescents may find it less threatening to look at situations and understand how others view them rather than recognize any possible consequences resulting from their own actions. Often, discussions with families provide some insight into the adolescents' behavior.

It is important to inform the adolescent that all communications with him are confidential and privileged. The only exception is a situation in which his life may be at stake. If that should occur, the professionals involved in his care will be informed.

Sensitive issues, such as sexuality, must be approached in a nonthreatening, nonjudgmental manner. Often the client's distress can be related to concerns about sexuality or fear of becoming HIV infected. The importance of education about abstaining from risky behavior is vital. Jody was 15 when she was admitted to the hospital for a fractured leg resulting from an auto accident. Jody explained that she had been having "a blast" at a party and had given no thought to her safety when driving home. At the party, she had also engaged in a casual unprotected sexual experience and was now anxious about the possibility of having contracted a sexually transmitted disease. The health worker then explained HIV testing to Jody and encouraged her to have that test as well as those for other diseases. They also spent time discussing the importance of delaying gratification as against being involved in impulsive (and unsafe) actions.

Helping adolescents view undesirable or dangerous behavior as harmful or destructive to themselves is no easy task. They usually have not matured in their thought processes, and find that concentrating on future consequences is difficult. They often view the possibility of problems endured by others as unlikely to happen to themselves because they believe themselves to be invincible and untouchable.

However, not all adolescents have as difficult a time as has been described. Youngsters who are exposed to warmth and openness in their homes, whose achievements are met with approval and affection, and who are encouraged to be independent move forward into adolescence with a minimum of anxiety, concern, and dread of the responsibilities of adulthood.

The adolescent may affirm or condemn the life represented by his parents. He picks up the subtleties of parental conflicts, ambivalence, and fear of failure. He rebels against being used to satisfy the unmet needs of his elders, the vicarious living through him by his parents. For example, Sally observes that her mother spends lots of money at the country club, on clothes, jewelry, and at the beauty parlor. The mother says that education is important, and regrets that she never had the opportunities open to her daughter. At the same time, the mother frequently mentions the costliness of Sally's education, accuses her of not understanding the value of money, and demands that she demonstrate her appreciation of the sacrifices being made for her. Yet, when Sally is home on vacation and wears old jeans, the mother ridicules her appearance and remains aloof. Sally feels that she is being thrifty by wearing old clothes, and wonders why her mother doesn't love her for herself, instead of looking at material aspects. She persists in being herself. Mother goes into a rage because of her own need to conform and impress others. Her insecurity is partially due to her concern about other people's reactions to her. Her perception of the situation is that Sally's behavior is hostile, and this leaves her frustrated. She threatens punishment. As a result, Sally feels misunderstood and withdraws in self-defense. She won't talk to Mother any more. At the time of her life that she most needs her mother, she becomes alienated from her. Sally feels that her mother's way of life is a hoax and lacks meaning. She is indignant because of the unfairness of standards preached but not practiced by her parents.

Parents may not have taken the time to know and understand their children because they have been preoccupied with their own interests, conflicts, and difficulties. Therefore, they will not know how to cope with the adolescent. They find it difficult to understand the meaning of new behavior patterns and almost impossible to accept the growth of their children's emotional independence and sexual and emotional investment in others.

During adolescence, one begins to think about possible occupations, the way one wants to earn a living, and the possible course of his life in regard to having a role in society. When jobs are scarce and the adolescent finds it impossible to find meaningful work, his sense of worth is lessened. He may feel that his driver's license and his Social Security card are society's only acknowledgment of his having grown up.

Many adolescents and their parents solve the lack-of-employment problem by using further education as a delaying tactic. Some teen-agers see college as an escape, or at least as an approved postponement of facing the adult world. In such a case, the student may find himself involved in intense scholastic competition which he cannot meet. He may be overwhelmed by all there is to learn, and unprepared for the lack of supervision or guidance in an environment less structured than that of his high school. Some find they are unable to develop their abilities or to meet parental standards. Others are bewildered, do not know what to study, and find the university gives them no direction in developing their talents. In large universities, students are often treated impersonally, and this may foster feelings of worthlessness. Dormitory life may also revive memories of infantile attachments to others of the same sex. Fears of intimate relationships when living closely together may throw an adolescent unsure of his identity into a homosexual panic. In short, college may really serve to intensify the adolescent's apprehensions and his feelings of inadequacy. All this may contribute to the current high suicide rate among college students.

The adolescent needs to reestablish trust and a sense of the worthwhileness of living in today's world. If his family is not available, he may resort to the health worker to help him experience understanding, love, and dependability. The adolescent needs to feel autonomous and have a real sense of commitment. He needs to feel secure and guided by people he can trust, people who will not retaliate when he attempts to work through pressures and problems, whether they stem from his childhood, present encounters, or future uncertainties. He needs time and understanding to resolve tensions set up by personal change, distrust of adults, and environmental chaos. He welcomes limits that offer security by protecting him from his own undesirable behavior, while allowing him to attain a measure of adulthood.

The adolescent is struggling to develop his strengths. He may be enjoying or fearing the budding of his adult status and physical being. He is groping with adaptations in school, thoughts of a career, his changing relationships with others, his social obligations, and his home responsibilities. An illness can interrupt or even destroy his choices, possibly ending all hope for the realization of his plans and dreams. He needs support from professionals in determining what options are realistically available to him and what his limitations are. His family also needs direction in evaluating their hopes for him, as well as in recognizing the pressures they are placing on him. Adolescence need not lead to constant turmoil if the youngster, family, and professional work together to assess and deal with the patient's valid needs.

Working with adolescents is challenging. Moreover, once their trust has been gained, the health worker has an enormous opportunity to share information, to help implement measures for behavioral change, and to provide support while the client learns to cope with new problems.

THE APPROACH TO THE ADOLESCENT

Immediate Intervention by the Adolescent

SELF-MANAGEMENT TECHNIQUES

Be aware of the normal bodily changes taking place during puberty. Recognize the need for establishing independent, responsible actions when leaving home for school or other areas. If hospitalization is needed, limit belongings brought to the hospital to whatever is necessary plus a few items that can be used for studies or enjoyment. Do not bring things of great value because others might "borrow" them. Be open to any suggestions by staff members who offer information on health matters. Ask all visitors to maintain decorum while visiting.

Professional Intervention

IMMEDIATE ACTION

Evaluate and document all physical or emotional complaints made during any contact with the adolescent. Do not ignore his or her statements, or be judgmental.

Establish rapport so that the adolescent will feel free to seek your help if needed in the future.

INTERMEDIATE ACTION

Understand the adolescent's need to mature. Whenever possible, include him in decisions that affect his care and treatment. Explain any procedures as completely as possible to alleviate his anxiety. Keep him informed about his progress during the treatment.

Do not impose your standards, beliefs or values on him. Do not moralize. Rather, allow him to share his opinions, accept what he has to say, and agree or disagree without becoming defensive. Recognize the problems that exist without being judgmental.

Recognize that adolescent problems involve family interaction patterns. The patient's preadolescent relationship with his parents has set the stage for the present pattern. Do not threaten to withdraw your support in order to force him to live up to parental expectations. Instead, help him assess his position, as well as that taken by his parents; offer him encouragement without taking sides. Praise and encourage him when he makes mature independent decisions. Show that you care.

Treat the adolescent with dignity and respect. Do not belittle or discredit his ideas, friends, or romantic relationships. Regard his difficulties seriously. Do not call attention to his clothes, hair style, or choice of foods. Avoid speaking of academic achievement as the only worthwhile endeavor in life. Encourage physical activity to diminish tensions and anxiety. Stress the individual's positive characteristics. Do not look at normal adolescent behavior as though it were abnormal.

LONG-TERM ACTION

Set limits that are fair, and enforce them consistently. Recognize the special needs of the adolescent to prevent antisocial behavior while encouraging his growth of self-control. Help him channel his energies constructively through prescribed limitations.

Unless you genuinely like and care about adolescents, do not work with them if you can avoid it. Whether you do or don't like them, however, recognize your own fears, insecurities, anxieties, and drives, and do not displace them onto the adolescent.

40

The Aged Person

What does it mean to grow old? Some of the meanings of aging can be discovered simply by taking time to become acquainted with the elderly. Not surprisingly, older people do not all feel the same way about aging. Those who enjoy their senior years see retirement as a time to pursue hobbies for which they had no time previously. They look forward to having fewer obligations, freedom to come and go as they please, time to sit and enjoy a good book.

Others feel that aging results in their no longer being needed. They see themselves as worthless because they are not earning a living. The decrease in their obligations is interpreted as an indication that no one wants them or cares about them. They have too much time on their hands, and do not know how to fill the many free hours that are available each day. Even when opportunities for activity are presented, they lack the energy and initiative to involve themselves.

The way one views his past life has much to do with the kind of person he is at, say, seventy. For instance, if a person feels he has had a comfortable life, with meaningful relationships, has accomplished some of his goals, and has achieved a sense of fulfillment within himself, he will tend to think of aging as a continuing, inevitable phase of life that has positive value. But if, in the past, the person viewed life as a hardship with many frustrations, and if his dreams and hopes have been unfulfilled, he will be likely to see his last phase of life as just another dead end.

By the same token, the aged person who has been active in his earlier years, has been a joiner, a doer, will usually continue to have an interest in being with others and participating with them in various activities. He will continue to be involved in the life around him, even if he physically cannot do as much as he once did. One lady, who had been a professional nurse for forty years, became a much-needed hospital volunteer who read books and wrote letters for incapacitated war veterans. Physiologically, she could no longer carry the work load of the average nurse. But through her volunteer service she continued to be in touch with her profession in a way which gave personal meaning to her life.

The individual who always tended to remain by himself, had little to do with other people, had few personal interests save watching television and dozing in an easy chair, day in and day out, will most likely follow the same routine as he ages. Excluding those who develop senile arteriosclerosis or Alzheimer's disease, people's personalities do not change drastically as their faces wrinkle. The same positive and negative facets of the personality are apparent, or perhaps they become more accentuated under the stress of advancing years.

An elderly gentleman was admitted to the hospital with a history of a year-long depression which dated back to the day he had sold his gardening business because he was no longer able to do the physical work that it required. From early youth onward, he had loved nature and the out-of-doors. Virtually his entire life had been spent working by himself, caring for grass, flowers, and plants. He enjoyed seeing the results produced by his marvelously green thumb. His work kept him so involved that he never felt a need to bother with anyone or anything else. Retirement took away the one thing upon which he had really depended. Even his family was not aware of how little he had been involved with them throughout their lives. In fact, they could not understand his being so unhappy in a situation which they thought would bring relief from work and responsibility. When the nursing staff attempted to engage the patient in various group therapies, he barely responded. Fortunately, one nurse who had a great deal of insight into his problem arranged for him to take care of the plants on the unit. She also talked to his relatives and together they contacted a nursery that could, indeed, use the services of an elderly gentleman gardener. The pay was negligible but that was immaterial compared with the importance of finding a way in which the patient could pursue the life style to which he was accustomed, and which made him happy.

The best way for the worker to find out how the aged patient sees himself and his past life, and how he feels about his future years, is to sit down and really listen to what he has to say. After all, he knows best what he really is all about, how he has managed all these years, what his habits have been, what works for him and what does not. For example, when an individual who is used to hot coffee and a pastry for breakfast, and has been enjoying it for seventy or so years, is suddenly faced with porridge, soft-boiled egg, and lukewarm coffee, he can be expected to lose his appetite completely. Any lectures by the young nurse on the subject of nutrition will be ignored or met with real anger.

The aging process affects the body's ability to maintain its immune system. Studies of immune cells, particularly the T lymphocytes, seem to indicate that areas known as telemeres (the specialized areas of genetic material on the ends of the chromosomes) become shorter as aging occurs. This has been interpreted as a sign of the ending of their ability to fight off invading pathogens. This may explain why some viruses (such as shingles), having been under control in the body for decades, suddenly proliferate.

Longevity is affected by a combination of genetic and environmental factors, including better nutrition, immunizations against diseases, and improved sanitation. The estimated maximum life span also appears to increase when there is a reduction in calories, perhaps due to the resultant lowering of metabolic activity accompanied by an increase in an antioxidant response. (These same effects are noted when animals hibernate and do not eat.) However, malnutrition is deleterious and should be prevented. In Dade county, Florida, a survey of the elderly poor by the Dade Alliance for Aging found that the risk factors for malnutrition included the taking of three or more medications each day, the inability to shop, cook, or eat (because of insufficient funds, illness that changed eating patterns, or swallowing problems related to dental or mouth status) and eating alone. Preventive measures might include referral to an organization, such as Meals on Wheels for delivery of meals to the homebound. For those able to leave home, the elderly might enjoy group expeditions to markets to purchase food or other household necessities or to attend senior social centers with meals served as part of the daily activities.

In 1890, the average age expectancy in Europe and the United States was 47 years. This increased to 75.5 years by 1993. The U.S. Census Bureau predicts that by the year 2030, 20% of the U.S. population will be elderly, with 8.8 million older than the age of 85. Some scientists believe the practical limit to life expectancy is 85 years, whereas others think survivors will reach 95 or 100, or even more.

Presently, Japan has the highest life expectancy in the world: 76.6 years for men and 83 years for women. There, nearly half of the disabled are older than age 65, with 20% of those older than age 80 requiring some level of care. The aging of the population has resulted in "children" of 70 years caring for their 90-year-old parents. There are inadequate placement facilities in Japan, with about 60,000 people on waiting lists to enter 3,000 homes. Admissions presently are limited to those who are bedridden or suffer from senile dementia. Community care and nursing homes are being increased but not sufficiently to meet the needs of a population that continues to age. The U.S. can learn from what has happened in Japan and use that information to formulate plans for our own growing numbers of aged.

The task ahead is to find ways to increase the proportion of life that will be free of diseases and disability. In a recent study at the Duke University for Demographic Studies, disability rates were unexpectedly found to drop by 14.5% between 1982 and 1994, with the greatest improvements occurring in those older than age 85, or those who were most severely disabled. Medicare costs have not dropped proportionately because more money has been expended for the treatment of heart problems, surgeries (including hip replacements, organ transplants, and eye care), and the development and use of prosthetic devices.

The American Academy of Orthopedic Surgeons stresses the importance of "moving for life," with the inclusion of physical activity as a way to slow the loss of muscle mass, to strengthen bones and joints, and reduce pain. Exercise has been found to improve mobility and balance, which, in turn, lessens the risk of injury from falls. Exercise also tends to improve the individual's mental outlook, as the capability for providing self-care increases, and the outlook for independent living increases.

Caretakers of the elderly often unintentionally contribute to increasing the chance of disability by rewarding dependent and compliant behavior. Mae was 90 years old when she entered an assisted living residence. She enjoyed being with others and taking her meals in the main dining room. One of her caretakers assumed that because of her age and some visual impairment, special attention was required. Without ascertaining Mae's actual needs, she was moved to a small room reserved for those requiring increased supervision at mealtimes. Mae became angry and agitated, and refused to eat in that area. A power struggle evolved between what the caretaker thought would benefit Mae and what Mae wanted. Not until her daughters intervened on her behalf was Mae allowed to return to the main dining room.

Once given the chance to maintain her freedom and dignity, Mae was able to use her habitual skills including socializing with the other residents at mealtimes as well as when walking and swimming. Allowed to join the others, she was no longer angry or agitated. She was the perfect example of the importance of recognizing the level of competency of the client. Unused skills may deteriorate to the point of being lost. It is important to encourage the use of all skills at whatever level they may be, regardless of the patient's age. The health worker should be alert to any actions on his part that may foster dependency because that will increase the patient's feelings of failure and helplessness. The patient who becomes dependent may believe he is unable to walk alone, travel independently, or even prepare food for himself. The aged person should be encouraged to do as much as he can for himself, even though he may require extra time and help to do so.

Some clients exhibit behavior that may be troublesome to the staff. The behavior should be regarded as a form of communication. For example, one client tended to wander away from the group at intervals. The health worker realized that this indicated the client's need for exercise. Rather than viewing the client as unwilling to remain with the group and be "good," a plan for regular exercise was instituted. The wandering then decreased significantly.

If the aged person is living at home, additional precautions may be needed. Safety is a major issue because falls or burns may result in permanent disability. In addition, medications may cause a problem as there is greater danger of a drug reaction. The drug may accumulate in the body or not be utilized correctly owing to organ failure. If there are any signs of a problem, the prescribing practitioner should be notified immediately. The individual as well as his caretaker should be made aware of possible interactions of food or other medications with the medication under question. For example, grapefruit juice may potentiate the strength of some drugs, causing the patient to show signs of an overdose. Some drugs may cause drowsiness, making it dangerous for the patient to engage in activities that require him to be alert.

The caregiver (particularly a spouse) should be encouraged to seek time away to lessen his own stress. Other family members or friends, or even a paid employee may be necessary to allow this. This is particularly important if the patient exhibits signs of dementia with a lessening of his cognitive functions. It is not unusual to hear patients accuse their caretakers of stealing possessions or imprisoning them. One elderly lady, cared for by her grandson, was unable to recognize him as he slept. She then called the police, stating that he was an intruder who had taken her money and jewelry. Fortunately, the grandson was able to prove who he was, and other relatives substantiated that nothing in the way of money or jewelry was missing.

Some staff members seem to have the attitude that older people have little need for privacy, few feelings, and no sexual ideas or urges. Patients tell us that the reverse is actually true. The older person enjoys a familiar, warm, well-lighted environment. He enjoys having a room of his own where he can keep his precious things and maintain a way of life that he can manage. He is sensitive, and needs attention to his individual needs. Many older people continue to enjoy an active sexual life. A sexual relationship is often thwarted by practical problems that beset the aged. Where, when, and with whom are not simple decisions when one has experienced loss of spouse, friends, and relationships, and has housing, transportation, and financial difficulties.

Health problems of the aged can interfere with sexual functioning. Atrophy of the vaginal wall with a resultant decrease in lubrication, prostatectomy, diabetes, heart disease, stroke, severe arthritis, emotional or physical difficulties may play a large role in the geriatric patient's inability to perform sexually. Individuals who see themselves as physically repulsive, with bodies that are no longer firm, often avoid any physical intimacy. Men frequently worry that they will cease to have erections, and may therefore go overboard proving their potency and virility through increased sexual activity. They may seek erotic magazines or motion pictures to stimulate their waning desires. Insecurity regarding the individual's own sexuality may give rise to undue jealousy and suspiciousness, if the spouse relates to others.

Health workers who recognize that they are anxious at the idea that old people have sexual relations would do well to examine the origin of their feelings. One health worker, who was very angry when she discovered two elderly patients in bed together, stated, "I could never picture my folks having sex. Everyone else, yes. But not *my* folks. If I weren't here, I'd swear they never did it." In the discussion that followed, the worker was able to see on a conscious level that these patients bore a resemblance to her own parents, and that she had transferred her negative feelings about sex onto them. On an unconscious level, she was not aware that her negative feelings stemmed from her childhood and were a defense mechanism to control the discomfort she felt when sexually attracted to her father. The health worker's understanding of the origin of her attitudes helped her to be less judgmental about her own parents' sexual love. In addition, she became more tolerant concerning feelings of sexuality among the aged.

Frequently, staff members shy away from the aged person, because they find the changes that occur repulsive: hesitant speech; occasional memory lapses; unsteady steps with the possibility of injury from falls; wrinkled, dry skin; thinning, white hair; impaired hearing and sight; a tendency to react negatively to change. Failing sensory and mental abilities are all reminders that a long life brings problems and imposes limitations. The nurse cannot turn the clock back thirty years and restore health and vitality to the aged patient, but she certainly can be aware of his needs, and incorporate them into her plan for his care.

Health workers may fall victim to the pressures of our culture which glorifies youth and seems to say that only the young are important. They may categorize all older people as fitting into a stereotype and be unable to see them as individuals. This attitude is reflected in the moans of a staff member who is told that her expected admission is a seventy-year-old lady. Before the patient has set foot on the unit, the nurse anticipates that her patient will be helpless, hopeless, and uninteresting—that she may need a great deal of extra attention, may make unnecessary noises, and be difficult and unrewarding to care for.

A pessimistic attitude on the part of the health worker is sometimes attributed to the idea that senility is rarely reversible. In many instances, it does progress as the individual continues to live. Even so, much can be offered to the aged in terms of therapy, including recreational therapy, occupational therapy, group therapy, and medications. Any or all of these may result in a lessening of distressing symptoms through improved contact with reality, increased motivation, and the reinforcement of appropriate behavior.

Frequently, it is depression, rather than senility, which causes patients to behave in a nonfunctional fashion. Involvement of the patient often decreases the depression and allows him to take part in life again. Additionally, use of certain medications (p. 76) may be useful.

Whether the patient is cared for at home or in a care facility, he requires stimulation. Clocks, pictures, photographs may help orient him to time and family. One nursing home scheduled regular visits by a nursery school group. Some elderly clients who were unresponsive to almost all other activities brightened immediately as the youngsters came to them, some sitting on the elders' laps and cuddling closely. The children were smiling and happy with these pseudograndparents. Both generations benefited from the meetings. In other nursing homes, residents have enjoyed visits from dogs, birds, or cats that responded to them. Music, shows, and other enjoyable activities help stimulate the elderly, increasing their alertness.

Projecting herself into the future may help the nurse to understand her elderly patients. Quickly, she will touch on not being active in nursing, her children grown and away, and perhaps limited savings. Her friends and relatives may have passed on; her health may be failing. But while she is projecting this image, she will also do well to keep in mind that somehow she will be able to cope and survive. She will realize her desire to make decisions about her dress, whom she wants to help her, and what she wants to do. She knows that she will not enjoy being ignored, treated in an offhand manner or as if she is "too old to know anything" because she has retired. Although she may expect to need a little assistance at times, she will not want to be treated as a child. She will expect others to accept her as she is and not impose unnecessary restrictions simply because of her age.

As the population ages, incidents of abuse of the elderly increase. Presently, there are almost 2 million cases yearly including those that are caused by physical injuries, psychological maltreatment, financial exploitation, or neglect. Unless professional caregivers are aware of these possibilities, the abuse may go unnoticed.

The possibility of physical abuse is often first noticed in the emergency room, when the elderly person is brought in for help. Usually the patient is accompanied by a "child," who may himself be older than age 60 and who answers any questions asked by staff members. He is unwilling to leave the parent's side and has quick answers for any queries. Bruises or broken bones may be explained by stories of a fall down a flight of stairs, whereas severe burns may be accounted for by a tale of a tea kettle having overturned onto the individual. The staff members may become suspicious as they notice a variation in the discolorations of bruises, indicating that they may have happened at different times. X-rays may demonstrate multiple fractures in various stages of healing, also an indication of injuries that have occurred at different times. All observations by the staff must be accurate and complete because there may be legal implications if the injuries are found to have been caused by another person. Photographs should be taken so that there is documentation as part of the record.

It is more difficult to discover abuse that results from psychological factors. The patient may appear fearful, unwilling to talk to any staff member, demoralized, and depressed. If the individual is physically, emotionally or financially dependent on a relative, there may be reluctance to report any abuse.

Another component of that is the pain associated with having to admit that someone who has been loved and trusted is now being abusive. Financial abuse is also a strong component of the relationship. If an adult child is angry, feeling that the parent has lived too long, and is now causing him to expend monies that he may have counted on for his own use, or for the expenses of his family, he may manipulate the available funds for his own benefit. This may result in inadequate health care, food or living conditions for the parent, who may not be aware of community resources available to help find a solution to the problem. If the patient is incapable of handling the necessary steps for protection, Adult Protective Services (a state agency) may be of help. Health workers should be supportive and nonjudgmental, even when the patient refuses to leave the abusive situation.

Abuse of the elder individual is not limited to those living with relatives. It also occurs in residences and nursing homes, where care may not be optimal. Some residents may require hospitalization as the result of an injury, bed sores, or dementia. At that time, the hospital staff may uncover evidence of serious abuse that should be reported to the authorities. Again, documentation must be complete and accurate in order to help the patient and protect the whistle blower from legal countercharges. It is important to offer support to the patient, to listen, to refer the individual to appropriate agencies for help, and to be available to answer questions that he may have.

THE APPROACH TO THE AGED PERSON

Immediate Intervention by the Patient or Caretaker

SELF-MANAGEMENT TECHNIQUES

Recognize any diminution in the ability for self-care. Have an emergency call system available if possible or a "buddy" system that includes others checking on the patient at regular intervals.

Professional Intervention

IMMEDIATE ACTION

Foster orientation by having clocks available, family photographs, familiar objects nearby. An identification bracelet or MediAlert bracelet should be worn at all times if the individual has medical problems or is on medication. *Be certain that food and fluid intake are adequate but not excessive.* Give the individual as much choice as possible about his diet, with whom and where he wants to eat.

Reinforce independence by having the older person do as much of his own care as possible. Plan sufficient time so that he does not feel rushed.

INTERMEDIATE ACTION

Encourage activities that the individual enjoys. Encourage visits from friends, family, and colleagues. Involve him with therapeutic groups to enlarge his scope of interests.

Have the individual become involved in tasks that will be helpful to him when he is alone. If possible, teach him to prepare simple foods, take his own medications, do his laundry, and keep his home clean.

LONG-TERM ACTION

Prepare the individual for living alone if necessary. Make lists of everyday tasks as well as telephone numbers of significant others (family, friends, and professional helpers).

Make plans for food delivery, including Meals on Wheels if available for delivery of cooked meals. The individual may need help in planning appropriate grocery shopping and meal preparation.

Plan appropriate supervisory visits by professionals to check on his physical and mental status. If deterioration occurs, have plans for additional care, either in the home or a residential facility that has been chosen in advance. Preplanning will give the patient a sense that he is in control of his own destiny.

Suggested Readings

INTERPERSONAL RELATIONS

Adler, M. M. (1995). Cultural diversity. *The Beth Israel Nurses, 7,* 9–12.

Aguilera, D. (1990). *Crisis intervention: Theory and methodology* (6th ed.). St. Louis: Mosby.

Aiken, L. (1995, September-October). Transformation of the nursing workforce. *Nursing Outlook, 43,* 201–209.

Aisenstein, T. (1995, November 27). For nurses new to home care. *The Nursing Spectrum* (Florida ed.). 12–14.

Anderson, J. (1990, May-June). Health care across cultures. *Nursing Outlook, 38,* 136–139.

Antai-Otong, D. (1997). Team building in a health care setting. *American Journal of Nursing, 7,* 48–51.

Bandman, E., & Bandman, B. (1990). *Nursing ethics through the life span* (2nd ed.). Norwalk, CT: Appleton & Lange.

Belluck, P. (1996, May 9). Mingling two worlds of medicine—some doctors work with folk healers in immigrants' care. *The New York Times,* pp. B1, 4.

Berger, J. (1996, March 24). Unneeded services inflating costs of home health care. *The New York Times,* pp. 1, 22.

Bernstein, N. (1997, September 15). On line, high-tech sleuths find private facts (access to private computer information). *The New York Times,* pp. A1, A12.

Bonczyk, K. (1997, June 2). Title VII—Sexual harassment. *Nursing Spectrum* (Florida ed.), *7,* 14–16.

Bond, M. L., & Jones, M. E. (1997). Creating culturally competent professionals. *Reflections—Sigma Theta Tau International* (2nd quarter), *23,* 18–19.

Brazino, J. (1997, February 24). Reinventing nurse extenders: The emergence of UAP. *Nursing Spectrum* (Florida ed.), *7,* 6–7, 17.

Bullough, B., & Bullough V. (Eds.). (1990). *Nursing issues in the nineties and beyond.* New York: Springer Publishing

Bunis, D. (1996, May 2). The nursing revolution: 2. Nurses fight back. *Newsday* pp. A7, 24–25.

Burgess, A. (1990). *Psychiatric nursing in the hospital and the community* (5th ed.). Norwalk, CT: Appleton & Lange.

Caplan, G. (1964). *Principles of preventive psychiatry.* New York: Basic Books.

Caton, C., Wyatt, R., & Felix, A. (1993, November). Follow-up of chronically homeless mentally ill men. *American Journal of Psychiatry, 150,* 1639–1642.

Clunn, P. (1996, 1st quarter). The nurse's kit for survivors: Care for care givers, families. *Reflections—Sigma Theta Tau International, 22,* 8–9.

Cohen, B., Levin, R., Bashoff, M., Ellis, E., Condie, V., & Gelfand, G. (1997). Educators' responses to changes in the health care system. *The Journal of the New York State Nurses Association, 28,* 4–6.

Craft, M., Bradford, K., Jost, K., Burton, D., & Rambo, A. (1996, 1st quarter). The many graces of Oklahoma nurses. *Reflections—Sigma Theta Tau International, 22,* 10–12.

Dibble, S. (1997). Celebrating diversity. *Reflections—Sigma Theta Tau International* (2nd quarter), *23,* 10–11.

Gianakos, D. (1997). Physicians, nurses and collegiality. *Nursing Outlook, 45,* 57–58.

Goldsmith, J. (1996, 1st quarter). Mending broken dreams (hurricane Andrew). *Reflections—Sigma Theta Tau International, 22,* 6–9.

Goleman, D. (1995, December 5). Making room on the couch for culture. *The New York Times,* pp. B5, B10.

Gregg, D. (1996, April). Choosing an HMO. *Harvard Health Letter,* pp. 9–12.

Grossman, D. (1996, July). Cultural dimensions in home health nursing. *American Journal of Nursing, 96,* 33–36.

Guy, R. (1995). Redefining the vision in rehabilitation nursing. *The Beth Israel Nurse, 7,* 6–8.

Habayeb, G. (1995). Cultural diversity: A nursing concept not yet reliably defined. *Nursing Outlook, 43,* 224–227.

Harding, A. (1995, December). Rehabilitation: Healing at home. *Harvard Health Letter,* pp. 6–8.

Huston, C. (1996, March-April). Unlicensed assistive personnel: A solution to dwindling health care resources or the precursor to the apocalypse of registered nursing? *Nursing Outlook, 44,* 67–73.

Kane, R. (1995). Expanding the home care concept: Blurring distinctions among home care, institutional care, and other long-term-care services. *The Milbank Quarterly, 42,* 161–186.

Kane, R. (1996). The future of group residential care. In Caring for frail, elderly people. *Policies in Evolution,* Organization for Economic Co-operation and Development. *Social Policy Studies N., 19,* 93–105.

Kayser-Jones, J., & Schell, E. (1997). The effect of staffing on the quality of care at mealtime. *Nursing Outlook, 45,* 64–72.

Kennedy, M., Schepp, K., & O'Connor. (1996). *Making a difference: Teaching self-management of psychiatric symptoms.* Paper presented at American Nurses Association Convention and Centennial Celebration, Washington, DC.

Kilborn, P. (1996, January 14). Veterans expand hospital system in face of cuts. *The New York Times,* pp. 1, 13.

Koyanagi, C. (1997, spring). Just what is "managed care"? *National Council of Jewish Women, 20,* 20–21, 30.

Lang, N. (1996, fall). Academic nursing practice: A case study of the University of Pennsylvania School of Nursing. *Penn Nursing, 1,* 17, 18, 36.

Leininger, M. (1992). Strange myths and inaccurate facts in transcultural nursing. *Journal of Transcultural Nursing, 3,* 39–40.

Leininger, M. (1991). *Cultural care diversity and universality: A theory of nursing.* New York: National League for Nursing Press.

Link, B., Phelan, J., & Bresnahan, M. (1995, July). Lifetime and five-year prevalence of homelessness in the U.S. *American Journal of Orthopsychiatry, 65,* 347–354.

Longman, P. (1997, August 11). Who is the victim (home care cost)? *U.S. News & World Report, 123,* 18–22.

MacKay, R., Hughes, J., & Carver, J. (Eds.). (1990). *Empathy in the helping relationship.* New York: Springer.

Mayotte, J. (1992). *Disposable people? The plight of refugees.* Maryknoll, NY: Orbis.

Minnick, A., Roberts, M., Young, W., Marcantonio, R., & Kleinpell, R. (1997, January-February). Ethnic diversity and staff nurse employment in hospitals. *Nursing Outlook, 45,* 35–40.

Morse, J., et al. (1996, 4th quarter). Nursing among diverse cultures. *Reflections—Sigma Theta Tau International,* pp. 6–27.

Mundinger, M. (1997). APNs can succeed best through strong partnerships with MDs. *APNSCAN, 15,* 1.

Ostrander, F. (1996, October). Management and evaluation: A how-to guide for home care nurses. *American Journal of Nursing, 96,* 16B, 16D, 16F, 16G.

Peplau, H. (1952). *Interpersonal relations in nursing* (pp. 17–42). New York: Putnam's.

Rabin, R. (1996, May 2). The nursing revolution: 1. New caregivers. *Newsday,* pp. A5, A28–29.

Robinette, A. (1996, July). Psychiatric consultation liaison nurses: Who are they? How can they help you? *American Journal of Nursing, 96,* 48–50.

Sarduy, I. (1997, March 24). The essence of customer satisfaction. *The Nursing Spectrum* (Florida ed.), *6,* 5.

Schoen, M. (1996, June 17). Managing legal risks in home healthcare. *Nursing Spectrum* (Florida ed.), 12–14.

Schraeder, C., Lamb, G., Shelton, P., & Britt, T. (1997). Community nursing organizations: A new frontier. *American Journal of Nursing, 97,* 63–65.

Stanley, J. (1997, March-April). Columbia School of Nursing signs managed care contracts. *Nurse Practitioner World News, 2,* 1, 3.

Travelbee, J. (1971). *Interpersonal aspects of nursing* (pp. 36–38). Philadelphia: Davis.

Ujhely, G. (1968). *Determinants of the nurse-patient relationship* (p. 93). New York: Springer.

Wells, S. (1996, October). Adding an "at home" path to your discharge plan. *American Journal of Nursing, 96,* 73–74.

Winslow, R. (1997, February 7). Nurses to take doctor duties, Oxford says. *The Wall Street Journal,* pp. 3–4.

SPECIFIC PSYCHIATRIC DISORDER

Anxiety

Goisman, R. (1997, May). Cognitive-behavioral therapy today. *The Harvard Mental Health Letter, 13,* 4–7.

Katon, W. (1993). *Panic disorder in the medical setting*. National Institutes of Mental Health, U.S. Department of Health and Human Services.

McNally, R. (1994). *Panic disorder: A critical analysis*. New York: Guilford.

Panic disorder (1995, February). *Harvard Women's Health Watch, 2,* 6.

Pollack, M., & Smoller, J. (1995, December). The longitudinal course and outcome of panic disorder. *Psychiatric Clinics of North America, 18,* 785–801.

Shear, M. K., Pilkonis, P. A., Cloitre, M., & Leon, A. (1994, May). Cognitive behavioral treatment compared with nonprescriptive treatment of panic disorder. *Archives of General Psychiatry, 51,* 395–401.

Stein, M., Walker, J., & Ford, D. (1996, February). Public speaking fears in a community sample: Prevalence, impact on functioning, and diagnostic classification. *Archives of General Psychiatry, 53,* 169–174.

Conduct Disorder

Brewer-Smyth, K. (1996, August 26). Preventing violence in the healthcare setting. *The Nursing Spectrum* (Florida ed.), *6,* 12–14.

Zollo, M., & Derse, A. (1997). The abusive patient: Where do you draw the line? *American Journal of Nursing, 97,* 31–35.

Personality Disorder

Sperry, Leon. (1995). *Handbook of diagnosis and treatment of the DSM-IV personality disorders*. New York: Brunner/Mazel.

Obsessive-Compulsive Disorder

Jenicke, M. A. (1993). Obsessive-compulsive disorder: Efficacy of specific treatment as assessed by controlled trials. *Psychopharmacology Bulletin, 29,* 487–499.

Jenicke, M. A. (1992). New developments in treatment of obsessive-compulsive disorder. In A. Tasman & M. Riba, (Eds.), *Review of psychiatry* (Vol 11). Washington, DC: American Psychiatric Press.

Obsessive-compulsive disorder: 1. (1995, November). *The Harvard Mental Health Letter, 12,* 1–3.

Obsessive-compulsive disorder: 2. (1995, December). *The Harvard Mental Health Letter, 12,* 1–3.

Obsessive-compulsive disorder. (1994, September). Washington, DC: National Institutes of Mental Health, National Institutes of Health.

Rapoport, J. (1991). Recent advances in obsessive-compulsive disorder. *Neuropsychopharmacology, 5,* 1–10.

Borderline Personality

Clarkin, J., Marzial, E., & Munroe-Blum (Eds.). (1992). *Borderline personality disorder: Clinical and empirical perspectives.* New York: Guilford.

Links, P. (Ed.). (1990). *Family environment and borderline personality disorder.* Washington, DC: American Psychiatric Press.

Paris, J. (Ed.). (1993). *Borderline personality disorder: Etiology and treatment.* Washington, DC: American Psychiatric Press.

Salzman, C. (1996, September). What drug treatments are available for borderline personality disorder? *The Harvard Mental Health Letter, 13,* 8.

Sansone, R., Sansone, L., & Wiederman, M. (1996, December). Borderline personality disorder and health care utilization in a primary care setting. *Southern Medical Journal, 89,* 1162–1165.

Depressive Disorder

American Psychiatric Association. (1993, April). Practice guideline for major depressive disorder in adults. *American Journal of Psychiatry, 150* (Suppl.).

Castonguay, L., Goldfried, M., & Wiser, S. (1996). Predicting the effect of cognitive therapy for depression: A study of unique and common factors. *Journal of Consulting and Clinical Psychology, 64,* 497–504.

Depression in primary care: Detection, diagnosis, and treatment (1993, April). Washington, DC: Public Health Service, U.S. Department of Health and Human Services.

Jermain, D. (1997, March-April). Affective spectrum disorders: How to recognize and treat depression. *International Journal of Fertility, 42,* 73–77.

Krupnick, J., Sotsky, S., & Simmons, S. (1996). The role of the therapeutic alliance in psychotherapy and pharmacotherapy outcome: Findings in The National Institutes of Mental Health treatment of depression collaborative research program. *Journal of Consulting and Clinical Psychology, 64,* 532–539.

Post, R. (Ed.). In *Review of psychiatry* (Vol. 9). Treatment of refractory mood disorders. Washington, DC: American Psychiatric Press.

Redmond, G. (1997, March-April). Mood disorders in the female patient. *International Journal of Fertility, 42,* 67–72.

Simon, G., VonKorff, M., & Barlow, W. (1995, October). Health care costs of primary care patient with recognized depression. *Archives of General Psychiatry, 52,* 850–856.

Suicidal Ideation

Block, S., & Billings, J. (1997, October). Psychiatry and assisted suicide. *The Harvard Mental Health Letter,* pp. 5–7.

Blumenthal, S., & Kupfer, D. (Eds.). (1990). *Suicide over the life cycle: Risk factors, assessment, and treatment of suicidal patients.* Washington, DC: American Psychiatric Press.

Courage, Godbey, Ingram, Schramm, & Hale. (1993). Suicide in the elderly: Staying in control. *Journal of Psychosocial Nursing, 31,*26–31.

Hendin, H. (1995, spring). Assisted suicide, euthanasia, and suicide prevention: The implications of the Dutch experience. *Suicide and Life-Threatening Behavior, 25,* 193–204.

Kowalski, S. (1993). Assisted suicide: Where do nurses draw the line? *Nursing and Health Care, 14,* 70–76.

Rich, E. (1997). Euthanasia and assisted suicide. *The Journal of the New York State Nurses Association, 28,* 8–11.

Stone, A. (1997, January). Physician assisted suicide and the psychiatric profession. *The Harvard Mental Health Letter, 13,* 4–7.

Tilden, V., Tolle, S., Lee, M., & Nelson, C. (1966, March-April). Oregon's Physician-assisted suicide vote: Its effect on palliative care. *Nursing Outlook, 44,* 80–83.

Zimbleman, J. (1994). Good life, good death, and the right to die: Ethical considerations for decisions at the end of life. *Journal of Professional Nursing, 10,* 22–37.

Brief Psychotic Disorder

Chen, Y., Swann, A., & Burt, D. (1996, May). Stability of diagnosis in schizophrenia. *American Journal of Psychiatry, 153,* 682–686.

Green, A., & Patel, J. (1996, December). The new pharmacology of schizophrenia. *The Harvard Mental Health Letter, 13,* 5–7.

Javitt, D., Zylberman, I., & Zukin, S. (1994, August). Amelioration of negative symptoms in schizophrenia by glycine. *American Journal of Psychiatry, 151,* 1234–1236.

Neumann, C., Grimes, K., Walker, E., & Baum, K. (1995). Developmental pathways to schizophrenia: Behavioral subtypes. *Journal of Abnormal Psychology, 104,* 558–566.

Szymanski, S., Lieberman, J., & Alvir, J. (1995, May). Gender differences in onset of illness, treatment response, course, and biological indexes in first-episode schizophrenic patients. *American Journal of Psychiatry, 152,* 698–703.

Phobia

Marshall, J. (1994). *Social phobia: From shyness to stage fright.* New York: Basic Books.

Electrostimulative Therapy

Fitzsimons (1995). Electrostimulative therapy: What nurses need to know. *Journal of Psychosocial Nursing and Mental Health Services, 33.*

SPECIAL CIRCUMSTANCES

Substance-Related Disorders

American Psychiatric Association. (1996, October). Practice guideline for the treatment of patients with nicotine dependence. *American Journal of Psychiatry, 153,* (Suppl.), 10.

Brent, C. (1997). Unexpected alcohol withdrawal. *American Journal of Nursing, 97,* 52–53.

Galanter, M. (Ed.). (1989). Psychoactive substance use disorders (alcohol). In *Treatments of psychiatric disorders: A task force report of the American Psychiatric Association.* Washington, DC: American Psychiatric Association.

Galanter, M., & Kleber, H. (1994). *The American Psychiatric Press textbook of substance abuse treatment*. Washington, DC: American Psychiatric Press.

Gerstein, D., & Harwood, H. (1990). *Treating drug problems* (Vols. 1 & 2). Washington, DC: National Academy Press.

Henning, S., Soyka, M., Mann, K., & Zieglgansberger. (1996, August). Relapse prevention by acamprosate: Results from a placebo-controlled study on alcohol dependence. *Archives of General Psychiatry, 53,* 673–680.

Larson, D. (1997). Smoking cessation: Counseling your patients. *Clinician Reviews, 7,* 57–60, 62–64, 67, 70, 73–75, 79–80.

Midanik, L., & Clark, W. (1995). Drinking-related problems in the U.S.: Description and trends, 1984–1990. *Journal of Studies on Alcohol, 56,* 395–402.

Miller, J., et al. (1995, January). A case-control study of cocaine use in pregnancy. *American Journal of Obstetrics and Gynecology, 172,* 180–185.

Orleans, C., & Slade, J. (Eds.). (1993). *Nicotine addiction: Principles and management*. New York: Oxford University Press.

Peele, S. (1991). *The truth about addiction and recovery: The life process program for outgrowing destructive habits*. New York: Simon & Schuster.

Peele, S., Brodsky, A., & Arnold, M. (1991). *The truth about addiction and recovery*. New York: Simon & Schuster.

Silverman, K., Higgins, S., & Brooner, R. (1996, May). Sustained cocaine abstinence in methadone maintenance patients through voucher-based reinforcement therapy. *Archives of General Psychiatry, 53,* 409–415.

Vaillant, G. (1995). *The natural history of alcoholism revisited*. Cambridge, MA: Harvard University Press.

Weathers, W., et al. (1993, February). Cocaine use in women from a defined population: Prevalence at delivery and effects on growth in infants. *Pediatrics, 91,* 350–354.

Woody, G., McLellan, T., Laborsky, L., & O'Brien, C. (1995, September). Psychotherapy in community methadone programs: A validation study. *American Journal of Psychiatry, 152,* 1302–1308.

Zuckerman, B., & Frank, D. (1992, February). "Crack kids": not broken. *Pediatrics, 89,* 337–339.

PSYCHOLOGICAL EFFECTS OF PHYSICAL ILLNESS

Cancer

Brody, J. (1997, February 12). Personal health: Children need special help when a parent has cancer. *The New York Times,* p. B12.

Brody, J. (1997, April 2). Personal health—with cancer, fatigue can be a bigger problem than pain. *The New York Times,* p. B12.

Calder, K. (1977, May-June). Managed care and cancer. *Coping, Living with Cancer, 11,* 14–15.

Dumas, M. A. S. (1996, April). What it's like to belong to the cancer club. *American Journal of Nursing, 96,* 4042.

Facing forward: A guide for cancer survivors. (1996). National Cancer Institute: National Institutes of Health. Bethesda, MD: U.S. Department of Health and Human Services.

Facione, N., & Facione, P. (1997, May-June). Equitable access to cancer services in the 21st century. *Nursing Outlet, 45,* 118–123.

Fink, D. (1991). *Guidelines for the cancer-related checkup.* Atlanta: American Cancer Society Textbook of Clinical Oncology.

Grinspoon, L., & Bakalar, J. *Marijuana: The forbidden medicine.* New Haven: Yale University Press.

Management of cancer pain. Clinical Practice Guideline, No. 9 (1994). Agency for Health Care Policy and Research, Public Health Service. Rockville, MD: U.S. Department of Health and Human Services.

Orenstein, P. (1997, June 29). 35 and mortal: A breast cancer diary. *The New York Times Magazine,* Section 6, pp. 28–33, 42–44, 52.

Poncar, P. (1994). Inspiring hope in the oncology patient. *Journal of Psychosocial Nursing, 32,* 33–37.

Phiffer, C. (1996, May-June). "Nobody but us really knows what it's like": A conversation with cancer survivor Linda Ellerbee. *Coping, 10,* 18–19.

Sanders, M., & Heitman, B. (1997, February 10). Common fallacies about cancer pain. *Nursing Spectrum* (Florida ed.), *7,* 14–16.

Simonton, O. C., Simonton S., & Creighton, J. (1992). *Getting well again.* New York: Bantam.

Sloane, M. (1997, March 24). Medical marijuana: The cannabis controversy. *The Nursing Spectrum* (Florida ed.), *5,* 6, 7, 11.

Taking time: Support for people with cancer and the people who care about them. (1996). National Cancer Institute: National Institutes of Health. Bethesda, MD: U.S. Department of Health and Human Services.

White, G., Griffith, C., Nenstiel, R., & Dyess, D. (1996, October). Breast cancer: Reducing mortality through early detection. *Clinician Reviews, 6*, 77–79, 83–84, 88, 90, 92, 94, 100–102.

Willette, J. (1997). Reflections: Walk with me. *American Journal of Nursing, 7*, 52.

Who plays God? (1996, May 3). WETA-TV. George Strait, host.

Coronary Heart Disease or Cerebrovascular Accident

Andreola, N., & Sloane, M. (1995, December). Post-stroke rehabilitation: New guidelines for consistent, quality care. *Nursing Spectrum* (Florida ed.), pp. 6, 7, 16.

Ashton, K. (1997, March 10). Nurses, women and heart disease: Making the connection. *The Nursing Spectrum* (Florida ed.), *7*, 14–16.

Crowe, J., Runions, J., Ebbesen, L., Oldridge, N., & Streiner, D. (1996, March-April). Anxiety and depression after acute myocardial infarction. *Heart and Lung, 25*, 98–107.

Frank, C., & Smith, S. (1990). Stress and the heart: Biobehavioral aspects of sudden cardiac death. *Psychosomatics, 31*, 255–264.

Gillyatt, P., & Husten, L. (1996). *Stroke: A Harvard Health Letter special report*. Boston: The Harvard Medical School Health Publications Group.

High blood pressure: Treat it for life. (1994). Washington, DC: National Heart, Lung and Blood Institute, National Institutes of Health. U.S. Department of Health and Human Services.

Jorgensen, R., Johnson, B., Kolodziej, M., & Schreer, G. (1996). Elevated blood pressure and personality: A meta-analytic review. *Psychological Bulletin, 120*, 293–320.

Kawachi, I., Sparrow, D., Vokonas, P., & Weiss, S. (1994, November). Symptoms of anxiety and risk of coronary heart disease: The Normative Aging Study. *Circulation, 90*, 2225–2229.

Linden, W., Stossel, C., & Maurice, J. (1996). Psychosocial intervention for patients with coronary artery disease: A meta-analysis. *Archives of Internal Medicine, 156*, 745–752.

Richman, E. (1996, April). Acute stroke intervention: Proactive strategies to preserve brain tissue. *Clinician Reviews, 6*, 79–94.

Diabetes

Bailey, B. (1996). Mediators of depression in adults with diabetes. *Clinical Nursing Research, 5,* 28–42.

Drass, J., & Peterson, A. (1996, November). Type II diabetes: Exploring treatment options. *American Journal of Nursing, 96,* 45–50.

Insulin-dependent diabetes. (1994). Washington, DC: National Institutes of Health, U.S. Department of Health and Human Services.

Noninsulin-dependent diabetes. (1992). Washington, DC: National Institutes of Health, U.S. Department of Health and Human Services.

The diabetes dictionary. (1994). Washington, DC: National Institutes of Health, U.S. Department of Health and Human Services.

Wang, C., & Fenske, M. (1996, September-October). Self-care of adults with non-insulin-dependent diabetes mellitus: Influence of families and friends. *The Diabetes Educator, 22,* 465–470.

Dementia

Brody, J. (1997, March 5). Alzheimer studies thwarted. *The New York Times,* p. B13.

Buntinx, F., Kester, A., Bergers, J., & Knottnerus, J. (1996). Is depression in elderly people followed by dementia? *Age and Aging, 25,* 231–233.

Caring for a person with memory loss and confusion (1995). Santa Cruz, CA: Journeyworks.

Early Alzheimer's disease: Recognition and assessment (1996, September). Agency for Health Care Policy and Research. (96-R123, pp. 1–5)

Hurley, A., Bottino, R., & Volicer, L. (1994). Nursing role in advance proxy planning for Alzheimer patients. *Caring,* 72–76.

Hurley, A., Volicer, L., Rempusheski, V., & Fry, S. (1995). Reaching consensus: The process of recommending treatment decisions for Alzheimer's patients. *Advances in Nursing Science, 18,* 33–43.

Kolanowski, A., & Whall, A. (1996, winter). Life-span perspective of personality in dementia. *Image: Journal of Nursing Scholarship* (Sigma Theta Tau International), *28,* 315–320.

LeNavenec, C.-L., & Vonhof, T. (1996). *One day at a time: How families manage the experience of dementia.* Westport, CT: Auburn House.

Mace, N. L., & Rabins, P. V. (1991). *The 36-hour day: A family guide to caring for persons with Alzheimer's disease: Related dementing illnesses and memory loss in later life*. Baltimore, MD: Johns Hopkins University Press.

Rader, J. (1996). *Individualized dementia care: Creative, compassionate approaches*. New York: Springer Publishing.

Silverman, H., Fry, S., & Armistead, N. (1994). Nurses' perspectives on implementation of the patient self-determination act. *Journal of Clinical Ethics, 5,* 30–37.

Simpson, C. (1996). *At the heart of Alzheimer's* (2nd ed.). Gaithersburg, MD: Manor Healthcare.

Abuse

Aggeles, T. (1996, October 21). Nursing DX: Sexual assault. *Nursing Spectrum* (Florida ed.), *6,* 6–7.

Devlin, B., & Reynolds, E. (1994). Child abuse: How to recognize it, how to intervene. *American Journal of Nursing, 94,* 2 6–32.

Draucker, C., & Petrovic, K. (1996, winter). Healing of adult male survivors of childhood sexual abuse. *Image: Journal of Nursing Scholarship* (Sigma Theta Tau International), *28,* 325–330.

Elder mistreatment: The nation's hidden problem. (1996, July-August). *NYSNA Report, 27,* 11.

Harrison, G., Mangweth, B., & Negrao. (1994, May). Childhood sexual abuse and bulimia nervosa. *American Journal of Psychiatry, 151,* 732–737.

Holtzworth-Munroe, A. (1995, August). Marital violence. *The Harvard Mental Health Letter,* pp. 4–6.

Lynch, S. (1997). Elder abuse: What to look for, how to intervene. *American Journal of Nursing, 97,* 27–31.

Quillian, J. (1996, April). Screening for spousal or partner abuse in a community health setting. *Journal of the American Academy of Nurse Practitioners, 8,* 155–160.

Sexton, J. (1996, May 12). As reports of child abuse rise, officials split up more families. *The New York Times,* pp. A1, 30.

Shea, C., Mahoney, M., & Lacey, J. (1997). Breaking through the barriers to domestic violence intervention. *American Journal of Nursing, 97,* 26–33.

Violence is still on the rise: OSHA urges "zero tolerance." (1996). *American Journal of Nursing, 96,* 69, 72, 73.

Wylie, M. (1996, March-April). It's a community affair (domestic violence). *The Family Therapy Networker, 20,* 5865–5896.

Sexual or Reproductive Disorder

Gabriel, T. (1996, January 7). High tech pregnancies test hope's limit. *The New York Times* (national ed.), pp. 1, 10, 11.

Hoffman, J. (1996, January 8). Egg donations meet a need and raise ethical questions. *The New York Times,* pp. 1, 7.

Lee, F. (1996, January 9). Infertile couples forge ties within society of their own. *The New York Times,* pp. 1, 7.

Lewin, T. (1997, April 5). Fearing disease, teens alter sexual practices. *The New York Times* (national report), p. 7.

Whitman, D. (1997, May 19). Was it good enough for us? (adult premarital sex). *U.S. News & World Report, 122,* 57–60, 62, 64.

Eating and Weight Disorders

Bemporad, J. (1996). Self-starvation through the ages. *International Journal of Eating Disorders, 19,* 217–237.

Brownell, K., & Fairburn, C. (Eds.). (1997, October). *Eating disorders and obesity: A comprehensive handbook.* New York: Guilford.

Eating disorders. (1994). Washington, DC: National Institutes of Health, U.S. Department of Health and Human Services.

Fairburn, C., Jones, R., & Peveler, R. (1993, June). Psychotherapy and bulimia nervosa. *Archives of General Psychiatry, 50,* 419–428.

Gordon, R. (1990). *Anorexia and bulimia: Anatomy of a social epidemic.* Cambridge, MA: Blackwell.

Hsu, L. K. (1990). *Eating disorders.* New York: Guilford.

Mitchell, J. (1990). *Bulimia nervosa.* Minneapolis: University of Minnesota Press.

Rorty, M., Yager, J., & Rossotto, E. (1994, August). Childhood sexual, physical and psychological abuse in bulimia nervosa. *American Journal of Psychiatry, 151,* 1122–1126.

Ross, C. (1994, March). Overweight and depression. *Journal of Health and Social Behavior, 35,* 63–78.

Yager, J. (Ed.). (1996). Eating disorders. *Psychiatric Clinics of North America, 19.*

Zerbe, K. (1993). *The body betrayed: Women, eating disorders and treatment.* Washington, DC: American Psychiatric Press.

Post-traumatic Stress Disorder

Barash, D. (1990). The San Francisco Earthquake: Then and now. *Perspectives in Psychiatric Care, 26,* 32–36.

Charney, D., Deutch, A., & Krystal. (1993, April). Psychobiologic mechanisms of post-traumatic stress disorder. *Archives of General Psychiatry, 50,* 294–305.

Clark, C. (1996, March 25). Post traumatic stress disorder: 2. Interventions. *Nursing Spectrum* (Florida ed.), pp. 12–14.

Hayes, G., Goodwin, T., & Miars, B. (1990, February). After disaster: A crisis support team at work. *American Journal of Nursing, 90,* 61–64.

Herman, J. (1992). *Trauma and recovery.* New York: Basic Books.

McNally, R., & Shin, L. (1995, June). Association of intelligence with severity of posttraumatic stress disorder symptome in Vietnam combat veterans. *American Journal of Psychiatry, 152,* 936–938.

Stanley, S. (1990, May). When the disaster is over: Helping the healers to mend. *Journal of Psychosocial Nursing, 28,* 12–16.

Tomb, D. (Ed.). (1994, June). Traumatic stress disorder. *The Psychiatric Clinics of North America, 17,* 2.

Postpartum Psychosis

Dalton, K., & Holton, W. (1996). *Depression after childbirth: How to recognize, treat and prevent postnatal depression.* New York: Oxford University Press.

Gilbert, S. (1996, May 1). Estrogen patch appears to lift severe depression in new mothers. *The New York Times,* p. 10.

Gotlib, D., Whiffen, V., Wallace, P., & Mount, J. (1991). Prospective investigation of postpartum depression: Factors involved in onset and recovery. *Journal of Abnormal Psychology, 100,* 122–132.

Hobfoll, S., Ritter, C., & Lavin, J. (1995). Depression prevalence and incidence among inner-city pregnancy and post-partum women. *Journal of Consulting and Clinical Psychology, 63,* 445–453.

Janssen, H., Cuisinier, M., Hoogduin, K., & deGraauw. (1996). Controlled prospective study on the mental health of women following pregnancy loss. *The American Journal of Psychiatry, 153,* 226–230.

Mercer, R. (1995). *Becoming a mother.* New York: Springer Publishing.

Robert, E. (1996, October 3). Treating depression in pregnancy. *New England Journal of Medicine, 335,* 1056–1058.

WuDunn, S. (1996, January 25). In Japan, a ritual of mourning for abortions. *The New York Times,* pp. 1, 5.

The Bereaved Person

Gifford, B., & Cleary, B. (1990, February). Supporting the bereaved. *American Journal of Nursing, 90,* 48–53.

Lawson, L. (1990, March-April). Culturally sensitive support for grieving parents. *American Journal of Maternal/Child Nursing, 15,* 76–79.

Chronic or Incurable Disease

Altman, L. (1997, May 6). Surviving with AIDS is one problem: Cancer is yet another. *The New York Times,* p. B. 10.

Brownlee, S., & Schrof, J. (1997, March 17). The quality of mercy. *U.S. News & World Report, 122,* 54–57, 60–62, 64, 65, 67.

Carson, V., Soeken, K., Shanty, J., & Terry, L. (1990). Hope and spiritual well-being: Essentials for living with AIDS. *Perspectives in Psychiatric Care, 26,* 28–34.

Curry, J., Douglass, S., rev. by Casey, K. (1996, May). HIV/AIDS Update '96-Florida. *Nursing Spectrum* (Florida ed.), pp. 14, 19–20.

Ferri, R., Witt, R., & Sharp, V. (1977). AIDS update. *Clinician Reviews, 7,* 83–86.

Lisanti, P., & Zwolski, K. (1997). Understanding the devastation of AIDS. *American Journal of Nursing, 7,* 26–35.

Libman, H., & Witzburg, R. (1996). *HIV infection: A primary care manual* (3rd ed.). Boston: Little, Brown.

Perry, S. (1990, June). Organic mental disorders caused by HIV: Update on early diagnosis and treatment. *American Journal of Psychiatry, 147,* 696–710.

Philips, H., Rachman, C., & Rachman, S. (1996). *The psychological management of chronic pain* (2nd ed.). New York: Springer Publishing.

Ungvarski, P. (1997, January). Update on HIV infection. *American Journal of Nursing, 97,* 44–52.

Ruppert, R. (1996, March). Caring for the lay caregiver. *American Journal of Nursing, 96,* 40–46.

Sherman, D. (1996, March). Taking the fear out of AIDS nursing: Voices from the field. *Journal of the New York State Nurses Association, 27,* 4–8.

Warren, M. T. (1992). Maintain identity in elderly couples with chronic illness. *Journal of Psychosocial Nursing, 30,* 8–11.

Terminal Illness

Baer, K. (1995, February). The final chapter: Death and dying. *Harvard Health Letter, 20,* 1–3.

Davis, A., Phillips, L., Drought, T., Sellin, S., Ronsman, K., & Hershberger, A. (1995). Nurses' attitudes toward active euthanasia. *Nursing Outlook, 43,* 174–179.

Fein, E. (1997, March 5). Talking around death. *The New York Times,* pp. A1, 14, 15.

Fein, E. (1977), March 6). Talking around death. *The New York Times,* pp. A1, 15.

Fein, E. (1977, May 4). A better quality of life, in the days before death. *The New York Times* (Metro), p. 39.

Kurukawa, M. (1996). Meeting the needs of the dying patient's family. *Critical Care Nurse, 16,* 51–57.

Jezewski, M. A. (1996). Obtaining consent for do-not-resuscitate status: Advice from experienced nurses. *Nursing Outlook, 44,* 114–119.

Lewin, T. (1996, June 2). Ignoring "Right to Die" directives, medical community is being sued. *The New York Times,* pp. 1, 14.

Mezey, M., Evans, L., Golub, Z., Murphy, E., & White, G. (1994). The patient self-determination act: A source of concern for nurses. *Nursing Outlook, 42,* 30–38.

Norman, M. (1996, January 14). Living too long. *The New York Times Magazine,* pp. 36–38.

Ray, M. (1996, May). Seven ways to empower dying patients. *American Journal of Nursing, 96,* 56, 57.

Scanlon, C. (1995–1996 winter). Understanding the moral life. *American Nurses Association Center for Ethics and Human Rights Communique, 4,* 1–3.

Shapiro, J. (1997, March 24). Death be not swift enough. *U.S. News & World Report, 122,* 34–35.

Smyth, M., & Singer, G. (1996, March). Ode to Mr. Keyes. *American Journal of Nursing, 96,* 54, 55.

Wiener, L., Aikin, A., Gibbons, M., & Hirschfeld, S. (1996). Visions of those who left too soon. *American Journal of Nursing, 96,* 57–59.

Wilkes, P. (1997, July 6). Dying well is the best revenge. *The New York Times Magazine, 6,* 32–38.

Written Testimony of the American Nurses Association before the Institute of Medicine Committee on Care at the End of Life 1996, June 10. ANA Policy Series.

Zerwekh, J. (1994). The truth tellers: How hospice nurses help patients confront death. *American Journal of Nursing, 94,* 31–34.

WORKING WITH DIFFERENT AGE GROUPS

The Young Child

Austin, J. (1990, March-April). Assessment of coping mechanisms used by parents and children with chronic illness. *American Journal of Maternal/Child Nursing, 15,* 98–102.

Children at risk. [Special issue]. (1997, July-August). *Natural History, 4,* 24–58.

Grandin, T. (1995). *Thinking in pictures: And other reports from my life with autism.* New York: Doubleday.

Lipkin, G. B. (1978). *Parent-child nursing* (2nd ed.), (pp. 206–221). St. Louis: Mosby.

Sherman, D. (1997, March). Death of a newborn: Healing the pain through Carper's patterns of knowing in nursing. *Journal of the New York State Nurses Association, 28,* 4–6.

Siegel, B. (1996). *The world of the autistic child: Understanding and treating autistic spectrum disorders.* New York: Oxford University Press.

Strauch, B. (1997, August 10). Use of antidepression medicine for young patients has soared. *The New York Times,* p. A1.

Wittert, D. (1996, October 21). Autism and the pervasive developmental disorders. *Nursing Spectrum* (Florida ed.), pp. 12–14.

Your child from birth to three (special ed.). (1997, spring-summer). *Newsweek.*

You and mental health: What's the deal. (1996). (Part of Caring for Every
    Child's Mental Health: Communities Together Campaign.) Children's
    Mental Health Services National Mental Health Services Knowledge
    Exchange Network, P.O. Box 42490, Washington, DC 20015.

The Adolescent

Coles, R. (1997). *The moral intelligence of children (how to raise a moral
    child)*. New York: Random House.
Roye, C. (1995). Breaking through to the adolescent patient. *American
    Journal of Nursing, 19,* 19–23.
Sandmaier, M. (1996, May-June). More than love. *The Family Therapy
    Networker, 20,* 21–33.

The Aged

Brayne, C., & Payhel, E. (1995). Cognitive decline in an elderly population:
    A two-wave study of change. *Psychological Study of Medicine, 25,*
    673–683.
Buchner, D. M. (1997). Physical activity and quality of life in older adults.
    Journal of the American Medical Association, 277, 64–66.
Foreman, M., & Zane, D. (1996, April). Nursing strategies for acute confu-
    sion, in elders. *American Journal of Nursing, 96,* 44–53.
How to age gracefully—without frailty or falls. (1996, February). *Consumer
    Reports on Health,* pp. 18–19.
Immunizations: Are you up to date? (1995, November). *Consumer Reports
    on Health,* pp. 126–128.
Kane, R., & Caplan, A. (Eds.). (1990). *Everyday ethics: Resolving dilemmas
    in nursing home life.* New York: Springer Publishing
Kolata, G. (1996, February 27). New era of robust elderly belies the fears of
    scientists. *The New York Times,* pp. 1, 10.
Lilley, L., & Guanci, R. (1996, November). Polypharmacy in elders.
    American Journal of Nursing, 96, 12.
Lee, M. (1996, July). Drugs and the elderly: Do you know the risks?
    American Journal of Nursing, 96, 26–32.
Navarro, M. (1996, August 7). Florida is leading the way in a big genera-
    tional shift. *The New York Times,* pp. A1, A10.

Olson, E., Chichin, E., & Libow, E. (Eds.). (1996). *Controversies in ethics in long-term care*. New York: Springer Publishing.

Patterns of aging—A special report. (1996, July 5). *Science, 273*, 42–80.

Stock, R. (1996, June 20). Living five score or more. *The New York Times,* p. C8.

Stock, R. (1996, April 18). Alcohol lures the old. *The New York Times* (home section), pp. 1, 2.

Stocker, S. (1996, September). Six tips for caring for aging parents. *American Journal of Nursing, 96*, 32–33.

Strength training. (1995, May). *Harvard Women's Health Watch, 2*, 2–3.

The new world of long term care for the elderly. (1996, July-August). *NYSNA Report, 27*, 1, 10.

Tillman-Jones, & Timberly, K. (1990, May). How to work with elderly patients on a general psychiatric unit. *Journal of Psychosocial Nursing, 28*, 27–31.

What is normal aging? (1997, June). *Harvard Women's Health Watch, 4*, 3–5.

Thomas, P. (1997). Longevity—biology isn't destiny—but it's part of it. *Harvard Health Letter, 22*, 1–3.

ORGANIZATIONS

American Gathering of Jewish Holocaust Survivors
122 West 30 Street, Room 201
New York, NY 10001

American Red Cross
17th and D Streets NW
Washington, DC 20036

Autism Society of America
7910 Woodmont Avenue, Suite 650
Bethesda, MD 20814

Disabled American Veterans
P.O. Box 14301
Cincinnati, OH 45214

National Alliance for the Mentally Ill
200 North Glebe Road, Suite 1015
Arlington, VA 22203-3754

National Cancer Institute
31 Center Drive
MSC 2580
Bethesda, MD 20892-2580

National Center for PTSD
Department of Veteran Affairs
VA Medical Center
White River Junction, VT 05009

National Depressive and Manic Depressive Association
730 North Franklin Street, Suite 501
Chicago, IL 60610

National Foundation for Depressive Illness
P.O. Box 2257
New York, NY 10116

National Mental Health Association
1021 Prince Street
Alexandria, VA 22314-2971

Vietnam Veterans of America
329 Eighth Street NE
Washington, DC 20002

For further information on computer web sites and toll-free numbers:

American Cancer Society
http://www.cancer.org
800-227-2345

American Diabetes Association
http://www.diabetes.org
800-342-2383

American Heart Association
http://www.amhrt.org
800-242-8721

Arthritis Foundation
http://www.arthritis.org
800-283-7800

World wide web health information site:
http://www.healthfinder.gov

Index

Springer Publishing Company

Developing Research in Nursing and Health
Quantitative and Qualitative Methods

Carol Noll Hoskins, PhD, RN, FAAN

"It is a clear and unencumbered 'snapshot' of essential information that can serve as a study guide for graduate students, a handy reference for researchers and faculty, and an 'instructor's manual' for teaching research. I would certainly use this guide...."

*—**Harriet R. Feldman**, PhD, RN, FAAN*
Dean and Professor, Pace University Lienhard School of Nursing

This handy volume is an excellent adjunct to traditional research texts and courses, and a boon to educators and researchers challenged to "know all" about the processes of research. Some of the important general features include:

- an outline format designed to highlight key information
- clarification of confusing and difficult information
- exemplars used throughout each chapter and in the appendices

This valuable guide stands out from traditional texts by offering a succinct overview of key sources of nursing and related literature; differentiation of the theoretical framework of quantitative and qualitative studies; a guide to abstracting research studies; clear presentation of the types, rules, and procedures of sampling; and a conceptual appproach to organizing descriptive and inferential statistics and qualitative data analysis.

Contents: Research in Nursing • The Research Question — Hypotheses • The Literature Review, Definition of Terms, and Theoretical Framework • Research Designs • Sampling in Qualitative Designs—Basic Issues and Concepts • Data Analysis and Interpretation—Qualitative Designs • Principles of Measurement • Development of Quantitative Measures

1998   130pp   0-8261-1185-8   softcover

536 Broadway, New York, NY 10012-3955 • (212) 431-4370 • Fax (212) 941-7842